PREDIABETES

ADVANCES IN EXPERIMENTAL MEDICINE AND BIOLOGY

Recent Volumes in this Series

A Continuation Order Plan is available for this series. A continuation order will bring delivery of each new volume immediately upon publication. Volumes are billed only upon actual shipment. For further information please contact the publisher.

PREDIABETES

Edited by

Rafael A. Camerini-Davalos

Diabetes Prevention Research Program
New York Medical College
Metropolitan Hospital Research Center
New York, New York

and

Harold S. Cole

Departments of Community and Preventive Medicine and Pediatrics
New York Medical College
Valhalla, New York
and Bronx Developmental Center
Office of Mental Retardation and Developmental Disabilities
  of the State of New York
Bronx, New York

PLENUM PRESS • NEW YORK AND LONDON

Library of Congress Cataloging in Publication Data

International Symposium on Early Diabetes (5th: 1988: Iguazu Falls, Argentina)
  Prediabetes.

  (Advances in experimental medicine and biology; v. 246)
  "Based on the proceedings of the Fifth International Symposium on Early Diabetes:
Prediabetes, held April, 1988, in Iguazu Falls, Argentina" — T.p. verso.
  Includes bibliographies and index.
  1. Prediabetic state — Congresses. I. Camerini-Davalos, Rafael A. II. Cole, Harold S.
III. Title. IV. Series. [DNLM: 1. Diabetes Mellitus — congresses. 2. Prediabetic State —
congresses. W1 AD559 v. 246 / WK 810 I6032p 1988]
RC660.A1I59   1988   616.4'62   88-32332
ISBN-13: 978-1-4684-5618-9   e-ISBN-13: 978-1-4684-5616-5
DOI: 10.1007/978-1-4684-5616-5

Based on the Proceedings of the Fifth International Symposium on
Early Diabetes: Prediabetes, held April, 1988,
in Iguazu Falls, Argentina

© 1988 Plenum Press, New York
Softcover reprint of the hardcover 1st edition   1988
A Division of Plenum Publishing Corporation
233 Spring Street, New York, N.Y. 10013

ORGANIZING COMMITTEE

Domenico Andreani

Rafael A. Camerini-Davalos, Chairman

Joseph Hoet

Ernst F. Pfeiffer

Felix E. Puchulu

J. Stuart Soeldner

PREFACE

Can the art of predictive medicine anticipate the development of diabetes? And if so, what can be done about it? How early is early enough to intervene effectively? With what therapeutic modality? Why?

Big babies are not an infrequent occurrence in mothers with normal carbohydrate metabolism for another 10, 20, or even 30 years. The abnormality present during pregnancy is now accepted as what is inherited with the diabetic predisposition, or what can be recognized as the diabetic susceptibility. It occurs before hyperglycemia, during the phase of dynamic resistance to diabetes, during the prediabetic period.

Prediabetes means before diabetes, and was applied for the first time by Marañon in Spain, to signify the stage before hyperglycemia. Foglia in Argentina used the term in 1944 for his pancreatectomized rats. We published the first paper on humans in 1951 (Camerini-Davalos, R.A., Landabure, P., and Serantes, N., Rev Med Cordoba 39: 187).

The term has been arbitrarily defined as the condition of those persons who are predisposed to hyperglycemia, but in whom no abnormalities of carbohydrate metabolism is demonstrable. From the definition, it is clear that the end of this stage is marked by the first detectable abnormality of carbohydrate metabolism. But when it does begin, if conception marks the "beginning" of the disease, how early in life is the disease trend manifest?

The Fifth International Symposium on Early Diabetes, sponsored by the Diabetes Prevention Research Program of the New York Medical College, held in Iguazu, Argentina, in April 1988, and from which this book evolved, attempted to answer some of these questions.

Rafael A. Camerini-Davalos

ACKNOWLEDGMENTS

To our Sponsors: Eleonora Abreu, Betasint, Pfizer International, Inc., Servier. Supporters: Argencard, SA, Bayer Int., Becton Dickinson Company, Diabetes Research Fund, Farmitalia Carlo Erba, Fundacion Grupo Universal, Novo Industria/s. Contributors: American Hoeschst Corporation, Ayerst Laboratories, Fundacion Bunge y Born, Fundacion Hermanos Agustin y Enrique Rocca, Hope for Diabetics Foundation, Nordisk, Laboratorios Rontag, S.A. and Miles-Sankyo, Ltd; we express our appreciation for the financial support which made this Fifth International Symposium of Early Diabetes possible.

The Editors

CONTENTS

PREDIABETES IN ANIMALS

IMMUNOLOGICAL MARKERS

PREDICTION OF DIABETES

PATHOLOGY OF PREDIABETES

POPULATION STUDIES

TREATMENT OF PREDIABETES

PREVENTION OF DIABETES

I.   PREDIABETES IN ANIMALS

HISTORY: THE DISCOVERY OF PREDIABETES IN ANIMALS

¶Virgilio G. Foglia

Instituto de Biologia y Medicina Experimental
Buenos Aires, Argentina

In 1940 diabetes was produced in the rat by removal of the pancreas. Surgical mortality during operation as well as during the following weeks was only 10 to 20% and the survival time of the rats ranged from 4 to 11½ months, maintained under standard diet (1). We were surprised to observe that even after 95% pancreatectomy, a few months elapsed before typical diabetes appeared.

DIABETES BY PANCREATECTOMY

In the rat the effects of 95% pancreatectomy developed in a progressive way through three successive stages.

First stage: Prediabetes

Latent, inapparent, transitory or prediabetes. We prefer to recognize this stage as prediabetes because for us it means anticipation of classic diabetes. From surgery to the appearance of glycosuria.

The daily food intake at the prediabetes stage of the rat was diminished and dental caries were found, probably produced by periodontal lesions which eventually caused the loss of many teeth. Spontaneous motility and volemia increased. (2). Number of erythrocytes increased in males but in females, plasma increased.

Glycosuria, polydipsia, polyuria or ketonuria was not observed. Fasting glycemia and glucose tolerance curves were normal as well as insulinemia (3). Normal fasting glycemia lasted 1 to 3 months in the prediabetic male and 4 to 6 months in females. Castration in both sexes shortened this period (2).

Sexual disturbances were marked. Sterility, giant fetuses, malformations, prematurity or death. The same facts were observed in the rat under alloxan diabetes.

In female rats, alterations in oestrus cycles were observed. These cycles shortened and the eggs collected in the oviduct were about 20% less than normals. All these facts led to diminution of fertility (4). In addition, pathological disturbances appeared in ovary and uterus easily seen

3

at histological examination. In cases of pregnancy, disturbances occurred in placenta and fetuses. Placenta was hemorrhagic and altered. Fetuses obtained from uterus between 18 and 21 days of pregnancy, showed high mortality, especially males (70% dead). In addition, they were big, weighing 8% more than normals while males at this stage showed disturbances in sexual behaviour accompanied by regressive lesions of the seminal line (5) and smaller response to gonadotrophins.

Regeneration lesions were observed in the pancreas remnant accompanied by cells degranulation (3). Kidney and liver (included fetal) were increased in size and weight. Muscle glycogen was also increased.

Modifying agents in prediabetes

It is well known that many factors are able to modify prediabetes both in its duration and in its pathology. In those rats having remnants larger than 5%, the appearance of later (more severe) stages is delay, for example, leaving a remnant of 20%, it takes up to 1 year to develop overt diabetes. Another important factor is the chemical composition of the diet used, poor or rich in carbohydrates (1).

Corticoids had different effects in accordance with substance and doses used; desoxycorticosterone was not active but cortisone was diabetogenic. Some factors anticipated the appearance of diabetes: for example, stress (injecting subcutaneously croton oil or producing bone fractures) (6). The same results were observed provoking infections in the rat with pyocianic bacillus (5) or with colibacillus (6). Androgens caused a similar effect in both sexes, more marked when administered at birth.

Diabetes appearance was delayed by ethionine because of pancreatic acini degeneration and new islets appearance, both in males and in females (3). Chloropropamide, thyroidectomy and radioactive iodine had a similar effect (5).

Second stage

The second stage of incipient diabetes was short and lasted one month, sometimes two. Fasting hyperglycemia and glycosuria appeared.

Third stage

The third stage of manifest diabetes showed all typical symptoms and ended with the animal's death between 7 and 11 months, generally by cachexia or paralysis. Carbohydrate metabolism disturbances were exaggerated with hyperglycemia, glycosuria, polyuria, ketonuria, liver and muscle glycogen decrease and body weight loss.

REFERENCES

1. Martinez, C., 1946, Influencia de la dieta sobre la diabetes de la rata. Rev Soc Argent Biol 22: 414-425.

2. Foglia, V.G., 1965, Prediabetes experimental. III Simp Panamer Farmac Terap Excerpta Med Intern Congr, Mexico, Series No. 127: 197-204.

3. Martin, J.M., Lacy, P.E., 1963, The prediabetic period in partially pancreatectomized rats. Diabetes 12: 238-242.

4. Foglia, V.G., 1970, Fetuses and newborns of 95% pancreatectomized female rats. In Early Diabetes, Camerini-Davalos and Cole, Eds., Academic Press, New York: 221-227.

5. Foglia, V.G., 1970, Experimental prediabetes. Proc VII Congr Intern Diabetes Fed Excerpta Intern Congr, Buenos AIres: 198-208.

6. Malgor, L.A., Foglia, V.G., Negro, Vilar A., 1963, Influencia de la pielonefritis experimental sobre el periodo de prediabetes de la rata. Rev Soc Argent Biol 39: 187-196.

HEREDITARY DIABETES IN THE KK MOUSE: AN OVERVIEW

¶A.S. Reddi[+] and R.A. Camerini-Davalos[++]

[+]Department of Medicine, UMDNJ-New Jersey Medical School, Newark, N.J.
[++]Department of Medicine, New York Medical College
Metropolitan Hospital Research Center, New York, New York

Diabetes and its complications cause increased morbidity and mortality in man. Despite numerous studies, the pathogenesis of these complications is poorly understood. This is partly due to the lack of large and well-controlled human studies. To this end, researchers have been forced to develop animal models of human diabetes. In such animals, the maintenance of controlled environmental conditions and selective breeding over several generations with a large number of offspring can easily be accomplished. This allows for extensive investigation in a relatively short period of time.

The Japanese KK mouse appears to be an ideal animal model for studying diabetes and its complications because: a) it develops spontaneous hereditary diabetes, preceded by a stage of prediabetes; b) it develops renal, retinal and neurologic complications similar to those seen in human diabetes; and c) it does not require either insulin or other medications for survival, thus allowing the investigator to study the natural cause of the disease without interference of drugs.

In this article, an overview of diabetes and its complications in the KK mouse is discussed in terms of:

1) Carbohydrate metabolism

2) Genetic transmission of diabetes

3) Microvascular complications

4) Complications of pregnancy

CARBOHYDRATE METABOLISM

The inbred strain of KK mice was first established by Kondo et al. (1)

This work was supported in part by the Diabetes Research Fund, New York, New York, and the Michael J. Bilotto Research Fund of Hope for Diabetics Foundation, New York, New York.

This paper is dedicated to the memory of Werner Oppermann.

TABLE I

PERCENTAGE OF HYPERGLYCEMIA (POST-GLUCOSE) in KK MICE IN CONSECUTIVE GENERATIONS

	(Percent)
F 6	87.5
F 7	68
F 8	87
F 9	56
F 10	46
F 11	79
F 12	80

in 1957 in Japan. In 1962, Nakamura (2) described spontaneous diabetes in these mice; earlier generations of which had been exposed to the atom bomb blast. Subsequently, several laboratories, including ours, used KK mice as a model for the study of genetic diabetes. Our colony of KK mice was obtained in 1965 from Smith, Kline, and French Laboratories, Philadelphia, which received them from Nakamura in Japan. Since then, these mice have been inbred for several generations. Our mice are neither obese or glucosuric.

Nakamura (2) reported that the hyperglycemic state of the KK mice resembles diabetes mellitus of the maturity-onset type in man. Later our group (3) and Iwatsuka et al (4) described the metabolic disturbance of KK mice as chemical diabetes, since the primary abnormality is impaired glucose tolerance with normal fasting blood sugar levels (Figure 1). These mice do not develop carbohydrate intolerance before 100 days of age, and thus they undergo a stage called prediabetes (Figure 1). During this stage, pretreatment of these mice with glucagon, growth hormone, and epinephrine impairs glucose tolerance to a greater degree than in Swiss albino mice, suggesting that KK mice are more sensitive to these hormones. Insulin values were found to be lower at 20 minutes following an oral glucose load only at 20 days of age. At 40 days of age, the fasting insulin levels were higher in KK mice and at 100 and 180 days the values were higher during the entire oral glucose tolerance test (Figure 1).

The percentage of mice with hyperglycemia (post-glucose values) varies considerably from generation to generation. This was demonstrated by the evaluation of 7 sequential generations of inbred KK litters (Table I).

Pancreatic insulin content was found to be greater in KK than in control mice. Histologic changes of the pancreas include hypertrophy and hyperplasia of islets, hypertrophy and degranulation of B cells, abundance of B-cell ribosomes, well-developed endoplasmic reticulum and enlarged Golgi areas of B cells, and diminution of the zinc content of insular cells. These findings suggest that enhanced synthesis and release as well as decreased storage of insulin within the islet occur in KK mice (5).

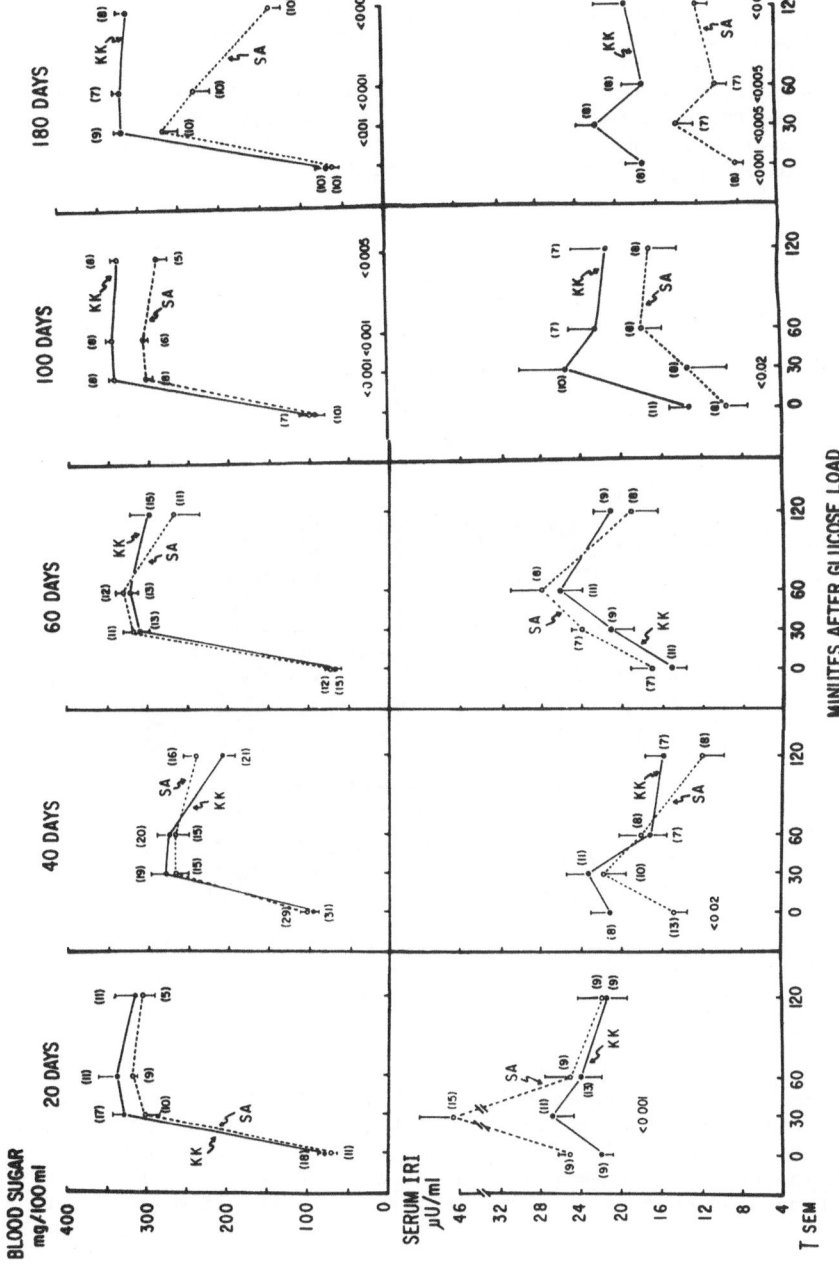

Figure 1. Blood serum and serum immunoreactive insulin (IRI) response to an oral glucose load in Swiss albino (SA) and KK mice at different age periods. Numbers in parentheses represent number of animals.

9

Light- and electron-microscopic studies of the anterior pituitary from 3-month-old KK mice showed hypertrophy and hyperplasia of growth hormone-secreting cells with an abundance of secretory granules. Consistent with the histologic findings, an increased amount of growth hormone in the pituitary was found on acrylamide gel electrophoresis (5).

Baseline glucose oxidation by epididymal adipose tissue was significantly decreased in older (7-11 months) KK mice, and addition of insulin to the medium failed to increase the oxidation. Although glucose oxidation was not impaired in diaphragm muscles of KK mice, the muscles' response to insulin was greatly reduced. Consistent with this peripheral insulin insensitivity is the observation that liver plasma membranes have decreased numbers of insulin receptors, which bind only 55 to 70% as much insulin per mg of protein as those of Swiss albino mice (5).

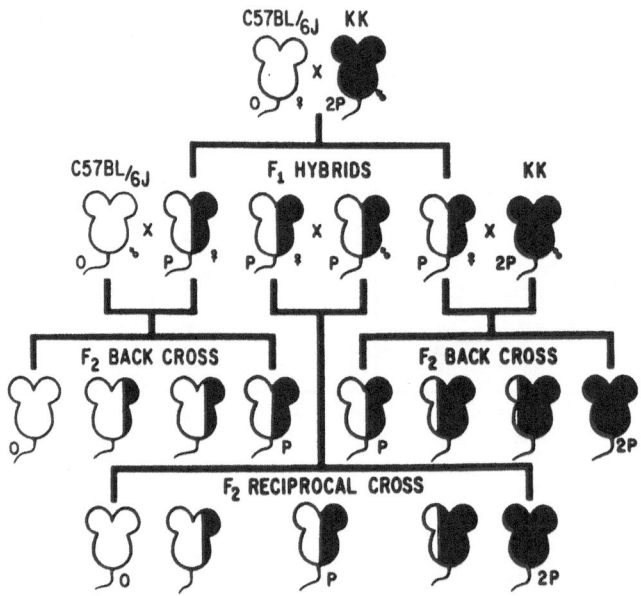

Figure 2. Mating procedure of female C57BL/$_{6J}$ and male KK mice.

KK mice were found to be relatively resistant to streptozotocin treatment, since the same dose of the antibiotic produced hyperglycemia in CBL mice. Phentolamine completely abolished the resistance, suggesting that the alpha-adrenergic system predominates in B cells of the KK mouse (5). All of these studies suggest that carbohydrate metabolism is altered in KK mice.

GENETIC TRANSMISSION OF DIABETES

The mode of inheritance of diabetes in KK mice is not clear. Nakamura and Yamada (6) and our group (5) using glucose tolerance as a criterion, suggested that the mode of inheritance is polygenic. On the other hand,

Butler and Gerritsen (7), using glucosuria as a genetic marker, explained the inheritance by proposing a single dominant gene with 25% to 75% penetrance. The presence or absence of glycosuria in KK mice from various laboratories appears to be due to selective breeding over several generations.

In order to understand genetic transmission of glucose intolerance to normal mice, we performed a mating procedure between normal control (C57-BL/6J) and KK mice, as shown in Figure 2. White indicates the CBL and black the KK gene dosage over the scale from 0 to 2 P. 0 stands for no KK or no diabetic gene dosage; 2 P indicates that both parents are of the KK species or that these mice carry 100% diabetic gene dosage. F2 backcrossing was performed by mating the FL hybrids with male CBL and male KK mice. The reciprocal F2 was obtained by mating the Fl hybrids with one another.

In Figure 3 the glucose areas of different types of mice at 5 weeks of age are plotted according to their postulated KK or no diabetic gene dosages from 0 to 2 P. By using this glucose area as the genetic marker for the diabetic syndrome, a line can be drawn from the left lower to the right upper side, indicating the increasing genetic potential for diabetes and providing support for the polygene theory as a mode of inheritance of diabetes in KK mice.

There was an increasing percentage of glomerulosclerosis from the backcross F2 (Fl x CBL) with 0.5 P or 25% gene dosage to the F2 type (Fl x KK) with 1.5 or 75% KK genes, indicating that there is a close correlation between the incidence of glomerulosclerosis and the average KK gene dosage (Figure 4). The observation of significant glomerular lesions in one-half of the hybrids (Fl x Fl) with 50% KK genes is further evidence for a positive relation between these two parameters. The findings suggest that the KK mouse inherits not only hyperglycemia but also glomerulosclerosis and that these characteristics can be genetically transmitted to healthy recipients by proper cross-mating.

MICROVASCULAR COMPLICATIONS

In addition to carbohydrate dysmetabolism, the KK mice develop human

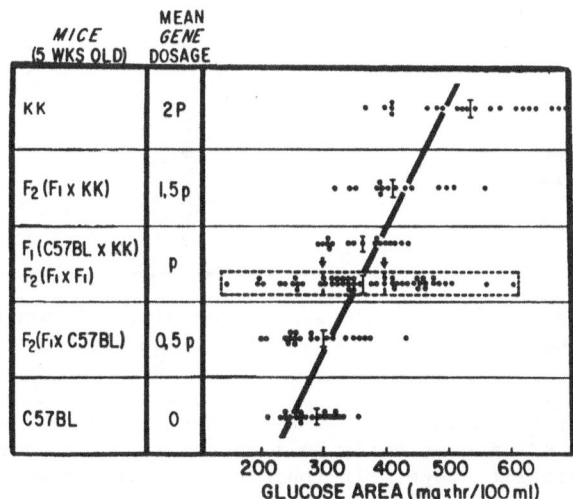

Figure 3. Tolerance to oral glucose after an 18 hour fast. Glucose area levels of KK, C57BL/6J and their hybrid offspring in relation to diabetic gene dosage.

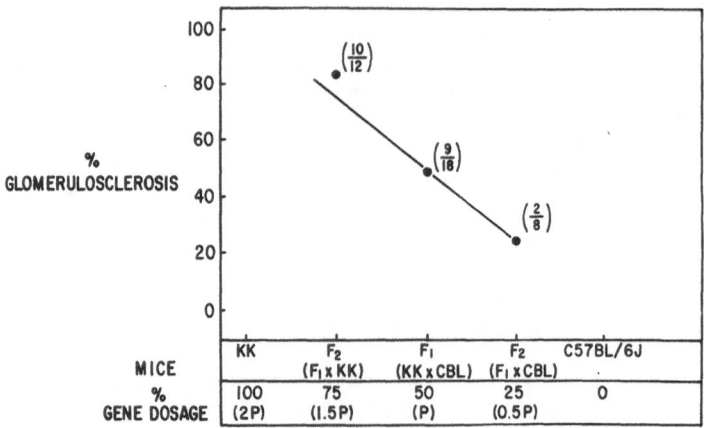

Figure 4. Percent decrease in glomerulosclerosis with decrease in mean gene dosage in hybrid mice derived from KK and C57BL/6J mice.

TABLE II

SIMILARITIES AND DIFFERENCES BETWEEN HUMAN DIABETIC PREGNANCY
AND PREGNANCY IN THE KK MOUSE.

	Human		KK	
	Yes	No	Yes	No
Maternal				
CHO intolerance in late pregnancy	X		X	
Fasting hypoglycemia	X		X	
Elevated serum insulin	X			X
CHO tolerance in consecutive pregnancies: decreased and improved	X		X	
Postpartum improvement of CHO tolerance	X		X	
Placental				
Small placenta due to maternal microangiopathy	X		X	
Placental hyperplasia	X			X
Fetal				
Macrosomia	X			X
Hydramnios	X			X
Intrauterine death	X		X	
Congenital anomalies	X		?	
Hyperinsulinemia	X		X	
Beta-cell hyperplasia	X		X	
Hypoglycemia due to fasting	?		X	

diabetic-like microangiopathy; glomerulosclerosis, retinopathy, and peripheral gnagrene due to small blood vessel disease (3).

Glomerulosclerosis: Diabetic glomerulosclerosis, which involves an excessive deposition of mesangial matrix, is a consistently demonstrable pathologic disorder in KK mice as early as 1 month of age, these kidney changes appear in the pediatric stage. In the older KK mice, the marked increase in the mesangial matrix results in the formation of glomerular nodules. Exudative-like glomerular lesions were also observed in some of these mice. Details of the kidney disease in the KK mouse are described elsewhere in this volume.

TABLE III

SUMMARY OF CERTAIN CHARACTERISTICS OF THE KK MICE
AND 4 DIFFERENT TYPES OF CONTROL MICE

Mice	Glucose intolerance	Hyper-insulinism	Obesity	Glomerular changes	Retinal changes	Neurologic changes
C57BL/6J	-	-	-	-	-	-
Swiss alb I	+	-	-	-	-	-
Swiss alb II	-	+	+	-	-	-
Yellow (A^y)	-	++	++	-	-	-
KK	++	++	-	+++	++	+

Retinopathy: Nakamura (1) reported that the thickness of the retina was reduced in KK mice. Later we reported retinal microaneurysms in these mice (Figure 5). Subsequently, these findings were confirmed by other investigators (5). In addition, elongation and constriction of veins, dilation of capillaries, and degeneration of intramural pericytes as well as tortuous, irregular, and strand-like capillaries were observed (5). These retinal lesions were more common in older animals. Electroretinogram (EGR) was subnormal in 7 to 20-month-old KK mice (9). About 27% of KK mice (18-20 months of age) showed atherosclerotic alterations with intimal thickening and new formation of connective tissue in the retinal arterioles. Electron-microscopic studies of the retinal capillaries revealed thickening of the basement membranes (8).

Administration of alloxan or IDPN (BB-iminodiproprionitrile) or both to 3-month-old KK mice cause protuberance and diminution of mural cells, proliferation of endothelial cells, and thickening of the capillary basement membranes. As to ERG findings, a significant decrease in amplitude in oscillatory potentials was observed. Ligation of carotid arteries also cause diminution in the number of mural cells (8).

Changes in the Optic Nerve: The optic nerve of KK and control DDY mice was examined with an electron microscope (9). Disorders of the myelin sheath, edematous change in the axon, and the tendency of enlargement and destruction of mitochondria were found in KK mice. In findings concerning the optic capillaries, the observed thickening of the basement membrane and reactive changes of the endothelial cells. Glial cells and pericytes did not show notable changes.

COMPLICATIONS OF PREGNANCY

It has been reported that pregnancy, when complicated by diabetes, exerts a profound influence on carbohydrate metabolism, fetus, and placenta in both humans and animals. We have extended these investigations to KK mice, where carbohydrate tolerance was studied in four consecutive pregnancies. Each female was mated with the same male, and similar environmental conditions were maintained throughout the experiment. In addition, the placental and fetal weights and composition were recorded (10). Table II summarizes similarities and differences between human diabetic pregnancy and pregnancy in our KK mice.

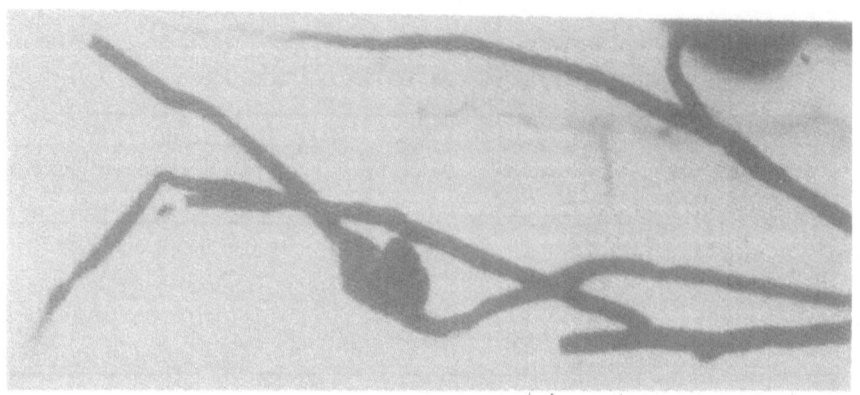

Figure 5. Microaneurysm in the retina of a 9 month-old KK mouse. Flat preparation with a modified in vivo silver nitrate perfusion technique.

SUMMARY AND CONCLUSIONS

Table III compares metabolic and morphologic characteristics of different species of control and KK mice. The C57BL/6J demonstrates no significant metabolic, clinical or histologic abnormalities. Our two highly inbred Swiss albino groups I and II also do not show significant glomerular lesions, although we found striking intolerance to glucose, hyperinsulinism, and obesity among them. Thus a genetic predisposition may be necessary in addition to various environmental factors to produce microangiopathy in KK mice. The yellow A^Y mouse is included in this table, since it is strikingly hyperinsulinemic and obese without concomitant vasculopathy such as the other mentioned control strains have.

In conclusion, the KK mice develop chemical diabetes preceded by a stage of prediabetes and also demonstrate renal, retinal and neurologic complications similar to those seen in human diabetes. Of particular interest is the development of mild to moderate glomerulosclerosis in the prediabetic stage; with progression to severe glomerulosclerosis and attendant proteinuria later in life. With proper back-crossing, both hyperglycemia and glomerulosclerosis can be transmitted to normal control mice, suggesting that a specific genetic background is necessary for the development of diabetes and diabetic-like microangiopathy. We therefore suggest that the KK mouse serves as an ideal genetic animal for the study of non-insulin-dependent diabetes mellitus and its complications for rational prevention and therapy.

REFERENCES

1. Kondo, K., Nozawa, K., Tomita, T., and Ezaki, K., 1957, Inbred strains resulting from Japanese mice. Bull Exp Anim 6: 107-12.

2. Nakamura, M., 1962, A diabetic strain of the mouse. Proc Jap Acad 38: 348-52.

3. Camerini-Davalos, R.A., Oppermann, W., Mittl, R., and Ehrenreich, T., 1970, Studies of vascular and other lesions in KK mice. Diabetologia 6: 324-329.

4. Iwatsuka, H., Matsuo, T., Shino, A., and Suzuoki, Z., 1970, Metabolic disturbance of KK mice in chemical diabetes. J Takeda Res Lab 29: 685-692.

5. Reddi, A.S., Oppermann, W., Velasco, C.A., Strugatz, L.H. and Camerini-Davalos, R.A., 1980, Diabetes mellitus in the KK mouse: Similarities and differences between genetic and other types of diabetes. In Secondary Diabetes: The spectrum of the diabetic syndromes, Podolsky, S. and Viswanathan, M., Eds., New York, Raven Press, 455-469.

6. Nakamura, M., and Yamada, K., 1963, A further study of the diabetic (KK) strain of the mouse. Proc Jap Acad 39: 489-493.

7. Butler, L., and Gerritsen, G.C., 1970, A comparison of the modes of inheritance of diabetes in the Chinese hamster and the KK mouse. Diabetologia 6: 163-167.

8. Morii, F., Hattori, M., Miyazaki, E., Fukuchi, S., and Tsukahara, I., 1974, Histological studies on congenitally diabetic KK mice., 1974, Folea Ophthalmol Jap 25: 372-389.

9. Miyazaki, E., Morii, F., and Yamashita, H., 1975, Histological studies on congenitally diabetic KK mice. Report 2. Electron microscope study findings concerning the optic nerve. J Jap Diab Soc 18: 101-104.

10. Reddi, A.S., Oppermann, W., Velasco, C.A., Strugatz, L.H., and Camerini-Davalos, R.A., 1975, Early genetic diabetes in the KK mouse. In Early Diabetes in Early Life, Camerini-Davalos, R.A. and Cole, H.S., Eds., New York, Academic Press: 413-425.

DEVELOPMENT OF MICROVASCULAR AND ISLET CELL ALTERATIONS IN RATS WITH

SPONTANEOUS NON INSULIN-DEPENDENT DIABETES

¶Gagliardino, J.S., Gomez Dumm, C.L., Semmino, Cristina
and Laguens, R.P.S.

CENEXA-Centro de Endocrinologia Experimental y Aplicada (UNLP-CONICET)
Facultad de Ciencias Medicas, Universidad Nacional de La Plata, Argentina

During the last few years, our group has been engaged in the study of ultrastructural and biochemical aspects of insulin secretion. In this regard, we have described the changes occurring in the size of several structures of the B cell (1) in the number of islet cell-tight junctions (2), in the islet cell plasma membrane Ca^{2+}-ATPase activity (3) and in the islet intracellular calcium distribution within B cells (4) in response to the glucose stimulus. We have also shown evidences on the existence of calcineurin in rat islets (unpublished data). All these data have been obtained from normal animals, therefore, we assumed that their study in a diabetic animal could provide some clues on the early detect of the B cell function.

The e Stilman Salgado (eSS) subline of rats, obtained in the Instituto de Investigaciones Medicas de Rosario from the eIIM line after several inbreedings (coefficient of inbreeding > 0.92), seemed to fulfill our main requirements(5). These rats develop spontaneously a non insulin-dependent diabetic syndrome of mild course that does not affect significantly their half-life span. The percentage of diabetic animals increases with age: 16.6% at 1 month and 90.5% at 10 months, being higher in male than in female rats at every age (5). Even when old animals can become obese, obesity would not be associated with the diabetic syndrome in young rats (5). However, food intake restriction can ameliorate the abnormal serum glucose levels obtained after the glucose load (6).

Studies performed in eSS rats at ages of 12 to 24 months using conventional histologic techniques, revealed a decrease in the endocrine pancreatic mass and a thickening of the glomerular basement membrane (7).

To further characterize the diabetic syndrome in the eSS rats, we report preliminary data on immunocytochemical and ultrastructural studies performed in the islets of eSS rats at different ages and on the appearance in these animals of structural and ultrastructural lesions in the kidney in the striated muscle and its capillaries and peripheral nerve fibers.

This work was partially supported with funds from CONICET and CICPBA from Argentina.

MATERIAL AND METHODS

Male eSS rats of different ages (1, 6 and 18 months) were studied, using age-matched male rats from the α subline as normal controls. All the rats were fed with a balanced commercial diet ad libitum. The animals were sacrificed around 09 a.m. by decapitation under slight ether anaesthesia. A blood sample was obtained previously from the retroorbital plexus for glucose and immunoreactive insulin (IRI) determinations.

The diagnosis of diabetes was assessed by the serum glucose levels measured in either the fasting state or after an oral glucose tolerance test (OGTT=2 g of glucose per kg body weight in 10% solution administered by gastric tube).

At the time of sacrifice, several organs were removed to perform the following studies

Light microscopy: Samples of the tail of the pancreas, kidney and straited muscle were fixed in Bouin's solution, dehydrated in graded alcohol concentrations and embedded in paraffin. For routine studies, sections were stained with hematoxylin-eosin.

Immunocytochemical studies: Pieces of the tail of the pancreas, previously processed as described above, were serially sectioned (1.5 μm) using a Reichert OmU2 ultramicrotome. Serial sections distant 21 um one from another were taken from every series and mounted on the same slide. Adjacent sections were mounted on other slides following the same pattern. Serial sections from three different levels of each block were then stained with hematoxylin-eosin and processed for immunocytochemical identification of insulin-,glucagon-,somatostatin-and pancreatic polypeptide-producing cells using the peroxidase direct method (8). For this purpose, our own insulin antiserum was used, while sera against glucagon, somatostatin and PP were kindly supplied by Dr. Lise Heding (NOVO Industria/s),Dr. Suad Efendic (Dept. Endocrinology, Karolinska Institute) and Dr. Ronald Chance (Eli Lilly). In each case, the specificity of the antisera was assessed by blocking the immunoctyochemical reaction with a previous absorption of the antisera with an excess of the corresponding hormone.

Volume density (Vvi) of the pancreatic islets as well as Vvi of each cell type were determined by the point-counting method (7). For such pur, pose, a 8 x 8 mm grid (289 intersections) was mounted in the eyepiece of the microscope.

Electron microscopy: Samples of the pancreas tail, kidney and striated muscle were fixed in 3% glutaraldehyde in phosphate buffer (pH 7.2), postfixed in 1% osmium tetroxide in the same buffer and embedded in araldite. Ultrathin sections were stained with uranyl acetate and lead citrate and observed in an Elmiskop I electron microscope.

Pancreatic insulin content: After removal, the pancreases were weighted and homogenized in tubes containing acidic ethanol. Insulin was further extracted (six times) with a graded mixture of acidic alcohol, and IRI concentrations were measured in appropriately diluted aliquots by radioimmunoassay using rat insulin as standard (kindly provided by Dr. Lise Heding).

Statistical analysis was performed using the Student's t-test for independent samples.

RESULTS

1. Blood glucose levels: Fasting glucose levels were within normal range

in control as well as in eSS rats, at every age-period studied. However, diabetic glucose levels were attained after the OGTT in the 6-and 18-months old eSS rats (Table 1).

TABLE I

OGTT IN eSS RATS

Serum glucose levels (mg/dl)

Age	0	30 min	60 min	120 min
6 months (7)	101.0±5.5	284.0±9.8	312.9±13.3	207.1±10.1
18 months (4)	117.5±9.6	308.0±26.9	416.0±42.4	293.5±28.9

Each value represents the mean ± SEM. Number of cases between parentheses.

2. Serum IRI levels: Although the non-fasting serum IRI levels were lower in 18-month-old eSS rats, they were not significantly different either from younger eSS rats or control rats of the same age.

3. Pancreatic studies

a) One-month-old-rats: light and electron microscopic studies performed in the eSS rats at this age did not differ significantly from the normal picture observed in the pancreas of the control rats of the same age. Conversely, insulin content was significantly higher in the former than in the latters (18.9+2.9 vs 3.3±0.4 mU/mg wet weight- 5 cases in each group).

b) Six-months-old rats: Light microscopic studies performed in the pancreases of the eSS rats showed remarkable changes compared to those corresponding to the age-matched control rats (Figure 1). The pancreatic islet structure looked disrupted and areas of fibrosis were commonly seen. A clear lymphocytic infiltration was not found, but a few zones with scattered lymphocytes could be observed near the endocrine cells. The immunocytochemical studies showed islets predominantly constituted by numerous well-granulated insulin-containing cell. These cells formed small groups or cords separated by abundant fibrosis. The frequent appearance of B cells surrounding pancreatic ducts and even forming part of the duct epithelium, suggested that an active regenerating process takes place at the level of the insulin-secreting cells. The rest of the islet cell populations were irregularly distributed in diabetic animals, opposed to the normal arrangement of A, D and PP cells in the islet periphery found in the pancreas from C rats.

The morphometric study (Table 2) showed that the Vvi of the endocrine pancreas, B cells and PP cells was significantly higher in diabetic rats compared to that of α rats (Table 2). On the contrary, the Vvi of exocrine pancreas and A cells was lower in eSS rats compared to that of α rats. No differences appeared in the Vvi of D cells.

TABLE II

Vvi OF PANCREATIC TISSUE AND ISLET CELLS IN   AND eSS RATS

Age		6 months		18 months	
Strain		α	eSS	α	eSS
Tissue Vvi	Exocrine	99.3±0.1	98.8±0.1 ↓ •	99.3±0.09	99.7±0.07 ↑ †
	Endocrine	0.7±0.04	1.2±0.1 ↑ •	0.7±0.09	0.3±0.07 ↓ †
Islet cell Vvi	B	74.1±2.6	83.3±2.9 ↑ §	60.2±2.9	41.3±1.9 ↓ §
	A	19.2±1.0	7.0±2.2 ↓ †	32.3±4.1	27.5±3.6
	D	5.1±1.0	4.9±1.3	6.6±1.3	31.2±7.9 ↑ †
	PP	1.6±0.7	4.8±0.3 ↑ •	0.9±0.005	--- ↓ †

Each value represents the mean ± SEM for the number of rats studied. § $P < 0.05$; • <0.02; † <0.01.

Pancreatic ultrastructure confirmed the findings described under the light microscope in eSS rats. Collagenous fibrosis occurred in most of the islets and occupied extensive zones around blood vessels and groups of insular cells. Among them, only B cells showed fine structural alterations which consisted of hypertrophy of endoplasmic reticulum, abnormal distribution of organelles and increased number of pale secretory granules.

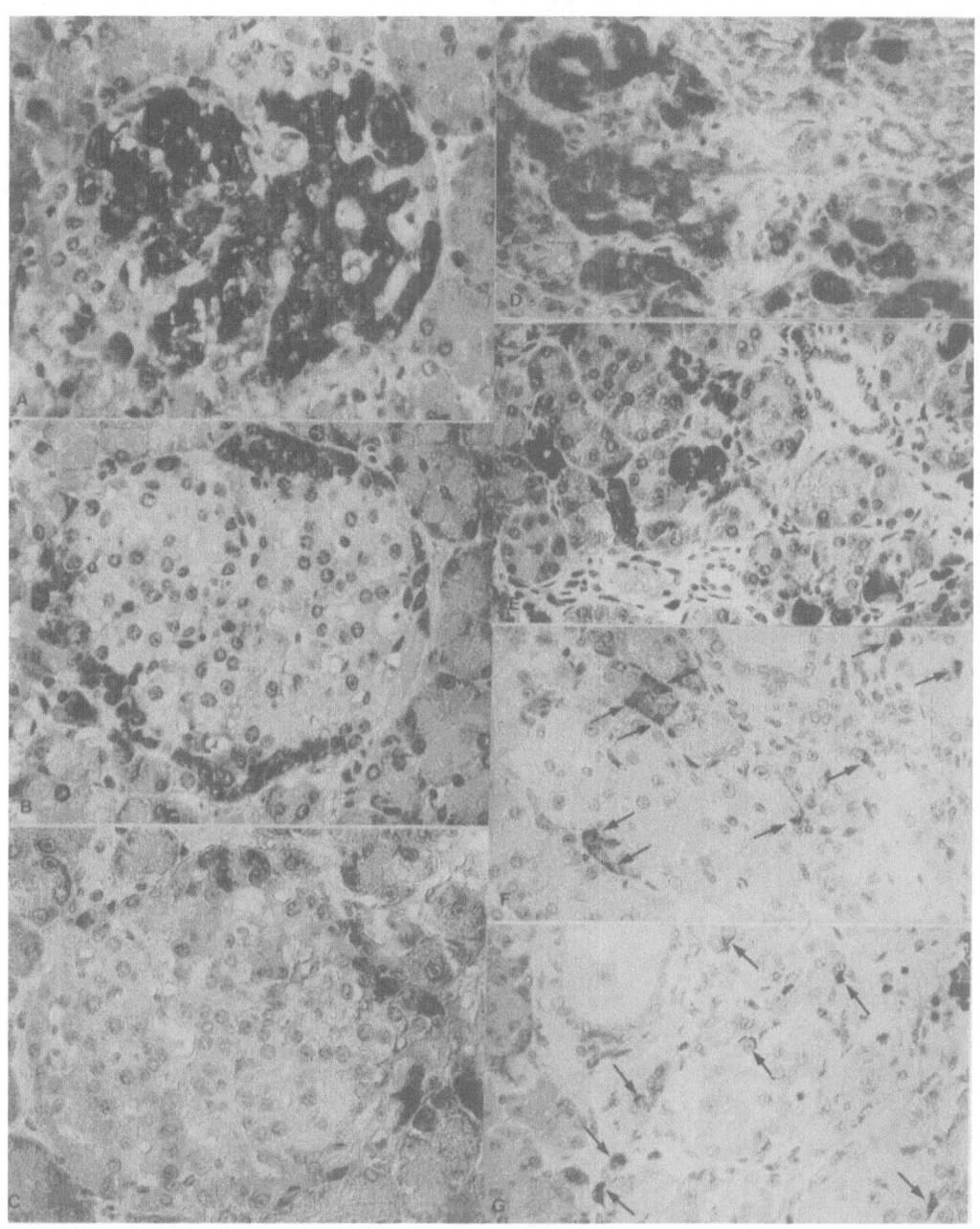

Figure 1. Left: Pancreatic islets from control rats, stained with A: insulin (6-months-old), B: glucagon (6-months-old) and C: somatostatin (18-months-old) antiserum. Right: Pancreatic islets from eSS rats, stained with insulin D: (6-months-old) and E: (18-months old), F: glucagon (6-months-old) and G: somatostatin (18-months-old) antiserum. The arrows point to specifically stained insular cells in F and G. (x 400).

The pancreatic islets from α rats showed normal ultrastructural features.

At this age, the pancreatic insulin content was similar in the eSS(3. 8±0.4 mU/mg W.W-5 cases) and in the α rats (4.0±0.4-4 cases). However, while control animals have similar pancreatic insulin content at the ages of 1 and 6 months, that parameter was significantly lower in the 6-months-old eSS rats.

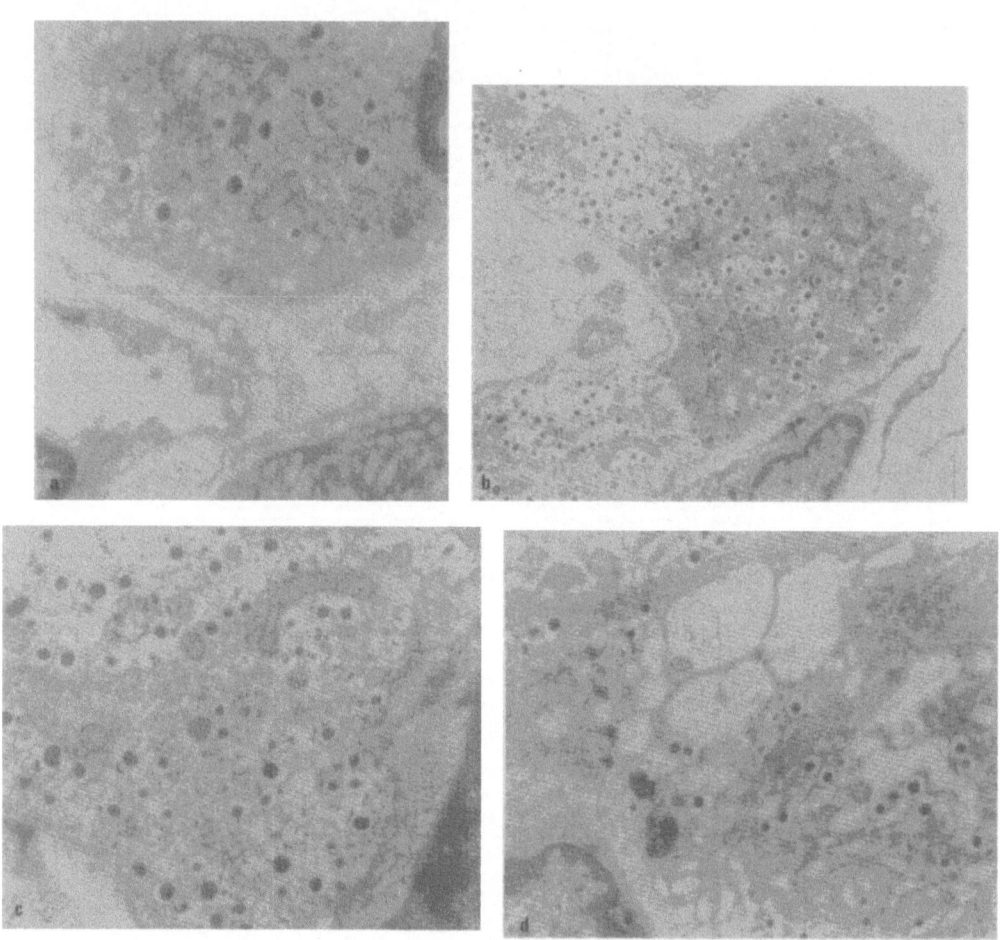

Figure 2. Ultrastructural aspects of endocrine tissue. a: normal B cell from a control rat. A blood capillary with its basement membrane can be observed in the upper left, (X 13,000); b: racket-shaped B cell from an eSS rat (18 months old) showing irregular distribution of secretory granules. Another abnormal B cell is seen in the lower left. A pronounced scarring of the stroma is also present, (X 6,500); c: detail of the B cell detectable in the lower left of b. Many secretory granules exhibit a broken limiting membrane. Small dense glycogen granules are scattered over the cell, (X 10,000); d: conspicuous dilation of the endoplasmic reticulum in a B cell from an eSS rat (6 months old), (X 8,000); (continued on next page).

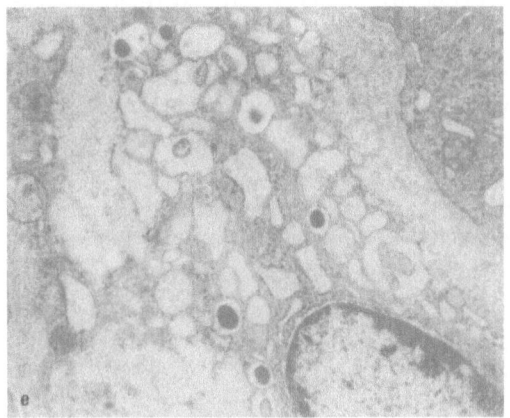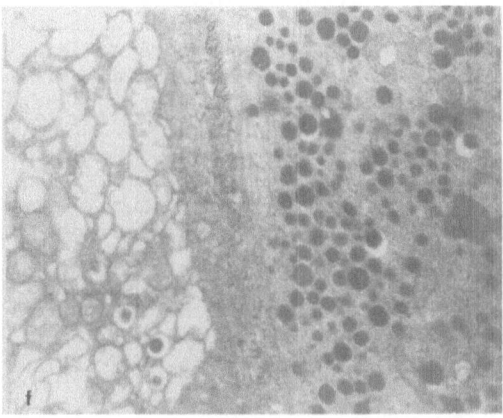

Figure 2 (continued). e: B cell from an eSS rat (18 months old) showing dilated cisternae of endoplasmic reticulum enclosing fine material. The surrounding collagen is not separated by a clearly detected plasma membrane (X 13,000); f: notice the contrast between a grossly altered B cell (left) and a normal A cell (right), (X 10,000).

c) Eighteen-months-old rats: The light microscopy showed that most of the pancreatic islets from eSS rats were abnormal. Their structure appeared distorted and a pronounced scarring of the stroma was frequently found.

Signs of probable regeneration of B cells were also seen together with an irregular distribution of islet cell populations, similar to the one observed in the 6-months-old eSS rats.

The morphometric analysis of the pancreas revealed conspicuous differences between eSS and α rats (Table 2). In the formers, the Vvi of the endocrine tissue, B cells and PP cells was significantly lower than that from control rats. Conversely, the Vvi of exocrine pancreas and D cells was higher in diabetic rats. No changes were found in the Vvi of A cells.

The electron microscopic studies of the pancreas from eSS rats showed striking ultrastructural changes in its B cells, while the other three types of islet cells maintained their normal fine structure. Many B cells presented distortion of the cytoplasmic organelles and contained abundant glycogen particles. The endoplasmic reticulum showed dilated vesicles containing finely granular or reticular material. Large bundles of collagen appeared surrounding single or grouped endocrine cells. Blood capillaries of the pancreatic islets revealed thickening of the basement membrane, which sometimes appeared multiple. The fine structure of islets from control animals was normal.

The insulin content of the 18-months-old eSS rats decreased significantly below the values found in these animals at 6 months (1.7 mU/mg w.w-13 cases).

4. Kidneys: Kidneys appeared severely damaged in 6-and 18-months-old eSS rats. Glomerular involoement was especially noticeable and mainly consisted of hypertrophy of mesangial tissue. No changes appeared in kidneys of 1-month-old ess rats or in those of control animals at any of the ages studied.

5. _Muscle blood vessels_: The elctron microscopic studies of skeletal muscle from 6-and 18-months-old eSS rats showed a diffuse increase in the thickness of capillary basement membrane. This finding coexisted with a quite remarkable number of pinocytotic vesicles in endothelial cells. No ultrastructural alterations of the skeletal muscle fine blood vessels were found in control rats.

6. _Muscle nerve fibers_: analysis of muscle nerve fibers revealed alterations in myelin ultrastructure, consisting of splitting of sheaths next to the axons. In the axoplasm, some large and heterogeneous lysosomes could also be found.

7. _Muscle tissue_: The ultrastructural studies of skeletal muscle from 18-months-old eSS rats showed, in some muscle cells, conspicuous breaking of the myofibrils, with lost of myofilaments.

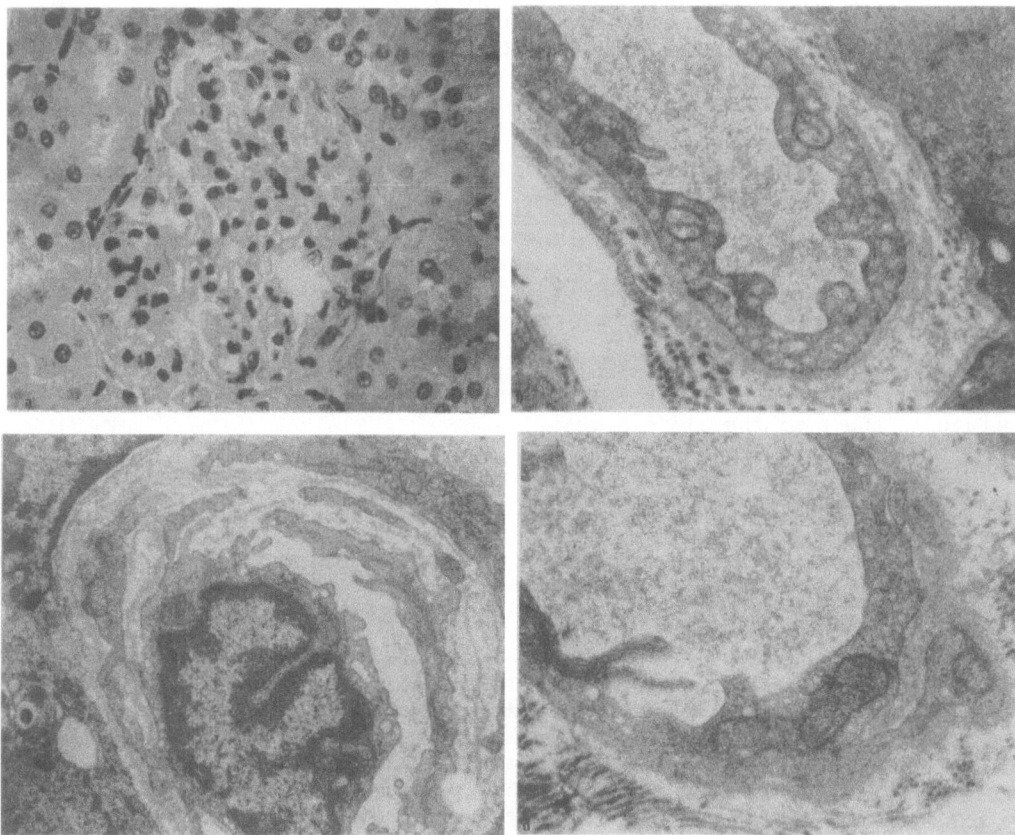

Figure 3. a: renal corpuscule from an eSS rat (18-months-old). The mesangial cells and matrix are increased, while the capillary lumen and Bowman's space are diminshed, (X 400). From b to d, ultrastructural changes in blood capillaries of eSS rats. b: capillary from striated muscle (6-months-old). There is a thickening of the basement membrane and a large number of pynocytotic vesicles, (X 22,000). c: capillary from a pancreatic islet (18-months-old). A multiple basement membrane is clearly seen. (X 12,000). d: capillary from striated muscle (18-months-old) with a diffuse thickening of the basement membrane and numerous pynocytotic vesicles. (X 8,000).

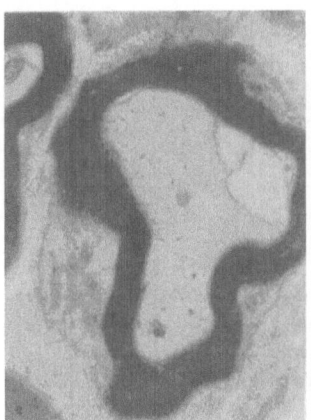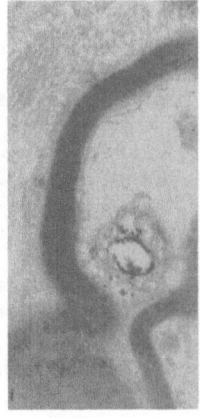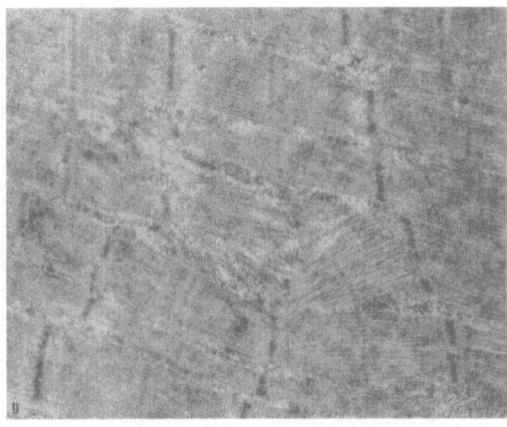

Figure 3 (cont.). e: electron microscopy of a nerve fiber from an eSS rat
(18 months old). Inner lamelae of the myelin sheath are splitted, forming
large vacuoles (X 12,000). f: the same case shown before. Heterogeneous
lysosome can be observed in the axoplasm of a mylinated nerve fiber. (X
12,000). g: ultrastructure of striated muscle from an ESS rat (18 month
old). A broken myofibril is clearly seen. (X 18,000).

DISCUSSION

Our results confirm the presence of a mild diabetic syndrome in adult
non obese (or slightly overweight) male eSS rats (5). Normal fasting glucose levels were found in all the animals tudied, regardless of the diabetic
levels found after the glucose load in the 6-and 18-months-old eSS rats.
Such abnormal values were higher in the latter than in the former group of
diabetic rats. However, no significant differences were found in the non-
fasting morning IRI levels either between the 6 and 18-months-old eSS rats
or when the diabetic animals were compared to their age-matched controls.

Clear-cut differences were observed between 6-and 18-months-old diabetic
rats in their endocrine pancreas volume density, islet cell population and
pancreatic insulin content. At 6 months, there was an increase in the endocrine pancreas, B cell and PP cell volume density together with a decrease in this parameter in regard to A cells. Conversely, at 18 months,
eSS rats showed a decrease in the endocrine pancreas and B cell volume density accompanied by an increase in the volume density of D cells. On the
other hand, no significant differences were found in these parameters in
the pancreas of either control or eSS rats at 1 month. No clear signs of
insulitis were seen at any of the age-periods studied. According to these
data, the endocrine pancreas might undergo an hyperplastic process at 6
months followed by a period of cell exhaustion accomplished at 18 months.
The progressive decrease in the pancreatic insulin content observed in the
eSS rats from 1 to 18 months, would suggests that the hyperplastic period
is an attempt of B cells to compensate for such a decrease. This effort
would lead to the final B cell exhaustion observed at 18 months. The
changes observed in the rest of the islet cell populations might only represent the consequence of the primary change in the B cell mass. Similar
behavior has already been described in the pancreas of other strain of rats
and human beings, with induced and spontaneous diabetic syndromes respectively (10).

The sequential appearance of normal, hyperplastic and hypoplastic islets in a relative short period, might render the subline of eSS rats suitable for the search for some early ultrastructural and biochemical defect in the islets, which leads to the establishment of the diabetic syndrome.

Regardless of the mild course of the diabetic syndrome in this model and the long period of normal fasting serum glucose levels, evident lesions in some tissues were already detected in the 6-months-old eSS rats. Such alterations affected the kidney, the striated muscle ultrastructure, as well as the myelin sheath of peripheral nerves fibers and the capillaries of pancreas and striated muscle. These lesions detected in the 6-months-old animals, become of greater magnitude in the 18-months-old eSS diabetic rats. Consequently, the peripheral alterations would appear together with the B cell lesion, being probably the morphological counterpart of the impaired metabolism which is characteristic of the diabetic syndrome. We do not know whether at this time the peripheral response to insulin is normal or significantly diminished. Such data would help to understand the pathogenesis of the peripheral lesions currently described.

The ultrastructural and hormonal alterations present in the endocrine pancreas, together with the peripheral lesions described, suggest that eSS rats might represent a suitable model to study different physiopathological aspects of the non insulin-dependent diabetic syndrome. It could also be used to test the effectiveness of different treatments to prevent the appearance of or to ameliorate the course of the islet and peripheral tissue alterations.

ACKNOWLEDGEMENTS

The authors wish to thank Dr. S.L. Rabasa and his coworkers for the kind provision of rats and unpublished information on the characteristics of the eSS rats; we also thank Mr. C. Bianchi, Lic., M.E. Garcia and R. Nieto for technical assistance and Mrs. S. Lunati for secretarial support. Labelled insulin for the insulin radioimmunoassay was kindly provided by Dr. Lise Heding (NOVO).

REFERENCES

1. Semino, M.C., Rebolledo, O.R., and Gagliardino, J.J., 1986, Quantitative ultrastructural changes induced by glucose in pancreatic B cells. Acta Physiol Pharmacol Latinoam 36: 447-461.

2. Semino, M.C., Gagliardino, E.E.P.de, and Gagliardino, J.J., 1987, Islet-cells tight junctions:changes in its number induced by glucose. Acta Physiol Pharmacol Latinoam 37: 533-539.

3. Gronda, C.M., Rossi, J.P.F.C., and Gagliardino, J.J., Effect of different insulin secretqgogues and blocking agents on islet cell Ca^{2+}-ATPase activity. Biochim Biophys Acta (accepted in press).

4. Gagliardino, J.J., Semino, M.C., Rebolledo, O.R., Gomez, Dumm, C.L., and Hernandez, R.E., 1984, Sequential determination of calcium distribution in B cells at the various phases of glucose-induced insulin secretion. Diabetologia 26: 290-296.

5. Tarres, M.C., Martinez, S.M., Liborio, M.M., and Rabasa, S.L., 1981, Diabetes mellitus en una linea endocriada de ratas. Mendeliana 5: 39-48.

6. Tarres, M.C., Martinez, S.M., Liborio, M.M., Picena, J.C., and Rabasa, S.L., 1986, Efecto del ambiente nutricional sobre la expresion del sindrome diabetico de las ratas eSS. Medicina 46: 429-434.

7. Martinez, S.M., Tarres, M.C., Liborio, M.M., de Robledo, H.A., Picena, J.C., and Rabasa, S.L, 1984, Modelo murino de la diabetes clinicamente benigna de los jovenes (MODY), Medicina. 44: 145-152.

8. Sternberger, L.A., Hardy, P.H., Cuculis, J.J., and Meyer, H.S., 1970, The unlabeled antibody enzyme method of immunochemistry. Preparation and properties of soluble antigen-antibody complex (horseradish peroxidase-antihorseradish peroxidase) and its use in identification of spirochetes. J Histochem Cytochem. 18: 315-333.

9. Weibel, E.R., 1969, Stereological principles for morphometry in electron microscopy. Int Rev Cytol 26: 235-302.

10. Orci, L., Baetens, D., Rufener, C., Amherdt, M., Ravazzola, M., Studer, P., Malaisse-Lagae, F., and Unger, R.H., 1976, Hypertrophy and Hyperplasia of somatostatin-containing D-cells in diabetes. Proc Nat Acad Sci (USA) 73: 1388-1342.

DEVELOPMENT OF DIABETES IN THE NON-OBESE NIDDM RAT (GK RAT)

¶Yoshio Goto, Ken-ichi Suzuki, Toshio Ono
Masayoshi Sasaki and Takayoshi Toyota

Third Department of Internal Medicine
Tohoku University School of Medicine, Sendai, Japan

We produce spontaneously diabetic rats from normal rats by repeating the selective breeding using glucose intolerance as the selection index. The rats are called GK rats and now we have the 37th generation. In this paper, characteristic features, insulin secretion and the effect of obesity will be presented.

BREEDING EXPERIMENT

In 1973, we performed oral glucose tolerance tests (2g per kilogram of body weight) in 211 Wistar rats. The grade of glucose intolerance was expressed as the sum of blood glucose values at five time points, i.e. fasting, 30, 60, 90, 120 min. after glucose administration. Of course, there were no diabetic rats among the conventional Wistar rats. The sums of blood glucose values (Σ BG) of the 211 rats were distributed between 380 and 740 mg/dl with a mean value of 558.8 ± 59.1 mg/dl (1).

For the selection, the two hour level was evaluated in addition to the sum (Σ BG). Of the 211, 18 rats were selected by the glucose tolerance test and mated, yielding 162 F1 rats. This procedure was repeated up to now. The distribution of Σ BGs shifted to the right (glucose intolerance or hyperglycemic zone) and all of the offspring had a diabetic glucose tolerance test after the 10th generation.

GLUCOSE INTOLERANCE AND INSULIN SECRETION

Glucose intolerance of the GK rats is found at 2 weeks after birth and it becomes prominent at 8 weeks. The intolerance does not become greater with age.

The plasma insulin response during oral or intravenous glucose tolerance tests showed a sluggish and delayed increase of insulin and the response was significantly less than that of normal Wistar rats (2).

The insulin response provoked by glucose stimulation in the isolated pancreas perfusion system, showed a lack of the first phase and a decreased second phase secretion. The insulin response to arginine stimulation, however, is normal.

The relationship between sum of the blood glucose values (Σ BG and the first phase insulin response, and the correlation between Σ BG and insulin content of the pancreas are shown in Figure 1. This result shows that glucose intolerance becomes manifest if the insulin content of the pancreas in less than 20 μ g per pancreas and GTT in frankly diabetic if the insulin content is less than 8 μ g per pancreas.

The values of GK rats are also indicated in the figure and it is clear that the values of GK rats deviate from the curves obtained in normal Wistar rats. This shows that the insulin secretion of GK rats is different from that of Wistar rats. In other words, insulin response to glucose is less in GK rats despite the relatively higher insulin content of the pancreas.

MORPHOMETRY OF THE ISLETS

The weight of the pancreas is not different from that of normal Wistar rats. The mean area of the islets of the GK rats was significantly less than that of normal rats at 16 weeks of age. The shape of the islets is round or oval until 8 weeks after birth, then it becomes irregular. Deformity rate of the islet was calculated by the following formula:

$$\text{deformity index} = \frac{L^2}{S \times 4\pi}$$

where S is area and L is circumference of the islet. In case of a circle, the index is 1.0 and it becomes greater with the grade of irregularity. The deformity index of the GK rats was not different than that of normal Wistar rats until 8 weeks after birth but it was significantly greater after 16 weeks. The morphometric studies were carried out to calculate the immunologically B and A cell numbers in each islet, and the results showed that the B and A cell numbers per islet were significantly less in the 16 week-old GK rats than those of the age-matched normal Wistar rats.

CHRONIC COMPLICATIONS

Nerve conduction velocity of the tail nerve of GK rats was significantly slower than that of age-matched normal Wistar rats and morphological studies of the nerves demonstrated many abnormalities. Sorbitol content of the sciatic nerves was significantly greater and myoinositol content was

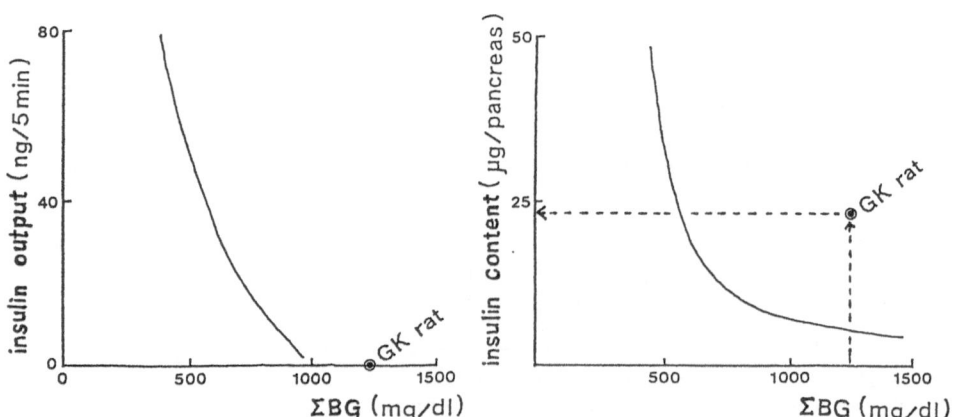

Figure 1. Correlation between glucose tolerance test (ΣBG) and insulin release or insulin content of the pancreas of the GK rat.

significantly less in GK rats than those in normal Wistar rats. Slowness of the nerve conduction velocity and abnormal sorbitol and myoinositol content of the nerves were improved by administration of aldose reductase inhibitors. Lower nerve fiber density was also improved by the inhibitors (3).

In Summary: the GK rat is a non-obese mild diabetic. Plasma insulin response to glucose is impaired but response to arginine is not. A decrease in size of the islets and B cell number is present. Shape of the islets becomes irregular and fibrous with aging. However glucose intolerance shows no aggravation with age. The glucose intolerance is augmented by sucrose feeding. Neuropathy and microangiopathy are present despite a mild glycemic state (4).

REFERENCES

1. Goto, Y., Kakizaki, M., Masaki, N., 1975, Spontaneous diabetes produced by selective breeding of normal Wistar rats. Proc Jap Acad 51: 80-85.

2. Goto, Y., Kakizaki, M., 1981, The spontaneous-diabetes rat: a model of noninsulin dependent diabetes mellitus. Proc Jap Acad 57,B: 381-384.

3. Goto, Y., Kakizaki, M., Yagihashi, S., 1982, Neurological findings in spontaneously diabetic rats. Excerpta Medica ICS No. 581: 26-38.

4. Suzuki, K., Sasaki, M., Ono, T., Abe, S., Toyota, T., Goto, Y., 1987, Recent findings on spontaneously diabetic GK rat. Diabetic Animals, 1: 125-133.

SPONTANEOUS DIABETES IN MACACA NIGRA: RELEVANCE TO HUMAN BEINGS WITH NIDDM

¶Charles F. Howard, Jr.

Oregon Regional Primate Research Center
Beaverton, Oregon

Classification of human diabetes mellitus based on a functional or pathological lesion has helped to clarify research issues and indicate research directions. However, there is increasing awareness of heterogeneity within each classification. An ancillary result of awareness of the heterogeneity is a greater focus on subgroups of individuals and attempts to define exact etiologies based on signs, symptoms, and secondary manifestations.

Older diabetic patients are generally classified as having NIDDM or Type II diabetes, and considered to have a functional lesion. One unresolved aspect of the current classification scheme is how a pathological lesion in the islets of Langerhans, in which there is cell loss and deposition of the protein amyloid, links with development of diabetes in older people. Identification of the lesion was reported almost nine decades ago. Subsequent work, mainly by pathologists, documented an increase in the prevalence of the insular amyloidotic lesions in older diabetics (e.g., 1,2); over age 50, more than 50% of diabetics have amyloid in the islets. The problem is to establish how this pathological lesion contributes to the development of diabetes in those who are generally viewed as having a functional lesion.

To further complicate interpretations, the lesion has been found in 2 to 16% of the population classified as nondiabetic; again most of these are older people. The recent isolation and characterization of a portion of the islet amyloid protein (3,4) has indicated a similarity to calcitonin gene related **peptide**. The source of amyloid and its function, if any, have not been established. However, these findings have reawakened interest in how this lesion relates to diabetes. Exact relationships between the lesion and expression of diabetes have been virtually impossible to explore in human beings.

Members of the monkey species Macaca nigra spontaneously develop impairments in insulin secretion and glucose clearance, and eventually become overtly diabetic. Impairments in this subset of monkeys occur as the islet cells deteriorate and there is concurrent deposition of amyloid (5); eventual loss of sufficient islet secretory cells leads to diabetes (hyperglycemia and insulin therapy). Four stages in the progression from non-diabetes to diabetes have now been established; each stage has distinct metabolic and hormonal characteristics, and the stages can be linked to changes

TABLE I

CLASSIFICATION OF MACACA NIGRA ACCORDING TO METABOLITE AND HORMONE
CONCENTRATION AND RESPONSE

Measure:	Nondiabetic	Hormonally impaired	Borderline diabetic	Diabetic	Units
IV-GTT[*]					
K	>2.0	>2.0	1.0-1.9	<1.0	%glucose clearance/min
ΔIRI	>150	26-150	25-130	<25	µU/ml
Fasting[†]					
Glucose	50-70	50-100	80-115	>140	mg/dl
Insulin	>25	>25	15-25	<15	µU/ml
Glucagon	600-1000	1000-2000	>2000-<1000	250-500	pg/ml
HbA_{IC}	2.1-3.1	--	3.0-4.0	7.1-9.2	% total Hb

[*]Glucose clearance (K) and insulin increment (ΔIRI) were calculated

from values taken during an intravenous glucose tolerance test (IV-GTT).

[†]Values measured after an overnight fast. HbA_{IC} = hemoglobin A_{IC}

in the islet morphology (6). Since the progression through the different
stages has been well established, it is possible to use these monkeys in
studies on the etiology of their diabetes.

Results gained from studies on Macaca nigra have also been used as
guides for examination of patients classified as having NIDDM. Our data
has allowed us to identify human beings who may also have the islet lesion.
These results provide the potential for identification of family members or
others at risk for the lesion and possible latent tendencies toward diabetes.

Progression of Macaca Nigra to Overt Diabetes

The four categories in the development of diabetes are summed in Table
I. Nondiabetic (ND) monkeys generally have metabolic and hormonal criteria
similar to those found in comparable human beings. Fasting blood glucose
(FBG) values in monkeys average about 50 to 70 mg/dl, values somewhat lower
than in human beings. The clearance of glucose (K = glucose clearance per
min) is > 2%/min, and the insulin increment secreted between 0 to 15 min
(Δ IRI) in an intravenous glucose tolerance test (IV-GTT) exceeds 150 U/ml.
Fasting glucagon (IRG) levels are higher in these monkeys than those found
in nondiabetic humans; the IRG molecular size is consistent with that of
pancreatic alpha cell origin. Architecture of the islets appears nearly
identical to that found in human beings.

The first signs of progression toward the hormonally impaired (HI)
stage are a decrease in the Δ IRI and an increase in IRG. The borderline
diabetic (BD) monkeys have further hormonal impairments (lower Δ IRI and

transiently elevated then lowered IRG) and glycemic changes become evident;
the K values drop to 1 to 2 %/min, and the postprandial glucose is elevated
by 10 to 20 mg/dl. Monkeys in the early phase of the BD stage will have
elevated IRG, but IRG levels decrease in the later phase. Diabetic (D)
monkeys have K values below 1 %/min, Δ IRI < 25   u/ml, IRG below 500 pg/ml,
and FBG > 140 mg/dl. Insulin therapy (Iletin II) is necessary for D monkeys.

A distinct advantage of using these monkeys to understand more about
the etiology of diabetes is that they can be experimentally manipulated in
ways not ethical or feasible for human beings. Biopsies of the pancreas
are taken every 4 to 5 years, without overall adverse affects on the monkeys, and at necropsy. Examination of the islets in tissue fixed immediately after removal provides information on the morphological status of
the islet cells, i.e., deterioration of membranes and cells, and appearance
of amyloid. Results are related to the metabolic status of each monkey at
that moment.

Islets of Langerhans of the HI monkeys will vary in their appearance;
some will have early basal lamina changes visible only by electron microscopy, whereas others will have up to 5 to 10% amyloid infiltration and concurrent loss of cells. Amyloid deposition in BD monkeys ranges from 20 to
50 % and D monkeys usually have more than 50 to 60% amyloid in the islets.

Changes in the islet cell populations explain many of the observed
metabolic /clinical changes (6). As beta cells decrease from an average
of 77 % in the ND down to 61% in HI monkeys, Δ IRI decreases; further cell
loss causes further decreases in ΔIRI and eventually there are substantially
lower levels of fasting IRI. Beta cells are less than 5% in the D monkey.
Alpha cells average 6% in the ND monkey and increase to 14% in the HI/early
BD stage as IRG increases; alpha cells comprise < 4% of the total cells in
the late BD stage, and ca. 2% in the D stage. Thus, the metabolic/clinical
stages are a reflection of changes in the islet cells. Whether amyloid is
primary or secondary to the islet lesion is not known. Certainly it can
serve as a marker of islet damage. However, it is the changes in the islet
cell populations that are the primary contributors to the metabolic abnormalities.

Islet Cell Antibodies

Since the deterioration of cells is similiar to what occurs in Type I
human diabetics, we examined blood for islet cell autoantibodies (ICAA) (7).
Our assay used Bouin's fixed, paraffin embedded baboon pancreas as substrate.
Although the assay utilizing frozen, unfixed pancreas and immunofluorescence
will detect some of the ICAA in monkeys, it is far less reliable than fixed
pancreas tissue for monkey ICAA. One reason may be differences in antigens
in this form of diabetes versus those in IDDM. When we washed frozen, unfixed pancreas sections with buffer and incubated the solution with ICAA+
sera, we found significant immunoreactivity. Results support some solubil-
ity of the antigens that cause ICAA formation in this particular form of
diabetes, and thus potential loss from frozen, unfixed tissues.

Blood from monkeys in all stages was examined; summation results are
presented in Table 2 (7). The HI plus BD monkeys had 90% as ICAA positive
(ICAA+). These two groups were significantly different from ND monkeys at
p < 0.01. A few of the ND monkeys tested positive. Most of the D monkeys
also had ICAA, but not as many as would have been expected for their metabolic stage.

TABLE II

ISLET CELL ANTIBODIES IN <u>MACACA</u> <u>NIGRA</u> OF VARIED
METABOLIC/HORMONAL STATUS

ICAA Reaction[*]	Metabolic/clinical stages[†]			
	ND	HI	BD	D
+	4	19	12	8
0	26	4	0	1

[*](+): Positive reaction with definite staining of islet

  cytoplasmic components, readily differentiated from

  unstained islet and acinar cells

  (0): Negative reaction with no or minimal differentiation of

  islets from surrounding acinar tissue.

[†] ND: Nondiabetic, HI: hormonally impaired; BD: borderline

  diabetic; D: diabetic

Most of the ND monkeys had no cell loss. Those ND with ICAA monkeys
might have been in the earliest stages toward the HI stage; certainly electron microscopic examination of islets revealed basal lamina changes in
a few of these monkeys prior to amyloid deposition. The HI and BD monkeys
have an active and progressive loss of cells. Presumably, there was continued release of antigens that elicited an immune response and resulted
in ICAA formation. The D monkeys, especially those in the later stages,
often had few cells of any kind; likely there would have been insufficient
release of antigens to sustain formation of ICAA.

Subsequent work on ICAA has revealed different stain patterns and
changes in these patterns with time (8). The most common ICAA is one
associated with the beta cells (B-ICAA), as determined by incubation with
ICAA and anti-insulin antibodies separately and appropriate double staining.
We have also identified staining patterns in which the ICAA reacted with
components in the alpha or D cells. The B-ICAA pattern is most prevalent;
the alpha/D staining can appeal alone or in conjunction of the B-ICAA pattern. The intensity of the B-ICAA pattern also varies with time. Results
support an episodic degeneration of different islet cells and release of
antigens that cause formation of different ICAA.

STUDIES ON HUMAN BEINGS

Sufficient evidence exists in the literature to document the high prevalence of the insular amyloidotic lesion in older human beings with diabetes (Table 3) (1,2). Much of our work linking the changes in the islet
with the metabolic/hormonal changes was accomplished by removal of pancreas
biopsies from monkeys at several times in their life and during different
metabolic stages. Although removal of pancreas samples from human beings
is generally not feasible, we have analyzed blood for ICAA from patients

TABLE III

AMYLOID IN THE ISLETS OF LANGERHANS OF HUMAN BEINGS*

	Diabetics		Nondiabetics	
Age Range	Numbers[†]	(%)	Numbers[†]	(%)
30 – 39	17/150	(11)	2/336	(1)
40 – 49	71/230	(31)	9/405	(2)
50 – 59	272/568	(48)	40/495	(7)
60 – 69	548/955	(57)	120/1215	(10)
70 – 79	406/633	(64)	149/995	(16)

* Composite statistics from several publications, including references 1 and 2.

† Number of cases with insular amyloidosis/total number of cases.

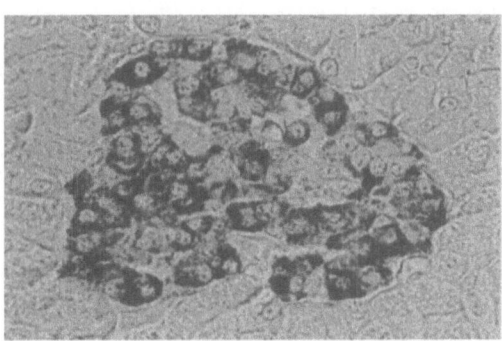

Figure 1. Pancreas from a neonatal baboon was fixed in Bouin's solution, embedded in paraffin, sectioned, deparaffinated and rehydrated. ICAA+ sera from an NIDDM patient was incubated at a 1:4 and 1:32 dilution, washed, then incubated with sheep anti-rabbit γ-globulin, rabbit peroxidase anti-peroxidase, and 3,3'-diaminobenzidine plus H_2O_2 to stain and visualize the reaction sites.

classified as having NIDDM by accepted criteria. A typical B-ICAA pattern observed with blood from an ICAA+ patient with NIDDM is shown in Figure 1.

Of 550 NIDDM patients over age 40 in which ICAA could be definitely scored as negative or positive, 139 (25%) were ICAA+; 62% of the ICAA+ patients were on insulin therapy whereas only 32% of the ICAA- patients received exogenous insulin (different at p < 0.01). There were no significant differences based on sex or ideal body weight. A control population of ORPRC employees and Red Cross blood donors were also examined; the only criteria for inclusion was to be over age 40 and have no known carbohydrate impairment or diagnosed diabetes in the individual or in the family. Only 14 of the 152 controls were ICAA+ (9%); results from controls and those with NIDDM are different at p < 0.01. These data are conservative, since patients with antibodies to insulin and those with the alpha/D pattern were excluded from statistical evaluations.

A few samples of pancreas have been available from autopsies of those on which ICAA had been assayed, and a few samples of blood plus pancreas were obtained from the National Disease Research Interchange. All of those with substantial amyloid (> 10%) were ICAA+, whereas those without amyloid were all ICAA-; a number of individuals with amyloid of < 1% gave equivocal ICAA intensity scores.

CONCLUSIONS

Macaca nigra progress through a series of metabolic/hormonal stages in which there are changes in islet cell populations and eventually development of overt diabetes. The presence of ICAA relates directly to the pathological lesion in the islets of Langerhans.

Older human beings classed as having NIDDM and who are ICAA+ may well have the insular amyloidotic lesion. Underlying causes for diabetes may relate to factors such as diet or obesity, but the islet lesion would cause further complications and would contribute to metabolic abnormalities. A small subset of human beings may have the insular amyloidotic lesion as their only contributor to diabetes. Monitoring human beings for the presence of ICAA can indicate cellular damage. These results support the presence of an insular amyloidotic lesion in about a fourth of the NIDDM population. Given that the ICAA data presented here have been deliberately kept conservative, that some insulin dependent older patients with long duration of diabetes may no longer have necrosing cells to release antigens (analogous to monkeys in the late D stages), and that there is likely episodic degeneration in which ICAA would not always be present in high titers, the actual percentage of those with a lesion could be significantly greater than indicated by these data.

Awareness of a pathological lesion as a part of the Type II classification requires rethinking the requirement that NIDDM be considered as arising only from a functional lesion. In the sense that there is loss of all islet secretory cells, then the Type I classification would be appropriate i.e., a pathological lesion contributing to diabetes. However, many of the patients we have studied are obese with signs and symptoms consistent for Type II diabetes. There is also a higher prevalence of ICAA+ patients on insulin therapy; this would be expected if ICAA arise from a pathological islet lesion. Depletion of beta cells would lead to a need for exogenous insulin. Others who have found ICA in older diabetic patients move from oral hypoglycemic therapy to a requirement for exogenous insulin (9,10).

Results reported in the literature on those who have islet amyloid, but who were considered as being nondiabetic (1,2), may be analogous to what occurs in HI and BD monkeys, which do not have hyperglycemia or glycosuria. Comparable people would have the islet lesion with the early changes in islet cells and some impairments in insulin secretion and glucose clearance, but the changes would not be severe enough to justify a diagnosis of diabetes; they would be considered as nondiabetic. Whether these people will become diabetic over time is as yet unknown. However, even minor impairments could contribute to the early stages of secondary complications.

A major value of monitoring NIDDM patients and their families for ICAA would be the potential for adapting therapy to this specific subgroup. Patients at entry might benefit from immediate insulin therapy rather than use of diet or oral agents. Residual beta cells in humans would be prolonged so that the person would not become insulin dependent as rapidly. Early results on a few HI/BD monkeys maintained on low doses of insulin indicate some amelioration of their metabolic abnormalities.

Macaca nigra have given definite insight into one further contributor to diabetes. They can be used to explore the potential for possible autoimmune reactions as an underlying etiology of the diabetes in these monkeys and in certain older human beings.

REFERENCES

1. Bell, E.T., 1952, Hyalinization of the islets of Langerhans in diabetes mellitus. Diabetes 1: 341-344.

2. Ludwig, V.G., Heitner, H., 1967, Zur Haufigkeit der inselamyloidose des pankreas beim diabetes mellitus. Zeitschrift Fur Die Gesmate Innere Medizin Und Ihre Grenzgebiete 22L 814-829.

3. Cooper, G.J.S., Willis, A.C., Clark, A., Turner, R.C., Sim, R.B., and Reid, K.B.M., 1987, Purification and characterization of a peptide from amyloid-rich pancreases of type 2 diabetic patients. Proc Natl Acad Aci USA, 84: 8628-8632.

4. Westermark, P., Wernstedt, C., Wilander; E., Hayden, D.W., O'Brien, T.D., and Johnson, K.H., Amyloid fibrils in human insulinoma and islets of Langerhans of the diabetic cat are derived from a neuropeptide-like protein also present in normal islet cells. Proc Natl Acad Sci USA 84: 38881-3885.

5. Howard, C.F., Jr., 1978, Insular amyloidosis and diabetes mellitus in Macaca nigra. Diabetes 27: 357-364.

6. Howard, C.F., Van Bueren, A., 1986, Changes in islet cell composition during development during development of diabetes in Macaca nigra. Diabetes 35: 165-171.

7. Howard, C.F., Fang, T-Y., 1984, Islet cell cytoplasmic antibodies in Macaca nigra. Diabetes 33: 219-223.

8. Fang, T.-Y., Van Bueren, T., Howard, C.F., Jr., 1988. Reaction patterns of islet cell autoantibody in Macaca nigra. Pancreas. In press.

9. Irvine, W.J., Sawer, J.S.A., Feek, C.M., Prescott, R.J., Duncan, L.J.P., 1979, The value of islet cell antibody in predicting secondary failure of oral hypoglycaemic agent therapy in diabetes mellitus. J Clin Lab Immunol 2: 23-26.

10. Maloy, A.L., Longnecker, D.S., Greenberg, E.R., 1981, The relation of islet amyloid ot the clinical type of diabetes. Hum Pathol 12: 917-922.

DISCUSSION

D. PYKE: I find this amyloid story confusing. Like you, I think, I don't know what it's doing there. You are talking about it in type 2 diabetes, but it had been found quite commonly in those, diagnosed early in life. Presumably those are type 1 cases, but that may be wrong.

C. HOWARD: The first report of amyloid by Opee in 1900 was in a 16 year old girl. Since that time all the statistics of reports of amyloid indicate that it occurs in greater prevalence with age, and at about age 30 is when it first begins to be noticeable to any statistical significance. The monkeys do not develop this lesion until past sexual maturity, at 7 or 8 years of age. This does not preclude being present in the type 1, but it is more common in type 2.

D. PYKE: Is it related to the known duration of diabetes, either in your animals or in humans?

C. HOWARD: That has not been established in humans. We do find that when these monkeys first begin the metabolic deterioration, if they live long enough, they will eventually have both diabetes and the amyloid, so there is a time component.

D. PYKE: And, does it get more intense the longer the diabetes?

C. HOWARD: That's right.

A. ROLLA: Can you tell us a little bit more about the nature of the amyloid you find? You said it's different from the other amyloids. And, a second related question. Did you find any evidence of amyloid anywhere else in the Macaque Nigra?

C. HOWARD: Let me answer the second question first. There is evidence often of systemic amyloids, but they are not concurrent. We have found this is true in both monkeys and in humans. There are reports in which they find amyloid in the pancreas and none elsewhere and also systemic amyloids may be found and none in the pancreas. In our solubilization procedure, we find that there are both soluble and insoluble amyloids. As to the basis of your question, "is there a difference", histochemically there appear to be no differences. Any number of proteins can be formed into an amyloid fiber. Why it is so insoluble nobody knows. The systemic amyloid, both immunoglobulin and amyloid, are soluble. Their molecular weights are about 20,000 or so.

A. NAJI: Dr. Howard, am I to understand that these animals are hyper-insulinemic? And, have you had a chance to look into the long term complications of these primates for microvascular disease?

C. HOWARD: First of all, they are not hyperinsulinemic. They become increasingly hypoinsulinemic over time. Now, we do have another subset of monkeys that is hyperinsulinemic. Interestingly enough, these monkeys will have some peripheral defects in the binding of insulin. There appear to be, as has been shown for type 1, some peripheral insulin resistance. But, they are not hyperinsulinemic.

Complications, yes. We looked at basal lamina of muscle capillary some years ago and we found significant increases. They do not develop micro-aneurysms. We have not looked at the kidneys, but they do develop atherosclerosis in the abdominal and thoracic aortas.

A. NAJI: And, are all the islets involved, or is this a patchy phenomenon?

C. HOWARD: In the case of the monkey, virtually all of the islets are involved.

J. BARBOSA: Dr. Howard, is there anything known about the genetics of your monkey model?

C. HOWARD: These monkeys come from the island of Sulowezi in the South Pacific. They come from a small portion of the island, and they seem to have inbred so that there is a high disposition towards it.

As to the genetics, we have no real factual information. Anecdotally, when we have bred diabetic or prediabetic males and females, we have a greater incidence in the offspring, but we don't have hard data on that. We think it is genetically monitored, genetically contributed, but we don't know specifically how.

II. IMMUNOLOGICAL MARKERS

INSULIN AUTOANTIBODIES IN PRE-DIABETES

¶ William J. Riley, Mark A. Atkinson and Noel K. MacLaren

Departments of Pathology and Pediatrics
University Of Florida College of Medicine, Gainesville, Florida

Evidence that insulin dependent diabetes mellitus (IDD) is an autoimmune disease has accumulated since autoantibodies to cytoplasmic antigens (ICA) in the pancreatic islet cell were first described a decade ago (1). In addition, other autoantibodies reactive to cell surface antigens of islet cells (ICSA) have been identified using various methods and sources of islet tissue (2-3). The frequencies of these islet reactive antibodies are highest near the time of diagnosis of IDD and fall progressively thereafter. Recently, several reports have observed that ICA can also present years before the onset of clinical diabetes and may, therefore, serve as markers for the autoimmune destruction of beta cells (4-5).

The invariable development of antibodies directed against exogenous, therapeutic insulin has long been recognized in patients with IDD (6). However, when sera from newly diagnosed IDD patients were assayed for insulin binding prior to initiation of insulin therapy, a significant number (18%) had serum proteins that bound to insulin in vitro. This increased insulin binding was found to be in the gamma globulin fraction of the serum proteins and were therefore described as insulin autoantibodies (INSAB) (7). This finding produced many question. Would the radio immunoassay (RIA) for INSAB be able to identify individuals at risk for the development of IDD similar to the ability of ICA? The significance of this question lay in the possibility of screening thousands of sera per week using a relatively simple RIA for INSAB instead of the more cumbersome and time consuming indirect immunofluorescent (IF) assay for ICA. To address this question we determined INSAB in sera from an ongoing prospective population study of high risk (relatives of proband with IDD) and low risk individuals (school children from Pasco County, Florida). Attempts to improve the original methodology of Palmer were also done (7).

METHODS

Patients

The patients evaluated in these studies were part of our ongoing study.

This work was supported by grants from the National Institutes of Health (1-RO-HD-19469-01 and RO-1-AM-36151-01) and the Clinical Research Center (RR-82). Dr. Riley is supported by a Research Career Development Award (KO4-AM-01421-01).

45

True reference ranges for these INSAB assays were obtained by using the entire population of one school (n = 295).

Laboratory studies

HLA typings were done by two color microcytotoxicity assay. ICA were determined by indirect IF as previously described (8). After an appropriate 3 day preparative diet and overnight fasting, 0.5 gm./kg. of 25% glucose was administered as a bolus over 2 to 4 minutes (5). Insulin concentrations were determined at -10, 1,3,5,10,30, and 60 minutes of the glucose bolus, using Cornign radioimmunoassay kits.

To analyze the effect of INSAB on the measurement of insulin in the standard radioimmunoassay, sera from 23 controls, 17 ICA+/INSAB+ and 12 ICA+/INSAB- individuals were analyzed for insulin both before and after PEG precipitation of any potential interfering immunoglobulins reactive with insulin.

Insulin Binding Assay

Two different procedures were developed, although the basic procedure for both methods was a modification of the assay kindly provided in detail by Dr. Jerry Palmer (7). In first method, 50 ul of ^{125}I porcine insulin (Serono lab # 62300, 2mCi/12.5 ml) using 6000 cpm/tube was used. In the second method, 200 μ l of 0.15 ng/ml ^{125}I A-14 purified monoiodinated human insulin (Eli LIlly Research Laboratories, Indianapolis, Indiana) having approximately 15,000 cpm/tube was used as the radioligand. The concentration of the ligand had been optimized to improve the discrimination between the control population and the patients with low titered INSAB from the first method. The nonspecific binding (NSB), and the total counts (TC) were recorded. The percent binding of the labeled insulin by the sera was calculated as follows:

$$\text{Radioligand \% Bound} = \frac{\text{CPM of sample} - \text{CPM of NSB}}{\text{CPM of TC}}$$

The intra-assay and inter-assay binding coefficients of variability were approximately 10% and 10% in first method and 10% and 25% in the second method.

RESULTS

Relatives of IDD were observed more frequently to have INSAB (as defined by insulin binding greater than 3 S.D. of the control population) by either method 3.5% in the first method vs. 4.3% in the second method. The comparison of the two methods for determining insulin binding demonstrated an increased number of newly diagnosed IDD patients with INSAB in the second method using an optimized concentration of the A14 monoiodinated ^{125}I as the ligand than the standard method, 38% vs. 67% respectively (p < 0.001). The differences in the mean insulin binding of the three groups are shown in Table I. In the second method using A14 monoiodinated ^{125}I insulin the mean insulin binding in the control population was lower. The relative difference of the mean insulin binding between the ICA+ and ICA- nondiabetic relatives was much greater in the second method (p < 0.05). The association of ICA with INSAB was more pronounced in the nondiabetic relatives of IDD using the mono iodinated ^{125}I insulin, however, that association with ICA was lost in the newly diagnosed IDD patients.

The relationship of INSAB and the HLA-DR phenotype of the patient is

TABLE I

COMPARISON OF 2 METHODS FOR INSULIN BINDING IN THREE PATIENT POPULATIONS		
PATIENT GROUPS	MEAN INSULIN BINDING ($\pm$ 1 S.D.) #1	#2
CONTROLS	1.68 $\pm$ 1.34	0.56 $\pm$ 0.39
RELATIVES OF IDD		
ICA-	1.81 $\pm$ 1.44	0.54 $\pm$ 0.49
ICA+	2.35 $\pm$ 2.28	1.95 $\pm$ 3.03
NEW IDD		
ICA-	2.27 $\pm$ 2.10	3.12 $\pm$ 3.48
ICA+	3.59 $\pm$ 3.02	3.21 $\pm$ 2.15

TABLE II

RELATIONSHIP OF HLA-DR PHENOTYPE TO MEAN INSULIN BINDING				
	NON DIABETIC PATIENTS[e]		INSULIN TREATED IDD	
HLA-DR PHENOTYPES	n	MEAN BINDING	n	MEAN BINDING
3/4	45	2.3	15	26.5
4/X*	107	2.1	15	34.2
3/X	81	2.0	9	19.8
X/X	53	1.8	4	20.3

* X = Non DR3 and Non DR4
[e] The non diabetic patients included all ICA+ and ICA-controls, relatives of IDD and IDD patients before insulin treatment.

shown in Table II. In patients untreated with insulin there was no difference in the mean binding among the various HLA-DR phenotypes; however, in patients treated with exogenous insulin, there was significant increase in the insulin binding in the HLA-DR4 phenotypes in comparison to the HLA--DR3 phenotypes ($p < 0.05$). The mean insulin binding of the HLA-DR 3/4 heterozygotes were between the DR3 (non DR4) and the DR4 (non DR3) IDD patients. The IDD patients in this analysis were similar with respect to duration of disease and type of exogenous insulin.

The effect of INSAB on the measurement of insulin in a standard radioimmunoassay is depicted in Figure 1. There was no difference in the insulin concentrations of the various groups of patients before and after PEG precipitation. The correlation coefficient was similar in controls (panel A, $r = 0.982$), patients with ICA and INSAB (panel B, $r = 0.990$) and patients with ICA without INSAB (panel C, $r = 0.993$), suggesting that INSAB did not interfere with the radioimmunoassay for insulin (Figure 1).

The use of INSAB in the prediction of impending IDD appears to be dependent on the age of the individual (Table III) and the concomitant presence of ICA (Figure 2). Patients with ICA under the age of 16 are more likely to develop IDD than are patients over 16 years of age (Table III) (p < 0.03). The presence of ICA and INSAB is significantly associated with diminished insulin responses to IV glucose (Figure 2). The mean first phase insulin response (sum of the 1 & 3 min. insulin concentrations) was significantly (p < 0.005) lower in the ICA+/INSAB+ patients (84 ± 34) than in the ICA+/INSAB-patients (183 ± 125). The insulin response of the control population was 243 ± 120.

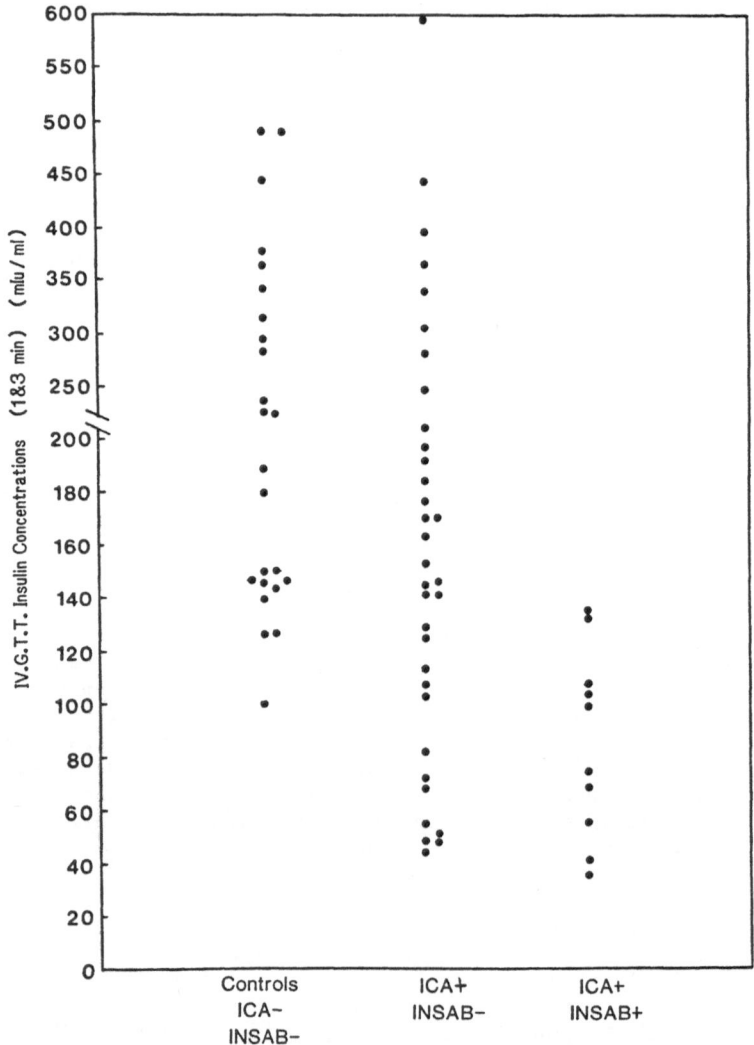

Figure 1. The first phase insulin release (sum of the 1 and 3 minute insulin concentrations) are plotted for the three groups: a control population, an ICA+ INSAB- group, and ICA+ INSAB+ group.

TABLE III

AGE AS A RISK FACTOR IN THE DEVELOPMENT OF INSULIN DEPENDENT DIABETES MELLITUS IN ICA+ RELATIVES OF IDDM			
AGE GROUPS	N	% ICA POSITIVE	RELATIVE RISK OF IDDM
< 10 YRS.	1136	4.3%	1.2
10-20 YRS.	1152	6.0%	1.7
20-30 YRS.	740	3.1%	0.8
> 30 YRS.	3172	3.1%	0.6

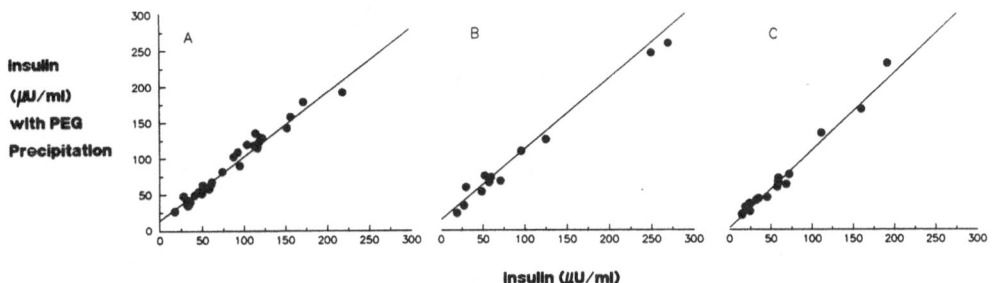

Figure 2.   The insulin concentrations with and without PEG precipita-
tation are plotted on the Y axis and the X axis, respectively. Panel A was a control population (r = 0.982), panel
B, an ICA+ INSAB- group (r = 0.990), and panel C, an ICA+
INSAB+ group (r = 0.993).

DISCUSSION

Palmer and colleagues first reported that some 20% of newly diagnosed
patients had IDD and IAA (7). In the comparison of the two methods in our
study, the frequency of INSAB in untreated newly diagnosed IDD patients increased from 38% to 67% by the use of an optimized concentration of Al4
monoiodinated ^{125}I insulin. A similar prevalence was found using an RIA
quantitated by specific displacement by radiolabeled insulin (9). However,
this assay using 0.15 ng/ml of Al4 ^{125}I monoiodinated insulin has practical
advantages in screening studies. The method of Soeldner is considerably
more labor intensive, requiring larger serum volumes (500 versus 200   1),
prolonged incubations (7 days versus overnight), extensive wash steps, and
increased counting time (18 minutes per sample versus 30 seconds).

The importance of insulin autoantibodies with respect to a possible
role in the autoimmune pathogenesis of IDD has not been established. However, the low autoantibody titers involved might support that they arise

as consequence of the islet autoimmunity rather than as its cause. Such appears to be the case in the evolution of pernicious anemia, where gastric parietal cell autoantibodies occur early in the course of the disease associated with atrophic gastritis (10). Autoantibodies to intrinsic factor however, are more likely to be found in patient with pernicious anemia the longer the duration of the disease.

Our results are similar to previous reports in which individuals with an HLA-DR4 phenotype were more likely to produce antibodies against exogenous insulin of either human or animal origins (6). On the other hand, patients with HLA-B8 and HLA-DR3 haplotypes were less likely to produce insulin antibodies in response to exogenous insulin. This difference in responsiveness has been used as an augument for two different types of IDD. However, the HLA-DR4 predominance was not found in individuals not exposed to exogenous insulin. Thus, these atuoantibodies to insulin may be different than those antibodies produced through immunization with exogenous insulin.

Notwithstanding, the important clinical question is whether INSAB could provide useful markers for subsequent IDD. Their association with ICA found in non diabetic individuals suggest that they might. However, prospective studies using INSAB as the screening assay need to be done to test the usefulness of INSAB alone. Nonetheless, an individual with both ICA and INSAB was found to have significant insulinopenia and thus more likely to develop IDD in the immediate future (5). Of importance is that this insulinopenia was not an artifact from the INSAB interfering with the insulin radioimmunoassay.

In summary, a modification of the INSAB assay resulted in increasing the number of newly diagnosed IDD with INSAB to 67%. INSAB were found frequently in non diabetic individuals who had been identified by the presence of ICA. The presence of INSAB in the sera did not interfere with the radioimmunoassay for insulin. Individuals with INSAB and ICA were more likely to demonstrate insulinopenia and thus be at risk for developing IDD.

REFERENCES

1. Lendrum, R., Walker, G., Cudworth, A.G., et al., 1976, Antibodies in diabetes mellitus. Lancet 2: 1273-1276.

2. Maclaren, N.K., Huang, S., Fogh, J., 1975, Antibody to cultured human insulinoma cells in insulin-dependent diabetes. Lancet 1: 997-999.

3. Lernmark, A., Freedman, Z., Hoffman, C., et al., 1978, Islet-cell surface antibodies in juvenile diabetes mellitus. N Engl J Med 229: 375-380.

4. Gorsuch, A.N., Spencer, K.M., Lister, J., et al., 1981, Evidence for a long pre-diabetic period in Type I (insulin-dependent) diabetes mellitus. Lancet 2: 1363-1365.

5. Srikanta, S., Ganda, O.P., Eisenbarth, G.S., Soeldner, J.S., 1983, Islet cell antibodies and beta-cell function in monozygotic triplets and twins initially discordant for Type I diabetes mellitus. N Engl J Med 308: 322-325.

6. Schernthaner, G., Borkenstein, M., Fink, M., et al., 1983, Immunogenicity of human insulin (Novo) or pork monocomponent insulin in HLA-DR typed insulin-dependent diabetic individuals. Diabetes Care 6: 43-48.

7. Palmer, J.P., Asplin, C.M., Clemons, P., et al., 1983, Insulin antibodies in insulin dependent diabetes before insulin treatment. Science 222: 1337-1339.

8. Neufeld, M., Maclaren, N.K., Riley, W.J., et al., 1980, Islet cell and other organ-specific antibodies in U.S. caucasions and Blacks with IDDM. Diabetes 29: 589-592.

9. Soeldner, J.S., Tuttleman, M., Srikanta, S., et al., 1985, Insulin dependent diabetes mellitus and autoimmunity: Islet-cell autoantibodies, insulin autoantibodies, and beta-cell failure. N Engl J Med 313: 893-894.

10. Riley, W.J., Toskes, P.P., Maclaren, N.K., Silverstein, J.H., 1982, Predictive value of gastric parietal cell autoantibodies as a marker for gastric and hematologic abnormalities associated with insulin dependent diabetes. Diabetes 31: 1051-1055.

SITES OF THE DEFECTS LEADING TO AUTOIMMUNITY

IN THE SPONTANEOUSLY DIABETIC BB RAT

Joanne Scott*, David C. Benjamin**,
John C. Herr[+], and Victor H. Engelhard**

Departments of Pediatrics*, Pharmacology*, Microbiology**
Anatomy and Cell Biology[+] and the Cancer Center

Although spontaneous hyperglycemic syndromes have long been recognized in a variety of species, only a very few appear to have an autoimmune pathogenesis. To date, the animal model most closely resembling human Type I diabetes mellitus is the BB rat (1,2, for reviews). The BB rat syndrome is characterized by a sudden onset of severe hyperglycemia associated with ketoacidosis, weight loss, and virtually complete pancreatic beta cell depletion, followed by death within a few days unless insulin is administered. Onset of hyperglycemia occurs in approximately 70 percent of diabetes-prone littermates, usually between 60 and 120 days of age. As in humans, susceptibility to diabetes is associated with the major histocompatibility complex (MHC). The BB rat also exhibits profound T-lymphocytopenia, antedating onset of diabetes and demonstrating a marked decrease in both T-helper/inducer (T_h/T_i) and T-cytotoxic/suppressor (T_cT_s) cell populations. As is typical of autoimmunity in other animals, BB rat lymphocytes show depressed responsiveness to concanavalin A (ConA) and to allogeneic stimulator cells in mixed lymphocyte reactions (MLRs). The autoimmune nature of the syndrome in BB rats is evidenced by the presence of an intense mononuclear infiltration of the pancreatic islets (insulitis) and the presence in serum of various autoantibodies, including antibodies directed against surface determinants of islet cells (1,2, for reviews).

Evidence that the diabetic syndrome in BB rats is T-cell-mediated stems from numerous observations, such as prevention of diabetes by neonatal thymectomy or by transfusions of peripheral T-cells from a diabetes-resistant line of BB rats. Injection of ConA-activated splenocytes has been shown to adoptively transfer diabetes in young diabetes-prone BB rats, or in lines of diabetes-resistant BB rats and MHC-compatible Wistar-Furth (WF) that had been pretreated with cyclophosphamide (1,2, for reviews).

Naji and co-workers reported that injection of bone marrow from normal rats into neonatal diabetes-prone BB rats greatly reduced the incidence of diabetes (3). The increased ability of such bone marrow-innoculated rats to subsequently mount alloantigen-specific MLRs was shown to be due to donor-derived T-cells. These results were interpreted as indicating that diabetes

These studies were sponsored in part by a Pilot Feasiblity Grant awarded by the University of Virginia Diabetes Research and Training Center, by a grant from the American Diabetes Association, by the National Institutes of Health grant R01-AM 34984, and by a grant from the Greenwall Foundation.

in the BB rat is at least partly due to a defect in a lymphoid stem cell precursor. However, it is well established that bone marrow contains a small population of mature T-cells; these T-cells most probably enter the bone marrow parenchyma as part of the normal recirculating lymphocyte pool. The studies by Naji and co-workers, therefore, did not specifically address the question of which lymphoid cell population was directly responsible for the prevention of diabetes and the restoration of lymphocyte responsiveness in inoculated recipients.

Taken together, the studies described above suggest the existence of multiple abnormalities in the BB rat: (a) the presence of ConA-responsive T-cells as effector or helper cells that augment onset of disease, and (b) the absence of a regulatory T-cell circuit that could prevent the disease. At issue is whether the impaired T-cell function in BB rats is obligatory for the expression of diabetes.

We wished to investigate how these defects in the T-cell compartment originate, and whether they result from an abnormal lymphoid stem cell within the bone marrow or from an abnormal T-cell differentiative environment. Our investigations involved three different approaches to the question: (a) neonatal bone marrow chimera studies, (b) adult bone marrow irradiation chimera studies, and (c) neonatal thymus transplantation studies.

NEONATAL BONE MARROW CHIMERA STUDIES

Naji and co-workers (3) had interpreted their earlier bone marrow chimera studies as indicative of a defect at the level of the bone marrow stem cell. We reasoned, however, that prevention of diabetes in those studies may have been due to co-transfer of mature T-cells in the inoculum, providing suppressor T-cells necessary for the control of autoimmune responses. A requirement for mature T-cells would suggest a defect in the T-cell differentiative environment (i.e., post-stem-cell) in BB rats. A defect in either the lymphoid stem cells or in the T-cell differentiative environment could account for the severe lymphopenia, the lymphocyte hyporesponsiveness, and the autoimmunity seen in BB rats. If the defect(s) in BB rats leading to diabetes and/or T-cell lymphopenia resides in the lymphoid stem cells, then transplanting only lymphoid stem cells from normal rats into neonatal BB rats should prevent the onset of diabetes and/or correct the T-cell abnormalities.

Procedures: As described previously (4), neonatal diabetes-prone BB rats (< 36 h old) were injected with bone marrow from MHC-compatible WF rats. One-half of the bone marrow recipients were given bone marrow that had been depleted of mature T-cells by treatment with anti-T-cell antibody plus complement. All animals were followed until onset of diabetes or until > 140 days of age. At time of sacrifice, the animals were also characterized with respect to lymphopenia, the distribution of T-cells among different functional subsets (by cytofluorographic analyses), and lymphocyte responses to mitogen and alloantigen.

Probability values (p) for differences in incidence of diabetes between experimental groups were calculated by χ^2-analysis. For leukocyte and lymphocyte counts, and for lymphocyte in vitro function, groups were compared by analysis of variance (with general linear model) accompanied by a Duncan's multiple-range test (α set at 0.05).

Results: Table I summarizes the results of our neonatal bone marrow chimera studies. As in the earlier study by Naji and co-workers (3), those animals receiving "whole" bone marrow, i.e., not depleted of mature T-cells, showed a decreased incidence of diabetes (p < 0.005 compared with

TABLE I

DIABETES INCIDENCE, LYMPHOPENIA, AND LYMPHOCYTE IN VITRO FUNCTION IN BB RATS NEONATALLY INJECTED WITH WF BONE MARROW

Animal Group	Incidence of Diabetes (%)[*]	Lymphocytes/μl	Mixed Lymphocyte Response[†]	Response to Concanavalin A[†]
BB controls	68	3,551 ± 539 (12)	2,865 ± 399 (5)	22,084 ± 2435 (15)
Neonates given untreated (whole) WF bone marrow	23[‡]	4,936 ± 786[§](16)	15,606 ± 4883[‖](6)	50,927 ± 8126[¶] (8)
Neonates given T-cell-depleted WF bone marrow	75[**]	3,053 ± 542 (11)	N.D.	N.D.

Animals are as described in the text. Lymphocyte data are expressed as means ± SEM; number in parentheses indicates number of rats examined. [*]Number of diabetics/total number of rats. [†]Spleen cells were plated in the presence of either ConA or allogeneic spleen cells, in medium containing 5% horse serum; responsiveness was assessed by subsequent incorporation of ^{3}H-thymidine. Results are expressed as means ± SEM of cpm ^{3}H-thymidine. [‡]$p < 0.005$ compared with BB controls. [§]$p < 0.02$ compared with BB controls, by analysis of variance. [‖]$p < 0.05$ compared with BB controls, by t-test. [¶]$p < 0.01$ compared with BB controls, by t-test. [**]NS ($p > 0.10$) compared with BB controls.

BB controls) and a restoration of lymphocyte _in vitro_ responsiveness ($p < 0.05$, $p < 0.01$, compared with BB controls, for MLR and ConA responses, respectively). The reduced incidence of diabetes in these animals, however, appeared to be unrelated to the extent of lymphopenia, as measured by peripheral blood lymphocyte counts (Table I) or splenic T-cell subsets (data not shown). Although a small improvement in lymphocyte counts was observed in these animals compared with BB controls ($p < 0.02$), they were still significantly leukopenic and lymphopenic compared with WF controls ($p < 0.006$, data not shown). In contrast, injection of T-cell-depleted bone marrow had no effect on incidence of diabetes, suggesting that mature T-cells in the inoculum were responsible for prevention of diabetes in our studies and in those of Naji and co-workers.

BONE MARROW IRRADIATION CHIMERA STUDIES

In a further attempt to determine the site of the defect(s) leading to diabetes and/or T-cell lymphopenia in the BB rat, a series of bone marrow irradiation chimeras were constructed using various combinations of normal or BB rat recipients and bone marrow donors (4). If the defect resides within the bone marrow stem cells, transplanting T-cell-depleted bone marrow stem cells from MHC-compatible normal rats into lethally-irradiated

TABLE II

DIABETES INCIDENCE, LYMPHOPENIA, AND LYMPHOCYTE IN VITRO FUNCTION
IN BB RAT BONE MARROW IRRADIATION CHIMERAS

Animal Group	Incidence of Diabetes (%)	Lymphocytes/μl	MLR (% of values for WF controls)[*]
WF rats injected with WF bone marrow (WF→WF chimeras)	0	7,647 ± 738 (5)	N.D.
WF rats injected with BB bone marrow (BB→WF chimeras)	0	7,974 ± 507 (5)	93 ± 4 (6)
BB rats injected with WF bone marrow (WF→BB chimeras)	0[†]	9,101 ± 904 (18)	93 ± 19 (10)
BB rats injected with BB bone marrow (BB→BB chimeras)	24[‡]	3,215 ± 299[§](19)	5 ± 5[§](16)
BB litter-matched controls	38	3,452 ± 359 (21)	2 ± 1 (13)

Animals are as described in the text. Lymphocyte counts are expressed as means ± SEM. Analyses were conducted at time of death, ∿150 days of age or within 2-3 wk after onset of diabetes. Number in parentheses indicates number of rats examined. [*]Spleen cells were plated in the presence of irradiated allogeneic spleen cells; results are expressed as the cpm incorporated ^{3}H-thymidine divided by the cpm ^{3}H-thymidine incorporated by WF lymphocytes, X 100. [†]$p < 0.007$ compared with BB→BB litter-matched irradiation chimeras. [‡]NS ($p > 0.5$) compared with litter-matched BB controls. [§]$p < 0.0001$ compared with WF controls (data not shown); NS ($p > 0.61$) compared with litter-matched BB controls.

diabetes-prone animals should prevent onset of diabetes and/or correct the T-cell abnormalities. Transplanting bone marrow stem cells from diabetic rats into irradiated normal rats should induce diabetes and/or lymphopenia.

Procedures: As described previously (5), the bone marrow recipients in this study were adults (37-44 days of age), and were given 800 rads whole-body irradiation immediately prior to bone marrow inoculation. Recipients were mildly anesthetized with methoxyflurane and given an intracardiac injection of 5 x 10^7 (excluding erythrocytes) viable T-cell-depleted bone marrow cells. Thirty-two diabetes-prone BB rats were inoculated with WF bone marrow and were designated WF → BB chimeras. Twenty-three WF rats were inoculated with bone marrow from overtly diabetic BB donors, and were designated BB → WF chimeras. Seven WF rats were given

TABLE III

T-LYMPHOCYTE SUBSET DISTRIBUTIONS IN BONE MARROW IRRADIATION CHIMERAS

Animal Group	Cell Type (% of Total)			
	T-cells (OX19$^+$)	T-cells (W3/13$^+$)	T_h/T_i (W3/25$^+$)	T_c/T_s/NK (OX8$^+$)
WF→WF chimeras (6)	43.1 ± 0.5	44.4 ± 1.7	28.1 ± 0.3	20.3 ± 0.5
WF→BB chimeras (13)	17.5 ± 2.2*	31.8 ± 1.5†	16.1 ± 0.9*	11.7 ± 0.9‡
BB→BB chimeras (15)	5.9 ± 0.6	25.5 ± 2.2	12.8 ± 0.9	9.2 ± 0.8

Rats are as described in the text and in Table 2; number in parentheses indicates number of rats examined. Spleen cells were analyzed on a fluorescence-activated cell sorter. Results are expressed as means ± SEM of the percent of total viable leukocytes with the indicated phenotype. *p < 0.003 compared with BB→BB chimeras; p < 0.001 compared with WF→WF chimeras. †p < 0.01 compared with BB→BB chimeras; p < 0.0001 compared with WF→WF chimeras. ‡p < 0.04 compared with BB→BB chimeras; p < 0.0001 compared with WF→WF chimeras.

WF bone marrow as irradiation controls, and were designated WF → WF "chimeras;" 21 diabetes-prone BB rats were given bone marrow from overtly diabetic BB rats, and were designated BB → BB "chimeras." Animals were sacrificed within a few weeks after onset of diabetes, or at > 140 days post-inoculation. At sacrifice, asessments were made of peripheral blood lymphopenia, splenic T-cell subset distributions, and lymphocyte in vitro responsiveness. In addition, a monoclonal antibody to the RT7.2 T-cell differentiation alloantigen (6) was used to document chimerism in the WF--BB animals.

Probability values (p) for differences in incidence of diabetes between experimental groups were calculated using the Fisher's Exact test. All other parameters were compared among the groups by analysis of variance (using a general linear model) accompanied by a Duncan's multiple range test (α set at 0.05).

Results: Table II illustrates the incidence of diabetes, lymphopenia, and lymphocyte in vitro responsiveness in the irradiation bone marrow chimeras and their litter-matched BB controls. As might be predicted, none of the 7 WF rats irradiated and injected with T-cell-depleted WF bone marrow (WF → WF chimeras) developed either diabetes or lymphopenia. In addition, none of the 23 WF rats irradiated and injected with marrow from overtly diabetic BB rats (BB → WF chimeras) developed diabetes or lymphopenia. Lymphocytes from the BB → WF chimeras demonstrated normal MLR responsiveness compared with WF controls. These results indicate that BB bone marrow stem cells can differentiate in an apparently normal fashion in an appropriate environment. In contrast, diabetes occurred in 24% of the BB → BB chimeras, an incidence not significantly different than the 38%

TABLE IV

INFLUENCE OF NEONATAL THYMECTOMY AND THYMUS GRAFTING ON INCIDENCE
OF DIABETES AND ON LYMPHOPENIA IN BB RATS

Animal Group	Incidence of Diabetes[*]	Leukocytes/μl	Lymphocytes/μl
Surgical "Shams" (S)	43% (12/28)	4,686 $\pm$ 515 (13)	2,944 $\pm$ 334 (13)
Thymectomized/thymus-grafted (TT)	30%[†] (13/44)	3,788 $\pm$ 203[†] (43)	2,543 $\pm$ 140[†] (43)
Completely thymectomized	50% (4/8)	4,309 $\pm$ 474 (8)	2,849 $\pm$ 273 (8)
Thymectomized only (T)	11%[‡] (3/27)	5,126 $\pm$ 412 (25)	2,806 $\pm$ 321 (25)
Completely thymectomized	0%[‡] (0/7)	3,625 $\pm$ 367 (5)	1,459 $\pm$ 113[§] (5)
WF controls (WF)	---	11,630 $\pm$ 631 (36)	10,528 $\pm$ 580 (36)

Animals are as described in the text; BB rat groups were litter-matched. Leukocyte/ lymphocyte counts are expressed as means $\pm$ SEM; number in parentheses indicates number of rats examined. [*]Number of diabetics/total number of rats. [†]NS compared with Group S, by analysis of variance. [‡]p < 0.01 compared with Group S, by analysis of variance. [§]p < 0.001 (by two-tailed t-test) compared with comparable animals (completely thymectomized) in Group TT.

incidence in litter-matched controls (p > 0.5). These latter results show that, if followed by immunologic reconstitution, irradiation per se does not significantly affect the incidence of diabetes. Lymphopenia and lymphocyte hyporesponsiveness in the BB → BB chimeras were comparable to untreated BB control rats. Onset of diabetes in the irradiated BB rats injected with WF bone marrow (WF → BB chimeras) was totally prevented. This group had normal lymphocyte counts and demonstrated normal MLR responsiveness, compared with WF controls.

Table III illustrates the distribution of T-cell subsets in the bone marrow irradiation chimeras. As one might predict, WF → WF chimeras and BB → BB chimeras demonstrated T-cell subset distributions essentially identical to WF controls and BB controls, respectively (data for untreated controls not shown). Surprisingly, WF → BB chimeras, in which diabetes was completely prevented, showed only partial restoration of their T-cell subsets, with all T-cell subsets still markedly decreased compared with WF → WF irradiation controls (p < 0.001).

NEONATAL THYMUS TRANSPLANTATION STUDIES

If the defect in the T-cell differentiative environment of the BB rat observed earlier resides in the thymus, transplantation of intact thymuses from neonatal MHC-compatible WF rats into neonatal diabetes-prone BB rats should prevent diabetes and lymphopenia, and should restore lymphocyte in vitro responsiveness, depending upon the level of control of the interaction of these different autoimmune parameters. Such a defect in the thymus might, however, be playing a dominant role, in which case animals receiving normal thymus grafts but retaining their own thymuses might still manifest the defect. In this study, consequently, we thymectomized the graft recipients immediately prior to transplantation. The results of these studies have been published in abstract form (7,8), and a manuscript describing these studies is currently under editorial review.

Procedures: Intact thymuses were removed from neonatal (< 3 d of age) WF rats and were grafted into the necks of 44 neonatal (< 2 d of age) diabetes-prone BB rats. Hypothermia was used as the anesthetic agent, in accordance with a protocol approved by the University of Virginia Animal Care Committee. The grafts were sutured in the vicinity of the thyroid gland to prevent descent of the graft into the superior mediastinum; this permitted us to later distinguish donor thymus vs. residual host thymus by position. Graft recipients were thymectomized immediately prior to transplant. Twenty-eight "Sham"-operated BB rats served as controls. An additional 27 BB neonates were thymectomized only. All three groups were litter-matched. All animals were followed until ≥ 195 days of age, or until onset of diabetes. At sacrifice, the neck regions of each rat were fixed for later histologic examination, to confirm the completeness of the thymectomies and the successful vascularization of the thymus grafts. In addition to expression of diabetes, the animals were characterized with respect to lymphopenia, as measured by leukocyte and lymphocyte counts in peripheral blood; with respect to the distribution of T-cells among different functional subsets, by cytofluorographic analyses; and with respect to lymphocyte responsiveness, by assessment of T-cell responses to ConA and to alloantigen.

Probability values (p) for differences in incidence of diabetes between experimental groups were calculated using the Fisher's Exact Test. All other parameters were compared among the groups by analysis of variance (using a general linear model) accompanied by a Duncan's multiple range test (α set at 0.05).

Results: Table IV illustrates the influence of neonatal thymectomy and thymus grafting on incidence of diabetes and lymphopena in BB rats. As one might predict, there was a marked reduction in incidence of diabetes in thymectomized-only rats compared with litter-matched "Shams." Diabetes developed in none of the thymectomized-only animals that had been completely thymectomized; a 15% incidence in partially-thymectomized animals was also significant (p < 0.01) compared with Shams. Thymus grafts, however, had no apparent effect on incidence of diabetes. The 30% incidence in thymectomized/thymus-grafted rats was a slight, but not statistically significant reduction compared with Shams; moreover, diabetes occurred in 50% of the thymectomized/thymus-grafted animals that had been completely thymectomized. Thymus grafting had no apparent effect on peripheral blood lymphopenia as measured by leukocyte counts and differentials, nor on splenic T-cell subset distributions (data not shown).

The grafting of a normal thymus did have, however, a striking effect on lymphocyte in vitro function. As shown in Table 5, splenic T-cells from thymectomized/thymus-grafted animals showed a marked increase in lymphocyte responsiveness, reaching normal MLR values in thymus-grafted animals that had been completely thymectomized. Even the partially-thymectomized thymus-grafted animals demonstrated near-normal lymphocyte responsiveness, significantly elevated above Shams (although still somewhat depressed compared with WF values). Of particular interest was the observation that

TABLE V

INFLUENCE OF NEONATAL THYMECTOMY AND THYMUS GRAFTING
ON LYMPHOCYTE IN VITRO FUNCTION IN BB RATS

Animal Group	Mixed Lymphocyte Response (cpm)	Response to ConA (cpm)
WF controls	51,974 ± 7,815 (26)	55,015 ± 3,295 (8)
Surgical "Shams" (S)	13,557 ± 3,442[*](12)	18,151 ± 3,129[*](8)
Thymectomized/Thymus-Grafted (TT)	37,003 ± 4,653 (32)	---
completely thymectomized	40,999 ± 8,943[†](6)	40,489 ± 4,031[‡](6)
Thymectomized only (T)	2,565 ± 748[*](22)	---
completely thymectomized	2,186 ± 481[*](4)	16,252 ± 4,403[*](3)

Rats are as described in the text and in Table 4; BB rat groups were litter-matched.
Number in parentheses indicates number of rats examined. T-cell-enriched spleen
cells were plated in the presence of irradiated allogeneic spleen cells or in the
presence of 10 μg/ml concanavalin A. Responsiveness was assessed by the subsequent
incorporation of ^{3}H-thymidine. Results are expressed as means ± SEM of cpm
^{3}H-thymidine. [*]p < 0.0001 compared with WF controls. [†]NS (p > 0.29) compared with
WF; p < 0.003 compared with Group S. [‡]p < 0.0001 compared with Group S; p < 0.0007
compared with WF controls.

diabetes occurred in lymphopenic animals with normal lymphocyte in vitro
function.

DISCUSSION

The experiments described in this paper were carried out to determine
whether the defects leading to autoimmunity and lymphopenia in diabetes-
prone BB rat reside at the level of the bone marrow stem cell or at the
level of T-cell maturation. If there is a defect in T-cell maturation,
does it reside within the thymic or postthymic compartments of the T-cell
differentiative environment?
In our neonatal bone marrow chimera studies, injection of MHC-compatible
bone marrow from normal (WF) rats into neonatal BB rats markedly reduced
the incidence of diabetes and restored lymphocyte in vitro responsiveness.
Injection of bone marrow depleted of mature T-cells had no effect on incidence of disease. These studies suggested a defect in the T-cell dif-

ferentiative environment in BB rats, i.e., either a thymic or postthymic defect.

In our bone marrow irradiation chimera studies, injection of T-cell-depleted WF bone marrow into lethally-irradiated 37-44 day old diabetes-prone BB rats completely prevented the onset of diabetes. In contrast, BB rats irradiated and inoculated with T-cell-depleted bone marrow from overtly diabetic BB rats developed diabetes with a frequency similar to untreated BB littermates. Comparing WF → BB chimeras with BB → BB chimeras, only their (donor) bone marrow stem cells differ; the T-cell differentiative environment is identical. These studies suggest, therefore, that prevention of diabetes in WF → BB chimeras was the result of the correction of a stem cell defect. On the other hand, neither diabetes nor lymphocyte abnormalities were induced in BB → WF irradiation chimeras. Comparing BB → WF chimeras with BB → BB chimeras, the (donor) bone marrow stem cells are identical, while their T-cell differentiative environments differ. Failure to induce diabetes and/or lymphocyte abnormalities in the BB → WF chimeras indicates that bone marrow stem cells from overtly diabetic BB rats can differentiate in an apparently normal fashion in an irradiated normal host. It appears, therefore, that the stem cell defect evidenced by the WF → BB chimeras is a necessary but not sufficient defect for diabetes expression in an animal with a normal T-cell differentiative environment. In WF → BB chimeras, T-cell subset distributions were only partially normalized compared with WF → WF chimeras. In these two chimeric models, the T-cell differentiative environments differ; the failure to completely restore the T-cell subsets in WF → BB chimeras could be interpreted as additional evidence for a defective T-cell differentiative environment in the diabetes-prone BB rat.

Taken together, these two bone marrow studies, and those of others, suggest that there are two defects in the BB rat leading to diabetes and/or T-cell lymphopenia. One of these occurs at the level of the bone marrow lymphoid stem cell while the other resides in the T-cell differentiative environment, either within the thymus itself or within the post-thymic compartments of T-cell maturation.

In our thymus transplantation studies, neonatal thymectomy prevented onset of diabetes, as predicted. The grafting of a normal MHC-compatible thymus, however, had no effect on either diabetes or lymphopenia. Thymus graft recipients developed overt diabetes at the same frequency as their non-grafted non-thymectomized littermates, and they remained lymphopenic. These results suggest that the defects responsible for the onset of diabetes and T-cell lymphopenia in the BB rat do not reside in the thymus. The defect in the T-cell differentiative environment suggested by our bone marrow chimera studies, therefore, apparently resides in the post-thymic compartment of T-cell maturation.

Surprisingly, however, thymus grafts had a striking effect on lymphocyte in vitro responsiveness. A dominant role played by the BB thymus in controlling lymphocyte dysfunction is suggested by comparing completely-thymectomized/thymus-grafted animals with only partially-thymectomized/thymus-grafted animals: the latter demonstrated only a partial normalization of lymphocyte in vitro function. These studies suggest that, at least in part, the in vitro lymphocyte hyporesponsiveness characteristic of diabetes-prone BB rats may result from a defect in T-cell maturation in the thymus. This thymic defect, however, does not appear to be responsible for the development of either the diabetes or the T-lymphocytopenia. Of particular interest was the observation that the expression of diabetes in lymphopenic BB rats is not dependent upon abnormal lymphocyte responsiveness; diabetes occurred in animals with normal response to alloantigen.

In summary, our bone marrow chimera and neonatal thymus transplantation studies suggest that there are two defects in the BB rat associated with diabetes and/or lymphopenia, one residing at the level of the bone marrow lymphoid stem cell and the other within the T-cell differentiative environment, apparently postthymic. There is a third defect in the BB rat, within the thymus, but this defect appears not to be responsible for the development of either the diabetes or the T-cell lymphopenia. Rather, the thymic defect appears to control the lymphocyte hyporesponsiveness characteristic of the diabetes-prone BB rat.

ACKNOWLEDGMENTS

We thank Dr. D.L. Greiner (University of Connecticut Health Center, School of Medicine, Farmington, Connecticut) for providing the monoclonal antibody RT-7.2. Mr. Paul McGill, from the University of Massachusetts (Worcester), performed all of the neonatal thymectomies and thymus transplantations. PZI insulin was generously donated by Eli Lilly (Indianapolis, Indiana).

REFERENCES

1. Rossini, A.A., Mordes, J.P., Like, A.A., 1985, Immunology of insulin-dependent diabetes mellitus. Ann Rev Immunol 3: 291-322. [Review].

2. Naji, A., Silvers, W.K., Barker, C.F., 1983, Autoimmunity and Type I (insulin-dependent) diabetes mellitus. Transplantation 36: 355-261. [Review].

3. Naji, A., Silvers, W.K., Bellgrau, D., Anderson, A.O., Plotkin, S., Barker, C.F., 1981, Prevention of diabetes in rats by bone marrow transplantation. Ann Surg 194: 328-338. ·

4. Scott, J., Engelhard, V.H., Curnow, R.T., Benjamin, D.C., 1986, Prevention of diabetes in BB rats. 1. Evidence suggesting a requirement for mature T cells in bone marrow inoculum of neonatally injected rats. Diabetes 35: 1034-1040.

5. Scott, J., Engelhard, V.H., Benjamin, D.C., 1987, Bone marrow irradiation chimeras in the BB rat: Evidence suggesting two defects leading to diabetes and lymphopoenia. Diabetologia 30: 774-781.

6. Greiner, D.L., Handler, E.S., Nakano, K., Mordes, J.P., Rossini, A.A., 1986, Absence of RT-6 T cell subset in diabetes-prone BB/W rats. J Immunol 135: 148-151.

7. Scott, J., Engelhard, V.H., Benjamin, D.C., 1985, The site of autoimmune defect(s) in the BB rat. Diabetes 34(Suppl. 1): 73A. [Abstract].

8. Scott, J., Benjamin, D.C., McGill, P., Engelhard, V.H., 1986, Thymus transplantation with and without prior thymectomy, in neonatal BB/Ch rats. Diabetes 35(Suppl. 1): 69A. [Abstract].

ASSAY FOR CYTOPLASMIC ISLET CELL ANTIBODIES USING TWO-COLOR

IMMUNOFLUORESCENCE AND RAT PANCREAS

¶Sergio A. Dib, Peter G. Colman, Francesco Dotta, Maura Tautkus,
Albert Rabizadeh and George S. Eisenbarth

Joslin Diabetes Center, Harvard Medical School, Boston, Massachusetts

A major problem in standardization of the islet cell cytoplasmic
antibody assay (ICA) is variation in sensitivity of the different human
pancreas substrates used in individual laboratories.

To circumvent this problem we have developed an assay which utilizes
Wistar-Furth rat pancreas as substrate, an anti-islet monoclonal antibody
(A2 B5) to identify islets and fluorescein conjugated protein A to identify
patient auto antibodies.

MATERIAL AND METHODS

ICA Assays: Our standard assay used frozen sections of normal human pancreas. Sections were covered first with 30µl of Trasylol (FBA, New York)
(diluted 1:2 in phosphate-buffered saline; PBS) and then with 30µl of serum
and incubated for 12h. at 4°C.

They were then washed with PBS and incubated with 40µl of fluorescein-
conjugated protein-A (1µg/ml;Sigma,St Louis, Mo) (FITC-pA). After a 20 min.
incubation, 10 µl of rhodamine-conjugated MoAb BISL-32 (Boehringer, Mannheim,
FRG) was added and 10 min. later, sections were again washed before incubation with rhodamine-conjugated anti-mouse Ig (Dako, Santa Barbara, Ca.) for
30 min. Finally, sections were washed with PBS, mounted with AFT systems
mounting medium (Behring), and read through a Leitz fluorescence microscope
(x25 and x10 oil immersion lens). All sections were read without knowledge
of the serum sample tested.

For the rat FITC-pA assay, frozen sections of 6-wk-old Wistar-Furth
rat pancreas were acetone fixed (5 min. at 20°C) immediately after section-
ing. Sera were absorbed overnight at 4°C. with acetone and methanol-extrated
rat liver powder and diluted 1:15 (vol/vol) in PBS plus 1% bovine serum
albumin(BSA) before use. Sections were covered first with 20µl of Trasylol
(diluted 1:2 in PBS) and then 20µl of absorbed serum and were incubated overnight at 4°C. They were washed with PBS and incubated for a further 30 min.
at room temperature with FITC-pA. After further washing with PBS, they were
incubated with MoAb A2B5 (diluted 1:100 in PBS-1% BSA) for 30 min. at room
temperature, washed with PBS, incubated with a 1:20 dilution of rhodaminated
anti-mouse Ig, washed, mounted and evaluated.

To further compare the fluorescence intensity with rat or human sections in the FITC-pA assay, specific islet fluorescence was quantitated, as previously described, by means of a Leitz MPZ compact photometer (Srikanta, S. et al Diabetes 34:300-5, 1985), for sera from 10 high-risk and 9 control subjects. At least 12 paired readings from islets and adjacent acinar tissue were obtained for each sample on both human and rat pancreas sections, and the mean specific islet fluorescence was obtained by subtracting the acinar background fluorescence from islet fluorescence. The mean intra-assay coefficient of variation for a standard ICA-positive serum was 14%.

Sera: Sera were obtained from 19 individuals (aged 6 - 68 yr) identified to be at high risk for development of type I diabetes by virtue of having a relative with type I diabetes and being cytoplasmic ICA positive with our standard assay (Srikanta, S. et al Diabetes, 34:300-5, 1985). Of this group, 5 have subsequently developed overt type I diabetes, and 7 others had no first-phase insulin secretion in response to intravenous glucose. All individuals were studied as out-patients.

Sera from 21 normal individuals (aged 13-62 yr) without diabetes and from 14 negative controls from ICA workshops were utilized as controls. In a further set of experiments, sera from 50 subjects from the offspring cohort of the Framingham heart study and 27 type I diabetics were assayed in parallel with rat and human pancreas substrate. Inter assay variation was assessed by including the same positive and negative control at a final dilution of 1:2 in each assay.

RESULTS

After the initial serial dilution studies (Fig-1, left panel) sera from control and high-risk individuals were studied at a 1:5 dilution via rat pancreas and assayed in parallel with our standard assay with human pancreas at a 1:2 dilution. Fifteen of 17 sera (88%) from high-risk individuals were positive with the rat pancreas compared to only 1 of 35 (28%) of sera from normal controls (Fig-1, right panel). The 1 positive normal control was subsequently read as negative on repeated assays, whereas hight-risk positives were repeatedly positive. With human pancreas, the same number of sera from the high-risk individuals were read as +w or greater and 1 of 22 controls as +w or lesser (Fig-1, right panel).

After developing the FITC-pA assay with rat pancreas substrate, we studied 27 type I diabetics and 50 controls from the offspring cohort of the Framingham heart study. Eleven of 27 (41%) type I diabetics were weak positive or stronger with both human and rat pancreas (Fig-2, left panel). Only 1 sample was weakly positive with rat but negative with human pancreas. Of 50 Framingham controls, 1 was +w with rat pancreas: all were negative with human pancreas (Fig-2, right panel).

Inter assay variation was evaluated by assaying the same positive and normal sera in multiple assays; the positive control was always read as positive (2-3+ on 1 occasion, 2+ on 3 occasions and 1+ on 1 occasion). The negative control was always read as less than +w (± 1 on 1 assay and negative on 6 assays).

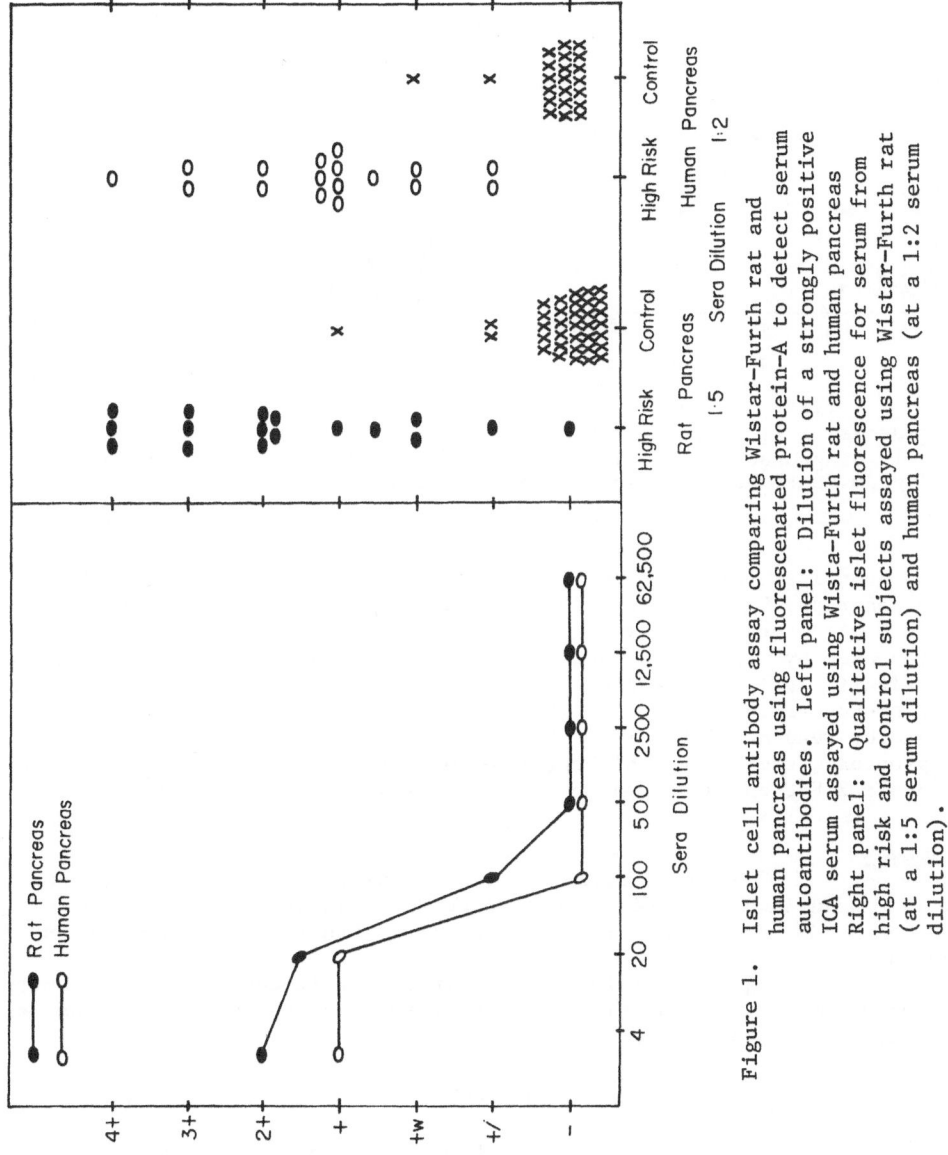

Figure 1. Islet cell antibody assay comparing Wistar-Furth rat and human pancreas using fluorescenated protein-A to detect serum autoantibodies. Left panel: Dilution of a strongly positive ICA serum assayed using Wista-Furth rat and human pancreas Right panel: Qualitative islet fluorescence for serum from high risk and control subjects assayed using Wistar-Furth rat (at a 1:5 serum dilution) and human pancreas (at a 1:2 serum dilution).

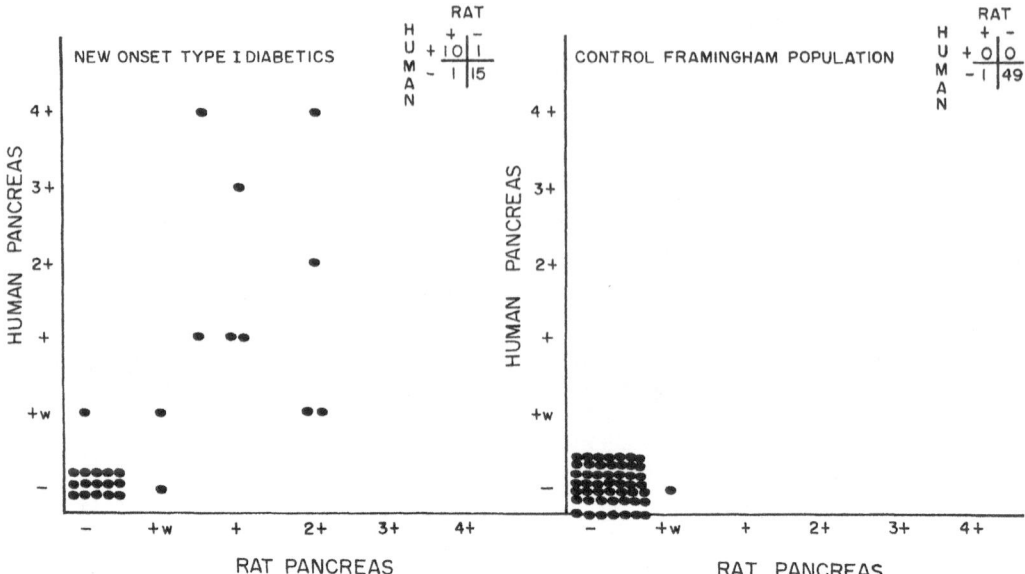

Figure 2. Islet cell antibody assay comparing Wistar-Furth rat and human pancreas using fluoresceinated protein-A to detect serum auto-antibodies in newly diagnosed Type I diabetics (left panel) and subjects from the Framingham Heart Study Offspring Cohort (right panel).

To quantitatively compare the fluorescent readings with rat versus human pancreas, 9 control and 10 sera from high-risk patients were studied via FITC-pA detect antibody binding with determination of specific islet fluorescence by means of a photometer. Readings on rat and human pancreas were significantly correlated throughout the entire range of specific islet fluorescence (r=.66, p < .01). The lowest control subject's sera gave a photometer reading of 2.1 ± 1.2 U (mean ± SE) on human and 5.6 ± 1.5 U on rat pancreas, whereas the highest ICA-positive subject's sera gave a reading of 23.6 ± 2.8 U on human and 35.2 ± 4.2 U on rat pancreas. (Fig. 3).

In summary:
          1. The great majority of sera which are islet antibody positive utilizing human pancreas can also be detected utilizing rat pancreas.
          2. End point titers are similar with rat and human pancreas substrates.
          3. Specific islet fluorescence quantitated using a photometer for sera from controls and high risk subjects on human and rat pancreas sections are highly correlated.

CONCLUSIONS

1. These observations suggest that Wistar-Furth rat pancreas expresses autoantigen(s) with similar immunocytochemical properties to the autoantigen(s) of human pancreas.
2. This information should facilitate biochemical characterization of "cytoplasmic" antigen(s) as well as comparison between surface (isolated rat islet cells) and cytoplasmic assays (frozen sections of rat pancreas).
3. A larger group of controls as well as islet cell antibody positive individuals will need to be studied to determine whether rat pancreas can substitute for human pancreas in screening all populations at high risk for Type I diabetes.

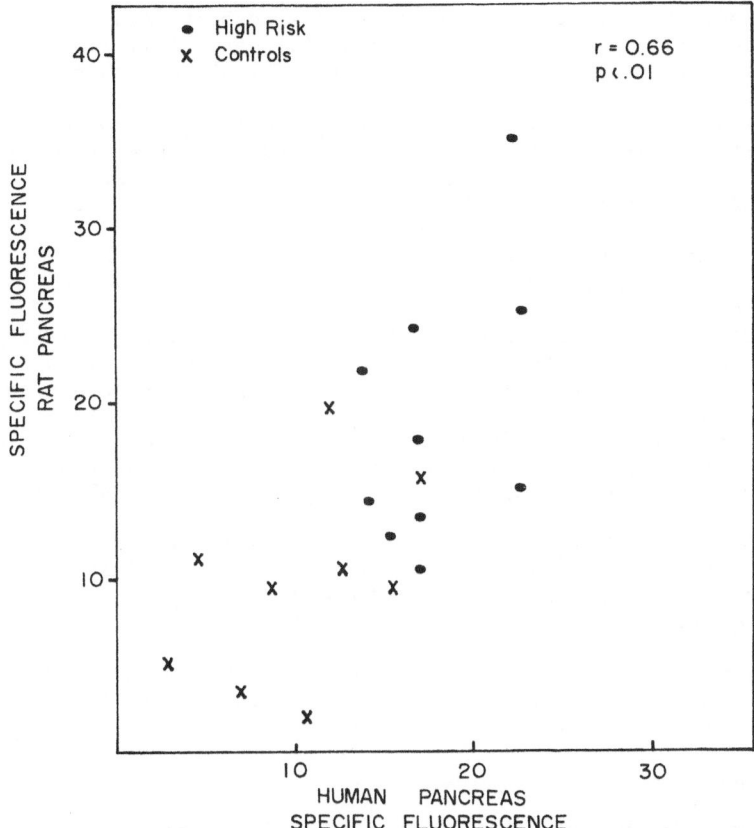

Figure 3. Comparison of specific islet fluorescence (quantitated using a photometer) using Wister-Furth rat and human pancreas for sera from control and high risk subjects.

DISCUSSION

J. BARBOSA: Dr. Scott, can you reconcile your work with what Dr. Rossini is saying about that RT6 population that seems to be vital in rat diabetes? And, also, the work of Dr. Like suggesting that natural killer activity seems to be vital. I have difficulty putting all these things together.

J. SCOTT: I don't think that anything that I've said and the concept that you just mentioned are mutually exclusive. I suspect that Dr. Greiner will be talking later about the RT6. But, he can correct me. It's my belief that the antigen is put on post-thymically.

D. GREINER: Yes, it is.

J. SCOTT: So, that is another example of different expression of post-thymic defect. The role of natural killer cells is being studied by several laboratories and the T-cell subsets that are generally shown as the oxate positive subset, which is cytotoxic suppressive or a natural killer cell. All of those are incorporated in the oxate positive. And, it has been shown that if you double the label you can account for all of the oxate positive cells as being natural killer cells, but there are essentially no cytotoxic suppressor cells in the peripheral blood of BB rats.

H. GLEICHMANN: At the international workshop on the standardization of ICA, it was obvious that complement fixing ICA are present in sera with high titered conventional ICA. And, I think that complement fixing ICA is not a subgroup of ICA.

D. KUMAR: Dr. Riley, when you classified your patients into two sub-groups, non-diabetic controls, children and adult, what's the clinical characteristics of these two subclasses? Age, height, weight?

W. RILEY: Age.

H. GLEICHMANN: Dr. Riley, what is superior, the combination and functional test with glucose, the insulin release plus ICA, or is the IAA positivity and ICA positivity superior to the other one? Can you exclude one of these tests or do you need all of them in order to define the patient at risk?

W. RILEY: I don't know if we can answer which one is the best. I think in the long run we're going to need all of them to really reach the point that all of us want where we can say with 100% assurity that this person is going to develop diabetes within a certain period of time so that we could intervene. But, I think that's the idea. I don't know if we could say which is the best or which is the worst. I think that the younger the children the more likely you're going to have the insulin antibodies, and I also think the progression tends to be much more rapid under 5 or so. So that it may be dependent on age rather than whether IVGTT or the insulin response and the insulin antibodies are better. It may be better in younger children with the insulin antibody but in the older adults it may be better if we look at the IVGTT.

DR. KUMAR: What's the age limit for the first group? That's your children.

W. RILEY: Well, we define it under 16, which is just past puberty.

G. GRODSKY: The question I'd like to direct to either Dr. Gale or to Dr. Riley is why do you think there are anti-insulin antibodies?

W. RILEY: I would suspect that the insulin antibodies probably are a secondary phenomena, you know, from say possibly a release of sequestered antigen in an area that's under an autoimmune attack, so there's a lot of autoreactive type cells there. I doubt the ICA has any pathogenic significance as far as causing the destruction itself. I think the structure probably was cellular mediated, probably not primarily antibody dependent.

E. GALE: I agree.

G. GRODSKY: Then, what about the possibility that these anti-insulin antibodies are not against insulin, but against a precursor of insulin? Is it possible that what you are seeing is an early form of insulin or some preform that's still absorbed and that then serves as an antigen? Have you ever attempted to see if your antibodies actually have preferential binding to something like proinsulin?

W. RILEY: We've tried proinsulin as far as setting up an assay, and we could not get it to work, although there has been one report in the literature that there are antibodies to proinsulin. I mean, your suggestion is a good one and we thought about that, but we never could get a proinsulin antibody assay developed.

S. EFENDIC: We have some preliminary data indicating that proinsulin levels are increased in siblings of type 1 diabetics. It's very preliminary.

I have a question, also. What is the incidence of other antibodies in your groups, let's say insulin receptor antibodies, antibodies against growth hormone, and so on?

W. RILEY: We've not looked for insulin receptor or growth hormone antibodies, but we've looked at other organ specific antibodies such as thyroid or gastroparietal cells or adrenal, and we find them in about the same frequency, at least in our ICA positive group, as we do in our diagnosed diabetic populations.

E. GALE: We haven't measured the antibodies you ask about, but we have looked at the other organ specific antibodies over many years with similar results. If you measure sequentially, as we have done, then the proportion goes up quite considerably. So, over 40%, for example, of the group have manifested thyroid microsomal antibodies with 10 years of follow-up.

We've looked at heterogeneity in terms of whether those who have multiple organ specific antibody response are different from those who do not. We have taken the two ends of the spectrum, those who have islet antibodies without any other auto-antibodies over many years and the other group, those who had persistent high titers of other antibodies over that time, and we can find no difference between them in terms of HLA typing or clinical behavior. And, so at least in these family study individuals, we see no evidence of type IA or IB diabetes. They all seem to behave the same.

CYTOPLASMIC ISLET CELL AUTOANTIBODIES:

PREVALENCE AND PATHOGNOMIC SIGNIFICANCE

¶Helga Gleichmann[+], Gian Franco Bottazzo[*] and Friedrich Arnold Gries[*]

[+]Clinical Department, Diabetes Research Institute, University of Dusseldorf
Federal Republic of Germany
[*]Department of Immunology, Arthur Stanley House
The Middlesex Hospital Medical School, London, U.K.

For many decades insulin-dependent diabetes mellitus (IDDM = Type I diabetes) has been regarded as a metabolic disorder with a typical <u>acute</u> clinical onset. In the past 15 years, however, there have been substantial changes in previously established concepts of the etiopathogenesis of Type I diabetes (1,2). Based on immunologic, genetic and epidemiologic studies it is apparent that the majority of patients with Type I diabetes have a long, clinically silent prediabetic period. This latency period, which can ante-date clinically overt manifestation of insulin-deficiency for up to several years, is featured by the presence of various autoimmune phenomena (2,3). Currently chronic autoimmune reactions are widely believed to play a key role in the progressive destruction of the insulin-producing beta-cells of the Langerhans islets, although a direct autoimmune attack has still to be proved.

Recently, Eisenbarth (3) has proposed Type I diabetes to probably re-sult from a sequelae of six major hypothetical stages. Briefly, in geneti-cally susceptible individuals (Stage I), an, as yet, unknown initiating factor (Stage II) could stimulate the development of a variety of immuno-logic abnormalities (Stage III). These phenomena precede a progressive loss of insulin secretion (Stage IV), until clinical diabetes becomes mani-fest (Stage V). At this point, some residual beta-cell function can still be traceable, but finally almost complete destruction of the beta-cells fol-lows (Stage VI). These conceptual changes have been developed from numerous investigations initially inspired by the detailed histological description of the insulitis morphology in the pancreas of IDDM patients (4), further stimulated by the observations of cellular immune reactions towards pan-creatic extracts (5) and supported by the description of circulating cyto-plasmic islet-cell antibodies (ICA) in IDDM patients (6). Prevalence of ICA were described first in Type I diabetic patients with other coexistent endocrine deficiencies and subsequently corroborated in diabetic patients without any other endocrinopathies (7). In epidemiologic studies ICA have been found in 50-85% of patients with newly diagnosed Type I diabetes (2).

The most stimulatory information, however, has emerged from prospective family (8) and twin studies (9) which have shown that individuals at risk to develop insulin deficiency can be identified by circulating ICA. Fur-thermore, determination of ICA has been applied in attempts to classify a subgroup within the adult diabetes syndrome with secondary oral hypoglyce-mic agent failure as having a retarded form of Type I diabetes, to evaluate

TABLE I

ICA AS MARKER OF IMPENDING INSULIN-DEFICIENCY IN PROSPECTIVE FAMILY STUDIES
OF UNAFFECTED FIRST DEGREE RELATIVES OF DIABETIC PATIENTS

Number members studied	Duration of study (years)	ICA-positive members		with IDDM		% (N) of members with IDDM		Reference
		N	%	N	%	ICA +	ICA -	
719	9	30	4.2	14	46.7	1.9 (14)	0.3 (2)	21
2,200	6	39	1.8	8	20.5	0.4 (8)	0.0	10
1,723	2	16	0.9	2	12.5	0.1 (2)	0.06 (1)	12

TABLE II

PREVALENCE OF ICA IN PROSPECTIVE STUDIES OF GENERAL POPULATIONS,
i.e. HEALTHY PERSONS WITHOUT A FAMILY HISTORY OF DIABETES

Number members studied	Duration of study (years)	ICA-positive individuals		with IDDM		Number of individuals with IDDM		Reference
		N	%	N	%	ICA +	ICA -	
2,512	6	10	0.4	0	0	0	0	10
1,112	4	6	0.5	0	0	0	0	22

TABLE III

PREVALENCE OF ICA IN APPARENTLY TYPE II DIABETIC PATIENTS AND INCIDENCE OF SECONDARY FAILURE TO THERAPY WITH ANTIDIABETIC DRUGS

N patients	N (%)		N (%) requiring insulin		Type and duration (years) of study	Reference
	ICA +	ICA –	ICA +	ICA –		
160	23 (14.4)	137 (85.6)	14 (60.8)	11 (8.0)	prospective (2)	15
106	17 (16.0)	89 (84.0)	10 (58.8)	2 (2.2)	prospective (3)	23
67	18 (26.9)	49 (73.1)	16 (89.0)	29 (59.2)	cross-sectional	16
154	22 (14.3)	132 (85.7)	9 (40.9)	32 (24.2)	prospective (2)	17
96	32 (33.3)	64 (66.6)	7 (21.8)	0 (0)	prospective (3)	24

the effect of immunomodulating drugs in patients treated close to the time of diagnosis and in post-transplantation monitoring of patients with islet or segmental pancreatic grafts.

Yet, despite the wider use and obvious diagnostic value of ICA measurement, until recently no efforts were made to standardize the test to enable inter-laboratory comparison. Data on the prevalence and pathognomic significance of ICA obtained in various population groups and approaches to standardize the ICA determination will be addressed.

Significance of ICA in Population Studies

In three independently performed family studies, as summarized in Table I, the percentage of ICA-positive unaffected first degree relatives of insulin-dependent diabetic patients varied between 0.9%, 1.8% and 4.2%, and the percentage of ICA-positive family members who developed diabetes with time varied between 12.5%, 20.5% and 46.7%, respectively; the overall incidence of first degree relatives who succumbed to diabetes was 0.2%, 0.4% and 2.2% in each of these family groups. It is noteworthy that in all these studies the overall incidence of the disease was higher in ICA-positive than in ICA-negative family members (0.1%, 0.4% and 1.9%, versus 0.06%, 0.0% and 0.3%, respectively). Thus, even though ICA have been demonstrated to be able to be predictive markers of forthcoming insulin-deficiency, their prevalence alone is not an including parameter. The obvious differences in the reported percentages of ICA-positive individuals in these family studies may be attributable at least to three variables: there was a different period of follow-up (2, 6 and 9 years, respectively), the prevalence of ICA could vary in distinct geographical populations and differences in the sensitivity of the ICA test may account for these apparent discrepancies. In two prospective studies conducted in a general population for 4 and 6 years, respectively (10), none of the ICA-positive individuals developed insulin-deficiency, as indicated in Table II. Here, the percentage of ICA-positive individuals was comparable, being 0.4% and 0.5% in the two groups.

It remains to be established whether all the identified persons with ICA will finally develop overt diabetes, since it has been shown that this immunological abnormality can in some instances precede functional impairment of the pancreatic beta-cells for at least a decade.

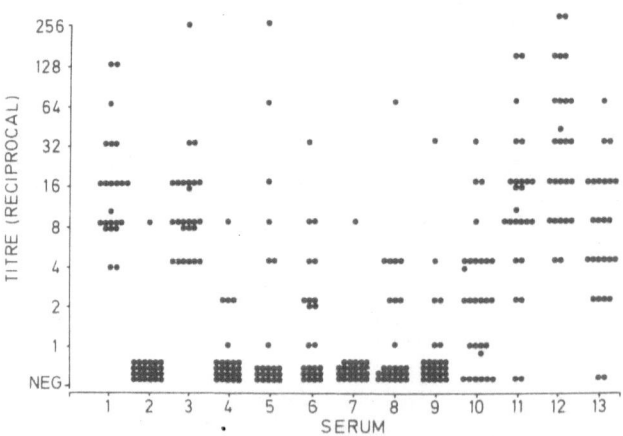

Figure 1.   End-point titres of ICA obtained by 24 laboratories according to a standard protocol with 13 coded sera. (Reproduced from Ref. 28 with permission of the Editor.)

Among adults who are classified as having non-insulin-dependent (Type II) diabetes according to clinical criteria, the presence of ICA may predict forthcoming development of secondary failure to treatment with oral hypoglycemic agents in the near future. The rate of beta-cell insufficiency indeed developed more rapidly in patients with ICA than in patients with Type II diabetes who were ICA-negative. As shown in Table III, the percentage of ICA-positive patients was approximately 15% in three reports and in two investigations, 27% and 33%. These differences are most likely attributable to the criteria determining the selection of the clinical material, especially in the latter studies. Type II diabetic patients who were ICA-positive required insulin therapy significantly sooner than those who were ICA_negative. The mean ± S.E.M. time interval since diagnosis of diabetes was 3.7 ± 0.9% in the former group and 8.4 ± 1.1 years, in the latter. A similar rapid decline in beta cell function was also observed in other studies by recording a faster decline of basal and stimulated C-peptide level in the patients.

Technical Aspects of ICA Determination

It is generally accepted that in the preclinical period of Type I diabetes circulating ICA might be relevant markers reflecting progressive beta-cell destruction. Since the first description of ICA (6) various methodic modifications have been introduced to improve the original indirect immunofluorescence assay. However, all the test procedures have different methodological designs and different degrees of sensitivity. Consequently, apparently independent, comparable studies have resulted in controversial data on the presence or absence of ICA in patients' sera. Several variables affect the determination of ICA including the concentration of antigenic determinants expressed in the pancreatic test substrate, use of different conjugates such as fluoresceinated protein A, monoclonal antibodies with specificity for islet cell determinants or immunohistochemical procedures. Furthermore, no methods have been developed to measure the absolute concentration of ICA in an individual's serum sample.

Despite the various technical modifications applied, until recently, no attempts have been made to standardize ICA determination. Standarization of ICA measurement, however, is a prerequisite to introduce ICA measurement as a reliable test to identify individuals at risk for impending insulin deficiency.

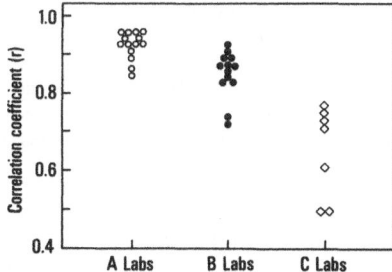

Figure 2.   Correlation coefficient of ICA determination of individual laboratory data obtained by using a coded reference standard in duplicate and by converting ICA end-point titres in arbitrary units. Laboratories are grouped according to a precision score. Group A was superior to Group B, and group C was found to have a low precision score. (Reproduced from Reference 27 with permission of the Editor.)

Standardization of ICA Determination

As demonstrated in Tables I and II, both the prevalence of ICA and the number of ICA-positive individuals who finally succumbed to diabetes varied markedly in the independently conducted population studies. In order to further evaluate the obvious diagnostic possibilities with confidence, since 1985 three international workshops were organized aiming at the standardization of the currently available assays for ICA determination. As reproduced in Figure 1, both discordance with regard to the presence or absence of ICA and a broad range of reciprocal ICA titres was obtained with coded sera analysed according to a standard protocol by individual laboratories. By applying calibrated standard curves to convert reciprocal ICA titres in arbitrary units the numerous variabilities of the different assay systems were overcome, thus permitting inter-laboratory comparison of results. As reproduced in Figure 2, availability of reference sera and determination of ICA in common units proved to increase intra- and interassay precision (reproducibility) and inter-laboratory concordance (11).

Currently profiency sera are being prepared to be distributed at regular intervals to laboratories performing ICA determinations. This envisaged Quality Control Programme is expected to continuously enable reliable and comparable ICA determinations.

DISCUSSION

Up to date ICA are the most extensively investigated abnormal immunological markers in the clinically silent prediabetic phase. Progress already achieved toward standardization of ICA determination by applying reference sera and by converting ICA titres in common units through standard curves by the individual laboratory will enable to pursue the following aims:

1. Assessment of the prevalence of ICA in various population groups, i.e. various ethnic groups, and in populations at risk for developing insulin-dependent diabetes.

2. Confident identification of individuals with impending insulin-deficiency.

3. Further elucidation of the pathogenic mechanism(s) resulting in continuous beta-cell destruction be it through cellular and/or humoral factors.

4. Tracing of environmental agents initiating the disease process.

Finally, it goes without saying that next to ICA additional immunological and functional abnormalities will be applied to ascertain individuals with impending insulin-dependent diabetes. Such investigations may contribute to develop therapeutical regimen to selectively arrest progression of the beta-cell destructive process.

REFERENCES

1. Kaldany, A., Busick, E.J., Eisenbarth, G.S., 1985, Diabetes mellitus and the immune system. In: Marble, A., Krall, L.P., Bradley, R.F. et al., eds. Joslin's Diabetes Mellitus. Lea & Febinger, Phila.: 51-64.

2. Bottazzo, G.F., Pujol-Borrell, R., Gale, E.A.M., 1987,Autoimmunity and Type I diabetes: Bringing the story up to date. In: Alberti, KGMM, Krall, L.P., Eds., The Diabetes Annual/3. Amsterdam, Elsevier Science Publishers B.V.; in press.

3. Eisenbarth, G.S., 1986, Type I diabetes mellitus. A chronic auto-immune disease. N Engl J Med 314: 1360-1368.

4. Gepts, W., 1965, Pathologic anatomy of the pancreas in juvenile diabetes mellitus. Diabetes 14: 19-33.

5. Nerup, J. Andersen, O.O., Bendixen, G., Egeverg J., Poulsen J.E., 1971, Antipancreatic cellular hypersensitivity in diabetes mellitus. Diabetes 20: 424-427.

6. Bottazzo, G.F., Florin-Christensen, A., Doniach, D., 1974, Islet cell antibodies in diabetes mellitus with autoimmune polyendocrine deficiencies. Lancet 2: 1279-1282.

7. Lendrum, R., Walker, G., Gamble, D.R., 1975, Islet cell antibodies in juvenile diabetes mellitus of recent onset. Lancet i: 880-883.

8. Gorsuch, A.N., Spencer, K.M., Lister, J., NcNally, J.M., Dean, B.M., Bottazzo, G.F., Cudworth, A.G., 1981, Evidence for a long prediabetic period in Type I (insulin-dependent) diabetes mellitus. Lancet ii: 1363-1365.

9. Srikanta, S., Ganda, O.P., EIsenbarth, G.S., Soeldner, J.S., 1983, Islet cell antibodies and beta-cell function in monozygotic triplets and twins initially discordant for Type I diabetes mellitus. N Engl J Med 308: 322-325.

10. Notsu, K., Oka, N., Note, S., Nabeya, N., Kuno, S., Sakurami, T., 1987, Islet cell antibodies in Japanese population and subsets with Type I (insulin-dependent) diabetes. Diabetologia 28: 660-662.

11. Bottazzo,G.F., Gleichmann, H., 1986, Immunology and diabetes workshops: Report of the first international workshop on the standardization of islet cell antibodies. Diabetologia 29: 125-126.

A NEW MARKER OF T LYMPHOCYTE ACTIVATION IN TYPE I DIABETES

John Cavanaugh, Neil E. Kay, Jaume Binimelis, Alberto de Leiva
and ¶Jose Barbosa

Division of Endocrinology and Metabolism, Department of Medicine
University of Minnesota and Division of Hematology and Oncology
Department of Medicine, Veterans Administration Medical Center
Minneapolis, Minnesota

Biological changes underlying T lymphocyte activation, are known to
be complex and are still poorly understood (1). Prominent in the early
activation-related phenomena (minutes to a few hours after the activation
signal) are the elevation of cytoplasmic calcium and changes in transmem-
brane electrical potential (TMP) (2-4). Resting T lymphocytes possess a
relatively constant TMP. However, following mitogen or antigen challenge,
T cell TMP changes over several minutes to hours with consecutive periods
of depolarization, repolarization and hyperpolarization (2). Selective
blocking experiments of the cell cation-transporting activity of the
membrane NA, K-ATP-ase, and the K and Na permeable channels, abrogate both
the TMP changes and T cell activation indicating a relationship between
them and suggesting that cell membrane depolarization is an integral part
of cell activation (2).

Peripheral blood and cerebral spinal fluid T lymphocytes expressing
Ia and Tac have been detected in increased numbers in various autoimmune
disorders, including insulin dependent diabetes (IDD) (6). Since IDD is
thought to be an organ specific autoimmune disease (6) we deemed it of
interest to study TMP in very early IDD patients and their nondiabetic
sibs.

METHODS

A. Patients and nondiabetic sibs. After obtaining informed
consent,30 cc of heparinized blood was drawn from 15 outpatients, aged 7
to 28 years, with IDD diagnosed 2 to 5 weeks previously. Similar blood
samples were also obtained from 21 normals aged 21 to 50 years, from 6
IDDs of duration greater than 5 years, from 3 non-insulin dependent
diabetics (NIDD) who were on insulin, and from 8 non-diabetic siblings
of IDD patients (ages 4 to 21).

Supported by NIH Grant AM20729, U.S.-Spain Joint Committee for
Technological Cooperation - Grant No. CCA 84/105, Eli Lilly and
Company, Indianapolis, Indiana, General Clinical Research Center
Program (RR-400) and Veterans Administration Merit Review Funds.

B. Methods. Mononuclear cells were separated from whole blood by density gradient centrifugation on Ficoll-Hypaque (Sigma Chemical Co., St. Louis, MO) within 3 hours of the time the blood was drawn. Cells were centrifuged again to remove platelets, and were washed twice with 0.01 M phosphate-buffered saline (PBS). T cells were separated by incubation for 10 minutes with 2-aminoethylisothiouronium bromide (AET)-treated sheep red blood cells (SRBC) and then the mixture centrifuged on Ficoll-Hypaque. SRBC were lysed with ammonium chloride-tris solution, and the T cells were washed twice with PBS and counted. Viability assessed by trypan blue exclusion was consistently > 95%. Between 94 and 98 percent of these cells formed rosettes with SRBC as assessed by microscopic examination using fluorescein diacetate.

Assessment of membrane potential. The method of TMP measurement was similar to that described by Shapiro et al. (5). After counting 3×10^5, T cells they were immediately placed in 1 ml PBS in a test tube. They were then refrigerated at 4° C until analyzed, which was never later than 3 hours after counting. 3,3'-di-pentyl-oxacarbocyanine (di-O-C$_{(5)}$(3)) was purchased from Molecular Probes Co., Eugene, OR. A 1 mM stock solution was prepared by dissolving the solid in dimethylsulfoxide (DMSO), and was kept wrapped in foil at 4 degrees C. A 5 micro M solution was prepared by mixing 10 microliters of the DMSO solution with 2 ml RPMI-1640 (GIBCO, Grand Island, NY). At the time of analysis, both the 5 micro M di-O-C$_{(5)}$(3) solution and the cell solution were warmed to room temperature. Ten microliters of the di-O-C$_{(5)}$(3) solution was then added to each tube with 3×10^5 T cells. The tubes were analyzed between 10 and 15 minutes later on a FACS 440 flow cytometer (Becton Dickinson, Mountain View, CA). The excitation wavelength was 488 nm and the emitted light was filtered with a dichroic filter at 535 nm, 15 nm band width. Seven to ten thousand cells were counted from each tube and data displayed, after selecting out dead cells by forward and 90 degrees scatter characteristics, in a plot of log fluorescence versus number of cells. The results are presented in the form of histograms of cell frequency (ordinate) against fluorescence intensity (abscissa). The majority of cells in each sample had similar fluorescence intensity, and were displayed as a peak. A minority of cells had a lower fluorescence, sometimes visible as a separate peak and sometimes displayed as a "shoulder" of the major peak (low %). From 0.5-10% of cells had fluorescence intensities greater than the major peak (high %) in some patients. Gates were placed to separate these three cell populations, and the percentage of cells in each subpopulation was determined by computer analysis. In addition, the mean fluorescence intensity for the entire sample was determined. The cells in the low-intensity group were considered to be relatively depolarized with respect to the cells in the main peak, and those in the high-intensity group were presumed to be hyperpolarized (5). The fluorescence intensity of the main peak was highly reproducible from sample to sample and from day to day.

Experiments using various concentrations of di-O-C$_{(5)}$(3), ranging between 2 and 20 lambda used to prepare the final solution did not significantly change the results in both normals or patients. Cells from normal control individuals were always run with each sample of diabetic (or prediabetic) cells.

The presence of islet cell cytoplasmic antibodies (ICAb) was determined by an indirect immunofluorescence technique described before (26). Statistical studies were done with the t-test for unpaired data or Wilcoxon rank-sum as appropriate.

RESULTS

Figure 1 shows four representative examples of histograms from the four groups of subjects studied. The newly diagnosed diabetic (Fig. 1, C) and the nondiabetic sib (prediabetic?) (Fig. 1, D) show a bimodel histogram with a prominent shoulder of depolarized T lymphocytes (lower fluorescence) as opposed to the long term diabetic on daily insulin (Fig. 1, B) and the normal individual (Fig. 1, A). The mean percentage of depolarized T lymphocytes in newly diagnosed diabetics (N=15) and in their nondiabetic sibs, (N=8) was significantly increased over normal controls and in diabetics on long term insulin treatment (Table I).

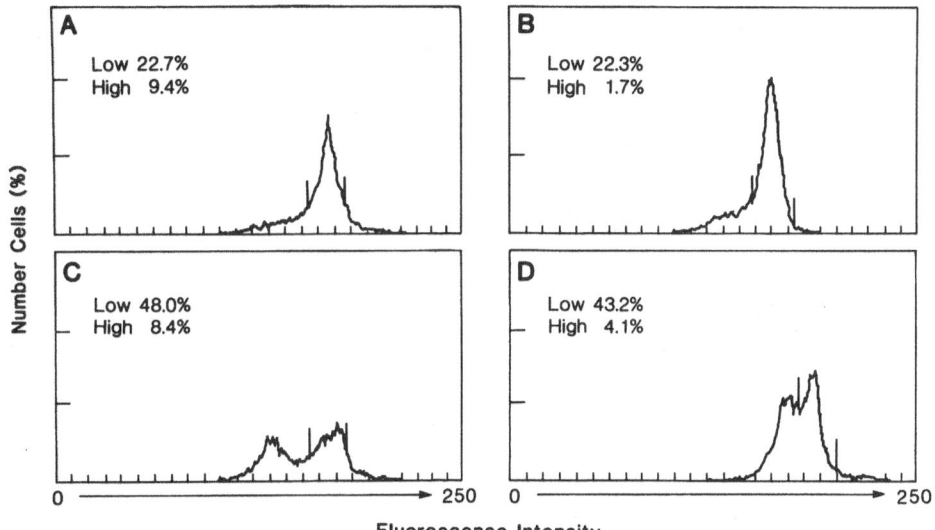

Figure 1. Fluorescence intensity profiles of isolated T lymphocytes exposed to 3,3'-di-pentyl- oxacarbocyanine iodide (di-O-$C_{(5)}$(3). Representative cells are shown for, A. Normal control; B. Long duration diabetic on insulin; C. Newly diagnosed diabetic; D. Nondiabetic sib of diabetic.

We further analyzed the relationship of TMP in T lymphocytes amongst our 4 patient groups by determining the percentage of T lymphocytes 2 to 3 standard deviations from the normal mean; Approximately 25% of patients had abnormal depolarization (Table 2). The total mean fluorescence was normal in all groups (Table 1).

In addition, there was no relationship between the percent of T cells depolarized and sex or age (or for the new diabetics duration of disease or insulin dose).

TABLE I

MEMBRANE POTENTIAL OF PERIPHERAL T LYMPHOCYTES IN EARLY INSULIN
DEPENDENT DIABETICS (IDD), THEIR NONDIABETIC SIBS (NDSD), LONG DURATION
DIABETICS (>5 YEARS), AND NORMAL CONTROL SUBJECTS. PERCENTAGE OF CELLS
WITH LOW, HIGH AND TOTAL FLUORESCENCE ARE SHOWN AS MEAN ± SD.

| | N | Fluorescence Intensity | | |
		Low %	High %	Total
New IDD	15	37.1 + 18.6*	4.5 + 2.8	157.1 + 8.9
NDSD	8	33.3 + 10.2*	2.3 + 1.3**	150.3 ± 10.1
Long term diabetics	9	23.5 + 4.7	2.8 + 1.4	153.5 ± 11.2
Normals	21	23.4 + 6.5	4.9 + 3.0	156.4 + 8.0

*New IDD and NDSD low % were statistically different from normals
(p<.004) and long term diabetics (p<.004).

**NDSD high % was statistically different from that in New IDD
(p<.02) and normals (p<.004).

TABLE II

NUMBER OF PATIENTS IN EACH GROUP WHOSE DEPOLARIZED (LOW
FLUORESCENCE) MEAN VALUE WAS GREATER THAN 2 SD and 3 SD FROM THE
MEAN VALUE FOR DEPOLARIZED CELLS IN THE NORMAL CONTROL GROUP (N=21).

	> 2 SD	> 3 SD
New IDD	4/15	3/15
NDSD	3/8	2/8
Long term diabetics	0/9	0/9

DISCUSSION

To our knowledge this is the first report showing that a number of patient at an early stage of an autoimmune disease, such as diabetes, have a large number of depolarized T lymphocytes in their peripheral blood. In addition, a subset of clinically normal sibs of these diabetic patients also carry a large percentage of depolarized T lymphocytes.

Two out of eight nondiabetic sibs showed a marked degree of T cell depolarization, (Table 2) but only one of these was positive for cytoplasmic islet cell antibodies, an immunological marker of prediabetes; overall there was no correlation between these antibodies and the degree of T cell depolarization.

The patients studied for TMP were also typed for HLA-DR and Tac antigen. Although a few patients had increased number of Ia+ T Lymphocytes, there was no correlation between this marker of activation and TMP (in preparation). This lack of correlation may reflect the fact that different activation markers relate to different stages of activation. While depolarization is necessary for activation and proliferation (2) it does not follow that all depolarized cells are activated. Depolarization may serve other functions in the resting cell as well as being the initial step in activation. Confirmation of this hypothesis would require detailed quantitative studies of cells at different stages of activation.

Several trivial explanations for these findings must be considered. If diabetics are treated daily with the foreign proteins bovine and/or pork insulin; such chronic stimulation could result in an increased number of activated T cells. This is unlikely, however, since the long term diabetics on insulin for many years (both IDD and non-insulin dependent diabetics) did not show increased depolarized cells and several of the normal sibs, never exposed to insulin, showed a degree of depolarization similar to that seen in early diabetics (Table 1).

Since mitochondria concentrates carbocyanine dye, mitochondria abnormalities could result in altered fluorescence as seen in the diabetics and their sibs. However, we know of no evidence suggesting that autoimmune T cells have abnormal mitochondria.

In conclusion, we describe in this report increased numbers of depolarized T lymphocytes in early diabetics and their nondiabetic sibs which may represent a new dimension of autoimmunity in diabetes. The possible relationship of the depolarized T lymphocytes to the pathogenesis of IDD needs to be determined.

REFERENCES

1. Williams J., Deloria D., Hansen J.A., Dinarello C., Loertscher J., Shapiro H., Strom T., 1985, The events of primary T-cell activation can be staged by use of sepharose-bound anti-T3 (64.1) Monoclonal antibody and purified interleukin. J. Immunol 135: 2249-55.

2. Witkowski J., Micklem H.S., 1985, Decreased membrane potential of T Lymphocytes in ageing mice: flow cytometric studies with a carbocyanine dye. Immunology 56: 307.

3. Kiefer H., Blumie A.J., Kaback H.R., 1980, Membrane Potential Changes During Mitogenic Stimulation of Mouse Spleen Lymphocytes. Proc Natl Acad Sci USA 77: 2200-04.

4. Waggoner A.S., 1979, Dye indicators of membrane potential. Ann Rev Biophys Bioeng 8: 47-68.

5. Shapiro H., Natale P., Kamentsky L., 1979, Estimation of membrane potential of individual lymphoctyes by flow cytometry. Proc Natl Acad Sci USA 76: 5728-30.

6. Jackson R. Morris M., Haynes B., Eisenbarth G., 1982, Increased circulating Ia-antigen-bearing T cells in type I diabetes mellitus. New Engl J Med 306: 785-88.

7. Barbosa J., Chavers B., Dunsworth T., Michael A., 1982, Islet cell antibodies and histocompatability antigens (HLA) in insulin-dependent diabetics and their first-degree relatives. Diabetes 31: 585-88.

DISCUSSION

J. SCOTT: Dr. Barbosa, I found your depolarization studies intriguing, and I realize that they're preliminary, but would you care to speculate on the specificity problem? Do you plan to look at the same phenomenon in children who have autoimmunity of other endocrine disorders or something like that?

J. BARBOSA: Yes, very definitely.

J. SCOTT: That especially interests me, because we have families and I'm sure everyone else does where one sib will develop diabetes, but the other sib will develop an autoimmunity against another endocrine gland. It may be a familial occurrence, but not necessarily diabetes specific.

J. BARBOSA: Oh, absolutely. I agree fully.

III.   PREDICTION OF DIABETES

STUDIES OF PREDIABETES IN THE SPONTANEOUSLY DIABETIC BB RAT

Kenneth L. Brayman, James F. Markmann,
Clyde F. Barker, and ¶Ali Naji

Department of Surgery, University of Pennsylvania
School of Medicine, Philadelphia, USA

It is now well established that human type I diabetes is a chronic autoimmune process characterized by a rather "silent" prediabetic stage of several months to years in duration. (1) An important issue in diabetes research is the identification during the prediabetic period of subjects at high risk of developing diabetes. Several immunologic and metabolic parameters have been studied to assess their reliability as predictors of future development of diabetes in high risk individuals. Even if the combination of several of these factors proves to be highly specific in defining the high risk individuals these studies require a lenghty follow-up period to ascertain their sensitivity and reliability in predicting impending diabetes.

The BB rat has proven to be a unique model in the study of the prediabetic stage and has resulted in definition of several immunologic events during this overtly "silent" period. The BB rat model of spontaneous diabetes was first identified by the Chappel brothers in a commercial colony of Wistar derived rats at Bio-Breeding Laboratories of Ottawa, Canada. The clinical features of diabetes in BB rats first reported by Nakhooda et al (2), include an abrupt onset of hyperglycemia between 60-120 days of age which is associated with severe insulin deficiency. The affected members are not obese and upon development of diabetes require daily administration of exogenous insulin to prevent ketoacidosis. Histologic examination of the pancreas at the onset of overt hyperglycemia reveals a diffuse mononuclear cell infiltration of pancreatic islets (insulitis) which constitutes a pathologic hallmark of the disease. Phenotypic analysis of the infiltrating cells in the insulitis lesion has identified a heterogenous population of lymphoid cells including T lymphocytes, B lymphocytes, macrophages and natural killer cells.

The susceptibility of the BB rat to develop spontaneous diabetes is associated with gene(s) of the major histocompatibility complex (MHC)(3). In BB rats serologic and mixed lymphocyte culture analyses of the MHC gene products has determined that all animals possess the Rtl^u haplotype at the MHC locus. The consistent onset of diabetes between 60 and 120 days of age in this model has allowed development of several protocols of immunotherapy and immunoprediction of the syndrome.

Immunoprediction of diabetes in BB rat

Since the BB rat is the closest animal counterpart of human type I diabetes mellitus available, this model has permitted study of the events occurring at the onset of hyperglycemia and evaluation of several immuno-logic events during the prediabetic stage in the normoglycemic BB rats (well before the onset of the overt diabetes). We have previously reported elevated levels of Ia+ positive T lymphocytes at the onset of diabetes in BB rats (4). The most striking increase was present shortly after the onset of the disease, with a subsequent decline toward normal with the progression of the disease. The frequency of Ia+ T lymphocytes appear to be independent of the blood glucose level or exogeneous insulin administra-tion. Elevated numbers of Ia+ T cells were present in spontaneously dia-betic BB rats before insulin therapy excluding the possibility that they were induced as a consequence to an immunologic reaction to heterologous insulin. That hyperglycemia per se was not responsible for the increased frequency of cells is indicated by the fact that streptozotocin diabetic BB rats were found to have normal circulating levels of Ia+ T cells.

Ia+ T cells were detected in T helper (W3/25+) and, in slightly fewer numbers, in the T cytotoxic (OX-8+) subset. The lack of subset specificity maybe pertinent to some of the salient features of BB diabetes. Certain W3/25+ cells are known to be required for antibody production by lymphocytes. Therefore the presence of elevated Ia+ T helper cells is consistent with the observation that the majority of diabetic BB rats have circulating anti islet cell surface antibodies.

In further studies, we determined the frequency of Ia+ T lymphocytes in diabetes prone BB rats to determine whether the elevated levels of these cells could predict the future development of hyperglycemia (5). Selecting the value of $\geq 4\%$ as elevated, the sensitivity of this assay in predicting diabetes was 85% while the specificity was 83%. This finding suggests that elevated levels of Ia+ T lymphocytes reflect an ongoing immune process and accurately predicts the likelihood of developing spon-taneous hyperglycemia when obtained from a high risk population. Employing a prospective study of diabetes prone BB rats we further characterized the temporal relationship between the appearance of Ia+ T lymphocytes and the onset of the insulitis lesion. Diabetes prone BB rats underwent prospective analyses to determine levels of circulating Ia+, "activated" T lymphocytes prior to 50 days of age. Pancreatic biopsies were obtained within 48 hours of lymphocyte sampling and histologically examined for the presence of lymphocytic infiltrate. It was noted that diabetes prone animals had an elevated level of Ia+ T lymphocytes prior to development of any visible insulitis lesion in the pancreas. Taken together these ex-periments suggest that an "abnormal" beta cell surface antigen may not be the initiating trigger for anti-beta cell autoimmunity, because one would expect the local cellular inflammatory response to either predate or closely coincide with the primary immune response.

In addition to using the prospective analyses of Ia+ T lymphocytes we investigated a much simpler assay of diabetes prediction based on enumera-tion of the peripheral blood lymphocytes. Using this approach we have been able to predict subsequent diabetes development in diabetes prone litters with 96% sensitivity and 100% specificity (6).

We have taken advantage of this finding to address a central issue with the studies of immune pathogenesis of type I diabetes. The question is whether in a diabetes susceptible host the initial abnormality resides at the level of the native beta cells or originates from a primary defect in immunoregulation. To address this issue, we employed islet allografts

to probe the immunologic status of diabetes prone BB hosts that were
either predicted to become diabetic or remain permanently normoglycemic.
In a group of diabetes prone BB rats tolerant of Wistar Furth antigens,
peripheral blood lymphocytes were assayed at 35 days of age. An inverse
relationship between the degree of lymphocytopenia and the propensity
for future diabetes was noted. Tolerant diabetes prone BB animals were
then divided into two groups, those predicted to develop diabetes
(lymphocytes < 3,800/mm^3) and those predicted to remain normoglycemic
(lymphocytes > 3,800/mm^3). All animals were subsequently injected with
streptozotocin to eliminate the majority of native beta cells of the
pancreas and subsequently had normoglycemia restored by transplantation
of isolated Wistar Furth islets. Since these diabetes prone BB hosts
were immunologically tolerant to Wistar Furth transplantation antigens
as manifested by their permanent acceptance of Wistar Furth skin allografts,
the islet allografts were therefore not threatened by rejection.

Results of these experiments are shown in Table 1 which indicates
that all animals which were predicted to develop diabetes had a spontaneous
recurrence of hyperglycemia following successful islet transplantation.
In contrast, all the recipients that had been predicted to remain normoglycemic, did so for greater than 100 days after islet transplantation.
These findings suggest that the absence of native of BB islets and the
substitution of islets from Wistar Furth origin did not interfere with
the initiation of autoimmunity. These results indicate that the propensity
for diabetes is not the result of an abnormal triggering factor inherent
in the beta cells of susceptible rats.

TABLE I

FATE OF WF ISLET ALLOGRAFTS IN PREDIABETIC BB RATS

Recipient*	Peripheral blood lymphocyte count +	Duration of posttransplant normoglycemia (days)
BB tol WF predicted to become diabetic	< 3800	8, 9, 13, 19, 31
BB tol WF predicted to remain nondiabetic	> 3800	8 x > 100

* After determination of lymphocyte count, animals were rendered
  chemically diabetic;islet allografts transplanted intraportally.
+ Peripheral blood drawn at 35 days of age.

In summary, the ability to define immunologically the prediabetic
state in the BB rat, prior to destruction of beta cells has important
ramifications. The sine qua non of autoimmune disease is the ability
to prevent or cure the illness with immunomodulation. As noted above,
various immunologic interventions have been reported to prevent or reverse
the diabetic condition of the BB rat. While the diabetes of the BB rat
syndrome and that of human type I insulin dependent diabetes may not be
identical, they are strikingly similar. Further investigations of the
prediabetic stage in this model would provide the basis for the discrimi-
nate use of immunotherapy in humans in an attempt to prevent the disease

Immunotherapy of prediabetic BB rat. Administration of polyclonal anti-rat lymphocyte serum (ALS) to prediabetic BB rats or animals with recent onset of hyperglycemia has been found to effectively prevent or reverse diabetes, respectively (reviewed in 4). Daily administration of another potent immunosuppressive agent, cyclosporine A, has been equally effective in preventing the development of diabetes in BB rats when administered during prediabetic period, commencing few weeks after birth. However, in contrast to ALS, cyclosporine has not been effective in reversing established hyperglycemia in this model. In view of the known toxicity occurring with cyclosporine administration it is of interest that administration of this agent in an intermittent fashion has also been effective in decreasing the incidence of diabetes (5). Unfortunately continuous immunosuppression is mandatory to prevent the autoimmune beta cell damage as discontinuation of these agents has been associated with relapse of diabetes.

Attempts at disease prevention utilizing monoclonal antibodies specific for rat T lymphocyte markers have also been successful. In particular, significant protection has been achieved by treating young prediabetic BB rats either with pan T lymphocyte monoclonal antibodies OX-19 or OX-8 which is specific for cytotoxic/suppressor T cells and natural killer cells (4). Administration of anti IL-2 receptor monoclonal antibody (ART-18) either alone or in combination with a short course of cyclosporine immunosuppression has also been effective in reducing the incidence of diabetes (6). Similarly, treatment with monoclonal antibody specific for class II MHC antigens (anti I-E) has also been noted to prevent the insulitis and onset of diabetes when administered to young diabetes prone BB rats (7). The role of macrophages in the immune pathogenesis of BB diabetes has been suggested by the finding that silica, an anti-macrophage agent, prevents diabetes in this animal model.

Interestingly several other protocols have also been reported to modify and prevent the onset of diabetes in BB rats. Chronic insulin injections, dietary manipulations and frequent phlebotomy during the prediabetic stage have all been noted to reduce the incidence of spontaneous diabetes.

REFERENCES

1. Eisenbarth, g.S., 1986, Type I diabetes mellitus: A chronic autoimmune disease. N. Engl. J. Med. 314:1360-68.

2. Nakhooda, A.F., Like, A.A., Chappel, C.I., et al., 1977, The spontaneously diabetic Wistar rat. Metabolic andmorphologic studies.
   Diabetes 26:100-112.

3. Colle, E., Guttmann, R.D., Seemayer, T., 1981, Spontaneous diabetes
   mellitus syndrome in the rat. Association with the major histocompatibility complex. J. Exp. Med. 154:1237-42.

4. Mordes, J.P., Desemone, J., Rossini, A.A., 1987, The BB rat. Diabetes
   Metab. Rev. 3:725-50.

5. Brayman, K.L., Amstrong, J., Shaw, L., Rosano, T., Barker, C.F.,
   Naji, A., 1987, Prevention of idabetes in BB rats by intermittent
   administration of cyclosporine. Surgery 102:235-41.

6. Hahn, H.J., Lucke, S., Kloting, I., Volk, H.D., Baehr, R.V.,
   Diamantstein, T., 1987, Curing BB rats of freshly manifested diabetes
   by short-term treatment with a combination of a monoclonal anti-
   interleukin 2 receptor antibody and a subtherapeutic dose of cyclosporin A. Eur. J. Immunol. 17:1075-78.

7. Boitard, C., Michie, S., Serrurier, P., Butcher, G.W., Larkins, A.P.,
   McDevitt, H.O., 1985, In vivo prevention of thyroid and pancreatic
   autoimmunity in the BB rat by antibody to class II major histocompatibility complex gene products. Proc. Natl. Acad. Sci. 82:6627-31.

8. Francfort, J.W., Barker, C.F., Kimura, H., Silvers, W.K., Frohamn, M.,
   Naji, A., 1985, Increased incidence of Ia antigen-bearing T lymphocytes in the spontaneously diabetic BB rat. J. Immunol. 134:1577-82.

9. Francfort, J.W., Naji, A., Silvers, W.K., Tomaszewski, J., Woehrle, M.,
   Barker, C.F., 1985, Immunologic studies of the prediabetic stage in
   the spontaneous autoimmune diabetes mellitus of the BB rat.
   Transplantation 40:698-701.

10. Brayman, K.L., Markmann, J.F., Barker, C.F., Naji, A., 1988, Immuno-
    prediction of diabetes and evaluation of pancreatic islet transplan-
    tation during the prediabetic period. Surgery Vol. 4;2 445-451.

CHEMICALLY-INITIATED HYPERGLYCEMIA:

STREPTOZOTOCIN-SPECIFIC T LYMPHOCYTE REACTIONS

¶Helga Gleichmann and Christiane Klinkhammer

Clinical Department, Diabetes Research Institute

University of Dusseldorf, Dusseldorf, F.R.G.

During the past 15 years ample evidence has been accumulated that immunological reactions are involved in the development of insulin-dependent diabetes mellitus, i.e. Type I diabetes. It is currently widely thought that insulin-deficiency results from a chronic, organ-specific autoimmune reaction ultimately resulting in beta-cell destruction. Despite abundant data on both humoral and cellular abnormal immunological patterns detectable during the clinically silent prediabetic period, to date unequivocal demonstration of a direct pernicious autoimmune lesion of the beta-cells is still missing (1). Based on epidemiological investigations, it is noted that environmental factors most likely trigger the disease process in susceptible individuals. In support of such an initiating event are the marked discordance rate of approximately 50% in identical twins (D. Pyke, Chapter 31), the increased frequency of children with Type I diabetes with the congenital rubella syndrome (2), and the enhancing and preventing effect of dietary constituents on the incidence of diabetes in the diabetes-prone BB rat (F.W. Scott, Chapter 34). In all these situations the participation of autoimmune signs is unquestionable, yet the beta-cell specific immunopathogenic pathway still remains to be defined.

A useful experimental model to analyse both the significance of an exogeneous initiating agent and the specificity of subsequently developing immune reaction(s) in the progressive destruction of the beta-cells was first described by Like and Rossini (3). When streptozotocin (STZ), a toxin produced by Streptomyces achromogenes, is injected intraperitoneally in subdiabetogenic doses on 5 consecutive days to male recipient mice, gradually increasing hyperglycemia can develop. Numerous observations indicated immunological reactions to be involved in the diabetogenic process, however, again the underlying mechanism(s) remained to be elucidated. We found that STZ can be a hapten in vivo evoking STZ-specific T cell reactions (4). STZ consists of a glucose moiety and a nitrosourea moiety, is a mixture of α and β anomers and under certain experimental conditions preferably exerts its effects on the beta-cells.

The multiple low-dose STZ model in mice appears to be relevant to human Type I diabetes because cell-mediated immune reactions are involved.

C. Klinkhammer is supported by the Deutsche Forschungsgemeinschaft (Gl 131/1-1), Bonn, F.R.G., and the Minister fur Forschung und Wissenschaft des Landes Nordrhein-Westfalen.

Furthermore, STZ may serve as model compound to trace constituents ubiquitously occurring in the environment such as nitrosourea or as food additive (5) which might initiate the process of continuous beta-cell injury in predisposed individuals. Such an approach is an essential research issue to enable development of disease-preventing precautions.

IMMUNITY TO STREPTOZOTOCIN

A. METHODS

In order to assess the effects of STZ on the immune system the popliteal lymph node assay (PLN) was applied. By this assay a direct, most likely subtoxic effect on the pancreatic beta-cells was avoided, thus permitting analyses of the effects on the immune system. For this purpose STZ or citrate buffer, the solvent of STZ, or alloxan or single cell suspensions were injected subcutaneously (s.c.) into one hind footpad leaving the contralateral side uninjected as control. The PLN assay was performed as previously described (6). Briefly, at the times indicated mice were sacrificed by cervical dislocation, the PLNs removed and their weights and/or cell numbers determined. The ratio of the measured parameter of the experimental over that of the contralateral control node was calculated and assigned PLN index. In normal mice the mean PLN index is 1.0 ± 0.3 SEM, a mean value of $\geqslant 1.5$ usually indicates an induced immune reaction.

For adoptive cell transfer experiments single cell suspensions of spleens were prepared by using sterile Hanks' balanced salt solution (HBSS), and depleted of erythrocytes by treatment with Tris-buffered ammonium chloride. Cell viability was determined by trypan blue dye exclusion and the cells adjusted to the desired concentration. Enrichment for T lymphocytes was obtained by passage of spleen cells through nylon-wood columns (4). Inhibition of cell mitosis was achieved by incubating 20×10^6 viable cells/ml with 50 mg mitomycin C for 30 min at $37°C$ with 5% CO_2, followed by three washes in HBSS.

For significance analysis the U-test of Wilcoxon/Mann/Whitney was used.

B. STZ-SPECIFIC T LYMPHOCYTE-DEPENDENT PLN REACTIONS

As seen in Table I, all six strains of mice studied developed a dose dependent PLN weight increase 6 days after s.c. injection of STZ. The PLN reaction comparable in both male and female recipients. A linear dose-dependency was observed in BALB/c, C57Bl/6, DBA/2 and C3D2 F1 recipients, a plateau of the reaction was already reached with the applied dosages in C57Bl/KsJ and C3H/Tif mice. By injecting 0.5 mg STZ into BALB/c, the peak reponse was measured on day 7, thereafter slowly declining to normal values around day 60.

As demonstrated in Table II, T lymphocytes were required for the STZ-induced PLN reaction. Only the heterozygous +/nu recipients mounted a significant (P<0.001) response to the s.c. injection of 0.5 mg STZ, whereas their nu/nu counterparts completely failed to do so. The PLN response was not prevented by 3-o-methylglucose injected s.c. at the time of administration of STZ. This observation contrasts the protective effect of 3-o-methylglucose on the diabetogenicity of STZ when given prior to the beta-cell toxin.

94

TABLE I

PLN WEIGHT INCREASE AFTER S.C. INJECTION OF VARIOUS STZ DOSES INTO INBRED STRAINS OF MICE

Strain	Sex	N	Dose of STZ (mg)	PLN index on day 6 ($\bar{x} \pm$ SEM)
BALB/c	♂	10	0.125	2.1 ± 0.3
		6	0.25	3.7 ± 0.9
		6	0.5	3.4 ± 0.6
BALB/c	♀♂	6	0.5	2.9 ± 0.7
C57Bl/6	♂	5	0.5	4.1 ± 1.2
		6	1.0	5.3 ± 0.9
C57Bl/6	♀♂	4	0.5	3.6 ± 0.7
C57Bl/KsJ	♂	5	0.125	3.7 ± 0.6
		4	0.25	3.0 ± 1.1
		4	0.5	3.0 ± 0.5
C57Bl/KsJ	♀♂	5	0.5	2.9 ± 0.9
DBA/2		10	0.25	4.0 ± 0.4
		10	0.5	7.0 ± 0.8
C3H/Tif	♀	10	0.25	4.1 ± 0.4
		10	0.5	3.6 ± 0.5
C3D2F₁	♂	10	0.25	4.0 ± 0.7
		10	0.5	6.3 ± 0.6

TABLE II

T-CELL DEPENDENCY OF STZ-INDUCED PLN WEIGHT INCREASE

Strains of mice ♂	N	Dose of STZ (mg)	PLN index on day 6 ($\bar{x} \pm$ SEM)	P*
BALB/c +/nu	11	0.5	5.2 ± 0.7	<0.001
BALB/c nu/nu	10	0.5	0.9 ± 0.1	
BALB/c +/nu	10	0.25	2.3 ± 0.4	<0.001
BALB/c nu/nu	10	0.25	0.8 ± 0.1	
C57Bl/6 +/nu	10	0.5	5.3 ± 0.5	<0.001
C57Bl/6 nu/nu	10	0.5	0.7 ± 0,1	
C57Bl/6 +/nu	10	0.25	5.2 ± 0.7	<0.001
C57Bl/6 nu/nu	10	0.25	0.8 ± 0.1	

* Wilcoxon-Test

Tables I and II reproduced with permission from Diabetes (Reference 4).

In further experiments we questioned whether the PLN response resulted from an antigen-specific reaction to STZ or a mitogenic effect on T lymphocytes. For this purpose BALB/c mice were injected s.c. either with NaCTR, i.e. the solvent of STZ, or with 0.5 mg STZ into one hind footpad. After 13 weeks, when the enlarged PLN had reverted to normal size, groups of mice received a second s.c. injection into the same footpad of either subimmunogenic doses of 0.1 or 0.05 mg STZ, or the solvent of STZ, or 0.5 mg alloxan (ALL). A secondary PLN response was measured only in those mice which had been both primed and challenged with STZ (Fig. 1). This significant (P<0.005) secondary response to 0.1 mg STZ developed in an enhanced and

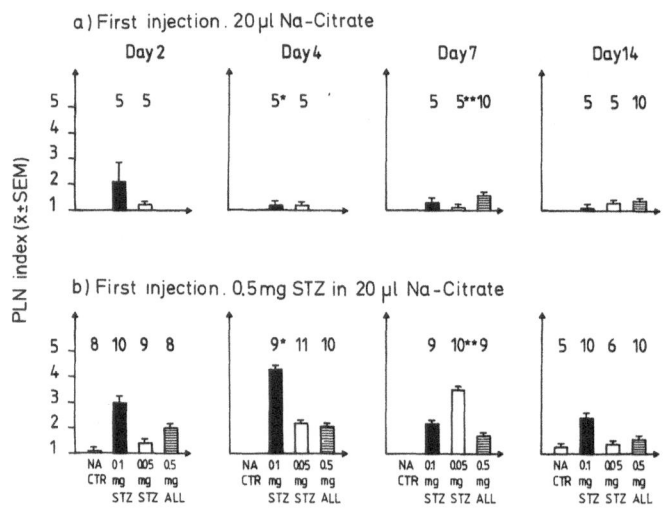

Figure 1. Kinetics of the secondary PLN response to STZ in BALB/c mice. First either sodium citrate (CTR), i.e. the solvent of STZ(a), or 0.5 mg STZ (b) was injected s.c. into one hind footpad. After 13 weeks groups of mice received a second s.c. injection into the same hind footpad of either the solvent or subimmunogenic doses (0.1 and 0.05 mg) of STZ or alloxan (ALL). The mean values ± SEM of the ratios of the PLN weights are illustrated. The numbers above the columns indicate the number of mice being used for the respective experiment. *, ** = P < 0.005. (Reproduced with permission from Diabetes (ref. 4)).

accellerated mode with a maximal response on day 4, the mean PLN index being 4.2 ± 0.4 SEM. A significant (P<0.005) secondary PLN response developed also upon an s.c. challenge with 0.05 mg STZ reaching a maximal mean PLN index of 3.6 ± 0.6 SEM on day 7. In contrast, challenging the STZ-primed mice with sodium citrate or alloxan, a diabetogen being structurally unrelated to STZ, failed to elicit a secondary PLN response. The alloxan-induced PLN response reflects a primary response, comparable to the reaction observed in recipients which had been primed with NaCTR (Fig. 1a). Furthermore, no secondary PLN reaction was generated to NaCTR in STZ primed mice (Fig. 1b).

C. ADOPTIVE CELL TRANSFER EXPERIMENTS

The results depicted in Figure 2 demonstrate that STZ-specific immunization can be induced also by the experimental scheme applied for induction of diabetes by multiple intraperitoneal (i.p.) injections of STZ. Spleen cell suspensions were prepared from mice which had received i.p. injections of 5 x 40 mg STZ/kg body wt or NaCTR. The cells were adoptively transferred into one hind footpad of syngeneic recipients which had been pretreated s.c. in the same hind footpad with either a subimmunogenic dose (0.1 mg) of STZ or NaCTR or alloxan (0.1 mg). A significant PLN weight increase was found on day 6 only in those mice which had received STZ 24 hrs prior to the transfer of spleen cells from STZ-treated donars. In contrast, neither spleen cells from NaCTR-treated donors injected into STZ-pretreated recipients nor spleen cells from STZ-treated donors transferred to solvent- or alloxan-pretreated mice resulted in A PLN reaction

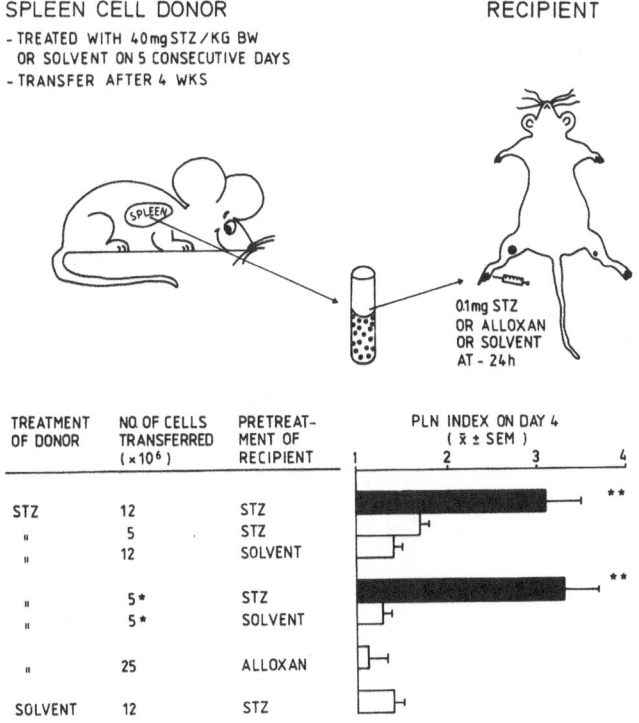

Figure 2. Experimental design of adoptive transfer of spleen cells and mean values ± SEM of the PLN weight indices. Spleen cells of BALB/c donor mice, which had received i.p. injections of either STZ or the solvent of STZ were inoculated s.c. into one hind footpad of syngeneic mice. The recipients had been pretreated s.c. with either a subimmunogenic dose (0.1 mg) of STZ or alloxan or solvent into the same footpad at 24 hr before the cell transfer. * = enriched for T cells, ** = P < 0.005 versus controls. (reproduced with permission from Diabetes (ref. 4)).

Sensitized T lymphocytes were required to mount this significant PLN enlargement in the adoptive cell transfer experiments. While 5×10^6 STZ-sensitized unseparated spleen cells failed to induce PLN weight increase (mean index 1.7 ± 0.1 SEM) in STZ-pretreated recipients, a significant ($p < 0.005$) reaction (mean index 3.3 ± 0.4 SEM) was found with 5×10^6 sensitized spleen cells enriched for T lymphocytes. The reaction of sensitized T cells was comparable to the reaction obtained with 12×10^6 sensitized unseparated spleen cells. Again no PLN reaction developed in solvent – or alloxan-pretreated recipients of both STZ-sensitized unseparated and for T lymphocytes enriched STZ-sensitized spleen cells. Spleen cells of solvent-treated donor mice also failed to mediate a PLN reaction in recipients which had been pretreated with STZ.

Sensitization of donor animals was demonstrable already 1 week after the last injection of STZ as summarised in Table 3 and developed independently of the metabolic disorder.

Mitomycin C treatment of STZ-sensitized spleen cells prior to the adoptive transfer completely abrogated mediation of STZ-specific PLN reactivity (4). This data indicates that STZ-sensitized proliferating cells, presumably T lymphocytes, are required to get stimulated upon re-exposure in vivo to STZ.

TABLE III

ADOPTIVE TRANSFER OF 25×10^6 SPLEEN CELLS AT VARIOUS TIME INTERVALS
AFTER PRIMING INTO BALB/c FEMALES

Priming of donors with 5x40 mg STZ/kg bw	Time interval between priming and transfer (weeks)	Pretreatment of recipients at -2h with	PLN index on day 6 ($\bar{x} \pm$ SEM)	
			Weight	Cell number
yes	1	solvent	1.7 ± 0.3	1.5 ± 0.2
yes		0.1 mg STZ	2.5 ± 0.3	3.5 ± 0.6[a]
no		0.1 mg STZ	1.5 ± 0.3	1.5 ± 0.3[a]
yes	2	solvent	1.4 ± 0.3	1.0 ± 0.2
yes		0.1 mg STZ	3.0 ± 0.5[b]	3.1 ± 0.4[c]
no		0.1 mg STZ	1.4 ± 0.3[b]	1.2 ± 0.04[c]
yes	4	solvent	1.3 ± 0.2	ND
yes		0.1 mg STZ	2.7 ± 0.2[d]	ND
no		0.1 mg STZ	1.0 ± 0.1[d]	ND

a = $P < 0.02$; b = $P < 0.005$; c = $P < 0.01$; d = $P < 0.001$; ND = Not Determined

DISCUSSION

Immunological reactions are involved in the development of insulin-deficiency in human Type 1 diabetes, in animal models with spontaneous diabetes (1) and in the murine model of low-dose streptozotocin administration (3,6). Although currently widely conceived that beta-cell destruction results from chronic, pernicious autoimmune reactions, a direct autoimmune attack of beta-cells still has to be proven. In addition to the abundant indirect evidence of an autoimmune pathway the well-known notion of environmental agents initiating the disease process warrants an avenue for future research to elucidate the mechanism(s) contributing to beta-cell failure.

The low-dose streptozotocin model appears to be a useful system to unravel the specificity of immunological reactions developing upon uptake of a beta-cell specific toxin. By applying the PLN assay we were able to demonstrate that STZ, which is not a mitogen for T lymphocytes, can elicit primary and secondary immune responses in mice in the absence of adjuvant. These immune responses required T lymphocytes and proved to be STZ-specific (Table 2 and Fig. 1). T cell-deprived nu/nu recipients completely failed to respond to s.c. injections of STZ with a PLN reaction whereas their euthymic counterparts consistently mounted a significant PLN weight increase. Both male and female recipients reacted to STZ to a comparable degree. An accelerated and enhanced secondary PLN response developed to subimmunogenic doses of STZ when given to STZ-primed recipients. By adoptive transfer experiments T lymphocytes prepared from spleens of donors treated i.p. with STZ were defined to mediate STZ-specific PLN reaction in syngeneic recipients pretreated s.c. with subimmunogenic doses of STZ.

A direct mitogenic effect of STZ on lymphocytes is highly unlikely because addition of STZ to lymphocyte cultures failed to induce cell proliferation (unpublished). Preliminary experiments, however, indicated that a primary lymphocyte reaction can be stimulated in vitro with syngeneic STZ-incubated stimulator cells akin to the reactions obtained with allogeneic stimulator cells (data not shown). Thus, STZ might be recognized as hapten in vivo and according to recently obtained data (not shown) also in vitro. The STZ-induced T cell-dependent PLN reactions were not inhibited by simultaneous injections of 3-o-methylglucose in contrast to the protective effect against the diabetogenic effect of STZ (7). These observations suggest that the immunogenic potential of STZ might be assigned to the nitrosourea moiety and that 3-o-methylglucose and streptozotocin bind competitively with a glucose recognition site on beta-cells.

Investigations with STZ-specific T lymphocytes are expected to elucidate whether T cell-dependent immune reactions akin to those obtained by using the PLN assay might be involved in the effect of STZ on the beta-cells of male recipient mice. It is conceivable that STZ attaches to class II molecules of the major histocompatibility complex of antigen-presenting cells in and around the pancreatic islets, rendering these cells immunogenic for autologous or syngeneic T lymphocytes. Thus, STZ could attach to Ia antigens expressed on the vascular endothelium and the ductular epithelium at the insular pole as well as to resident dendritic-like cells adjacent to the capillaries within the islets (8). Subsequent T cell-dependent immune reactions with specificity for these STZ-modified cell structures might be reflected by infiltrations with mononuclear cells in and around the pancreatic islets, leading secondarily to beta-cell destruction in some animals. It is also possible that either STZ-specific T lymphocyte reactions toward STZ-modified beta-cells are induced resulting in direct immunological beta-cell destruction or activation of autoreactive T lymphocytes for unaltered beta-cells. At present none of the proposed immunopathogenic pathways are mutually exclusive and require further analysis.

The recent reports on the diabetogenicity of either class I or class II expression on beta-cells in transgenic mice (9, 10) without lymphoid cell infiltrates suggest that rather intracellular mechanism(s) than pernicious autoimmune reactions are operative in the induction of the process of diabetes development. Thus the lymphoid infiltrates described as insulitis in man and animals might represent a non-specific inflammatory reaction as a consequence of beta-cell necrosis rather than its cause.

Further analysis of the role of STZ-induced immune reactions in the process of gradually developing hyperglycemia and assessment of the immunogenic potential of STZ-derivatives and their diabetogenic potential are expected to disclose environmental structures with the capacity to trigger progressive beta-cell failure in predisposed individuals.

ACKNOWLEDGEMENTS

We are grateful to Prof. Dr. F.A. Gries for his continuous support and interest in our work.

REFERENCES

1. Barbosa J, Bach, FH, 1987, Cell-mediated autoimmunity in Type 1 diabetes. In Diabetes/Metabolism Reviews. 4: 981-1004. John Wiley and Sons.

2. Ginsberg-Fellner, F., Witt, M.E., Fedun, B., Taub, F., Doberson, M.J., McEvoy, R.C., Cooper, L.Z., Notkins, A.L., Rubinstein, P., 1985, Diabetes mellitus and autoimmunity in patients with congenital rubella syndrome. Rev Infect Dis 7: 170-5 (Suppl 1).

3. Like, A.A., Rossini, A.A., 1976, Streptozotocin-induced pancreatic insulitis: new model of diabetes mellitus. Science 193: 415-7.

4. Klinkhammer, C., Popowa, P., Gleichmann, H., 1988, Specific immunity to the diabetogen streptozotocin: cellular requirements for induction of lymphoproliferation. Diabetes 34: 74-80.

5. Helgason, T., Jonasson, M.R., 1981, Evidence for a food additive as a cause of Ketosis-prone diabetes. Lancet 2:716-20.

6. Gleichmann, H., 1981, Studies on the mechanism of drug sensitization: T cell-dependent popliteal lymph node reaction to diphenylhydantoin. Clin Immunol Immunopathol 18: 203-11.

7. Ganda, O.P., Rossini, A.A., Like, A.A., 1976, Studies on streptozotocin diabetes. Diabetes, 25: 595-603.

8. Farr, A.G., Anderson, S.K., 1985, In situ ultrastructural demonstration of cells bearing Ia antigens in the murine pancreas. Diabetes 34: 987-90.

9. Allison, J., Campbell, I.L., Morahan, G., Mandel, T.E., Harrison, L.C., Miller, J.F.A.P., 1988, Diabetes in transgenic mice resulting from overexpression of class I histocompatibility molecules in pancreatic cells. Nature 333: 529-33.

10. Sarvetnick, N., Liggitt, D., Pitts, S.L., Hansen, S.E., Stewart, T.A., 1988, 1988, Insulin-dependent diabetes mellitus induced in transgenic mice by ectopic expression of class II MHC and interferon-gamma. Cell, 51: 773-82.

DIABETIC LYMPHOCYTES TRANSFER AND BETA CELL FUNCTIONS

¶J.C. Basabe,* L.E. Fabiano de Bruno* and M. Arata*

*Fundacion Laboratorio de Investigaciones Pediatricas (FLIP)
Hospital General de Ninos "Dr. Pedro de Elizalde "
Buenos Aires, Argentina

There is now consensus that the immune system is involved in the pathogenesis of insulin dependent diabetes mellitus (IDDM) in man and animals. This destructive autoimmune process may occur over a long-lasting period and only when a sufficient number of beta cells are destroyed does clinical evidence appear.

Although the precise triggering events that initiate autoimmune IDDM are unknown, there is evidence to support that T lymphocytes, macrophages; interleukin 1 (IL1) or 2 (IL2) and free radicals could be important as autoimmune effectors (1-2). The role of T cells in the pathogenesis of Type I diabetes is supported by several major arguments,however the mechanism of T cell action remains to be elucidated.

To help to establish that a disease is a cell-mediated immune process, passive transfer to unaffected host, using effector cells, and immune modulation, should be demonstrated. Studies utilizing peripheral mononuclear blood cells (PMBC) or splenocytes from IDDM patients, multiple low doses streptozotocin (m l d STZ) induced diabetic mice and spontaneous models of autoimmune IDDM such as BB rats and NOD mice, showed that disease can be transferred (2).

Clinical manifestation of IDDM is the end point of a prolonged period where immune events are only merely indicators of ongoing autoimmune reactions, which does not necessarily indicate the state of aggression of islet cell destruction.

Since immunologic abnormalities give poor information related to when IDDM is likely to develop or to the time course of the beta cell mass reduction, endocrine function was also studied. Of all the tests performed, first phase insulin (I) secretion (I determined at 1+3 min post 0.5 g/kg glucose IV.) showed to be the most useful approach to detect alteration of beta cell function (1). Response to IV. glucose appears to be lost earliest while a significant response to glucagon or arginine remains and seems to be a possible way to assess residual beta cell mass during the prediabetic period (3). Taken together, immunologic and hormonal data, makes it possible to identify individuals with a high risk of developing overt IDDM.

The present report studies immunologic and hormonal parameters in the prediabetic period after passive transfer of PMBC or splenocytes. Lymphocytes (ly) from IDDM children and from inbred (F?+27) C57Bl/KsJ diabetic mice (by m.l.d STZ), were transferred to athymic mice and to syngeneic mice respectively.

MATERIALS AND METHODS

Lymphocytes transfer

Recipients: For IDDM children Ly = male athymic nude mice, BALB/c, aged 8 weeks, from the Comisión Nacional de Energía Atómica were used. For C57Bl/KsJ diabetic mice (m.l.d. STZ) ly: syngeneic mice from the Centro Nacional de Genética Médica.

Donors: IDDM children: Ly were extracted from peripheral blood of the following groups:

1) Controls: children without endocrine or autoimmune diseases or familiar history of diabetes (males and females 6 to 15 years old).

2) Newly diagnosed: children with IDDM prior to I therapy or under treatment for up to one month (males and females 6 to 15 years old).

3) Long standing: children with IDDM under I treatment during 4 to 31.4 months (males and females 5 to 19 years old).

4) Remission: children with IDDM without I administration during 15 or more days, without glycosuric and ketonuria, with fasting normoglycaemia (males and females 6 to 16 years old).

Transfer procedure

1) From man to mouse: It was performed according to Buschard et al. (4). The Ly fraction was separated by a "Hypaque-Ficoll" gradient. Each mouse was injected with 6×10^6 cells intraperitoneally. Cells from each child were injected into four to five nude mice. Transfer was considered positive when at least four animals developed hyperglycaemia.

2) From mouse to mouse: The technique described by Rossini et al. was utilized (5). Spleen cells were isolated by shredding the spleen with steel wire mesh followed by two washes in Hanks buffer. Each recipient mouse received IP. an aliquot of 5×10^7 live nucleated cells.

Trapping of syngeneic diabetic Ly in normal mouse pancreas: Splenic Ly from C57Bl/KsJ mice undergoing diabetes by m.l.d.STZ were isolated, labelled with ^{51}Cr and injected IV. into normal syngeneic mice. After 24 hours the radioactivity in several organs was measured. Control Ly suspensions were prepared in the same way from normal syngeneic mice. The percentage of radioactivity in each organ was calculated as :

$$\% \text{ radioactivity} = \frac{\text{c.p.m. in organ}}{\Sigma \text{ c.p.m. of all organ studied}} \times 100$$

Ly effect on I response of dispersed rat islet cells: was performed as described by Debray-Sach et al. (6). The I secretion was stimulated by glucose 16.5 mmol/l and theophylline 5 mmol/l. Wistar rat islet suspension was obtained as Ono et al. (7). The results were expressed as net basal and net stimulated release (uU/5 $\times$ 10^3 cells/5 min) or as

$$\text{Secretion index} = \frac{\text{(net stimulated release)} - \text{(net basal release)}}{\text{(net basal release)}} \times 100$$

Perifusion of pancreas slices: the technique described by Burr et al. (8) was used.

Insulin was determined by radioimmunoassay (9) using rat insulin standards and porcine ^{125}I insulin as a tracer. The sensitivity of insulin assay was 5 uU/ml, the results were reproductible with a coefficient of variation of 8.96%.

Statistical analysis of the data was performed with Student's t test for unpaired samples and with one way Anovar and Newman Keuls test. Results are given as mean ± SEM.

RESULTS

LY-TRANSFER FROM CHILD TO MOUSE

a) <u>Blood glucose</u> in experimental mice transferred with Ly from newly diagnosed IDDM was higher than in control mice, at 8, 15, or 24 days after Ly injection (p 0.001 at all times studied). Ly from longstanding IDDM or IDDM in remission did not modify blood glucose levels.

b) <u>Ly effect on I response of dispersed rat islet cells</u>: When incubated in the presence of Ly from newly diagnosed IDDM, glucose-theophylline-induced I secretion was significantly inhibited, when compared with controls (uU/5 x 10^3 cells/5 min 8.11 ± 1.29, n = 9 vs 25.89 ± 1.64 n = 15 respectively; p < 0.001. Secretion index 179.05 vs 617.81 % respectively). Ly from long standing IDDM also impaired secretion by dispersed rat islet cells (13.03 ± 2.47, n = 13 uU/5 x 10^3 cells/5 min, p < 0.01 secretion index 231.29%.

c) <u>I secreted by perifused pancreas slices from BALB/c (nu/nu) mice</u>: pancreas from athymic animals transferred with Ly from children with recently diagnosed IDDM clearly secreted a diminished first and second phase of I when compared with controls (areas under the curve, uU of I secreted by 100 mg wt.; first phase (min 3 to 6): 542 ± 16, n = 16 vs 978 ± 40, n = 12, p < 0.05 respectively). Pancreas from mice transferred with Ly from long standing IDDM showed an impaired first phase of glucose-induced I release (area under the curve 756 ± 38, n = 12, p < 0.02). I secreted by pancreas slices from mice injected with Ly of diabetic children in remission, was no different from controls.

d) In a separate set of perifusions we studied the I response to glucose in pancreas from mice transferred with Ly from the same four children, before, during and after the remission period. First phase I secretion of pancreas slices from mice transfered with Ly from children in pre or post remission was significantly inhibited (I. secretion, uU/area under the curve, pre-remission: 694 ± 14, post-remission: 710 ± 36, control: 918 ± 37; p < 0.02 for both groups).

e) In new experimental PMBC from children with long standing IDDM or long standing in remission were <u>cultured in the presence of Con A</u> (10 ug/ml x 10^6 cells) for three days.

Ly from children with long standing IDDM cultured with Con A augmented the inhibitory effect on first phase glucose-stimulated I secretion when transferred to nude mice (uUI/area under the curve; Ly long-standing 683

± 22, n = 12 vs Ly Con A long standing = 471 ± 33, n = 12, p ≤ 0.05). On the other hand, Ly from children in remission cultured with Con A, did not produce any change in the pattern of insulin secreted by the recipient mice pancreas (uU/area under the curve, 1st phase: 946 ± 66, n = 4).

Comments

Ly from recently diagnosed and long standing IDDM showed anti beta cell autoimmunity, indicated as inhibition of stimulated insulin secretion from dispersed islets cells. This immune aggression significantly inhibited the glucose-stimulated first phase I secretion from perfused pancreas slices of transferred mice. However, only Ly from the recently diagnosed group produced hyperglycemia. Lymphoid cells cultured with the lectin Con A, increased the inhibitory effect of long standing and then hyperglycemia appeared. This indicated that blood glucose levels could be related to the magnitude of the immune aggression and to the I secretion impairment. The alteration in the I secretion pattern persists for at least 60 days after diabetic Ly injection.

Transfer of Ly from children with longstanding diabetes during the remission period failed to induce any change in the pattern of I secreted by the perifused pancreas slices, even when previously cultured with Con A. During post remission period, Ly inhibitory effect on 1st phast I secretion, appeared again.

In preliminary results we observed that Ly from children in remission had no effect on the I response of dispersed rat islet cells to glucose theophylline stimulus.

LY TRANSFER FROM C57B1/KsJ MOUSE TO SINGENEIC MOUSE

a) Trapping of singeneic diabetic (m.l.d. STZ in C57B1/KsJ mice) Ly in normal mouse páncreas: diabetic and normal splenic lymphocytes were labeled with ^{51}Cr injected to normal syngeneic mice and radioactivity counted after 24 hrs. When comparing the lodging of normal and diabetic Ly in different organs, no differences could be seen in any of them, except pancreas. It could be observed in pancreas that % radioactivity was 0.70 ± 0.14 when animals were injected with control Ly and 1.07 ± 0.11 (p < 0.01) when injected with diabetic Ly.

Effect of diabetic (m.l.d. STZ) Ly on I response by dispersed rat islets cells to glucose and theophylline stimulus: Ly from diabetic mice inhibited the stimulated I secretion (I uU/5 x 10^3 cells/5 min; control Ly: 28.33 ± 0.33, n = 7, diabetic Ly: 8.30 ± 0.60, n = 7, p < 0.001).

Diabetic Ly transfer did not alter blood glucose levels of syngeneic recipients mice during the first three weeks after injection.

Temporal study of hormonal and immunological parameters. a) Seven days after Ly transfer: Ly from mice transferred with diabetic Ly clearly inhibited I response to glucose/theophylline, when incubated with dispersed rat islets cells (uUI/5 x 10^3 cells/5 min, control Ly; 30.5 ± 0.57, n = 7 vs diabetic Ly; 16.88 ± 0.95, n = 6, p < 0.01). However perfused slices of pancreas from recipient mice injected with control or diabetic Ly, showed a similar pattern of I secretion when stimulated by 16 m mol/1 glucose or with arginine/glucose (20/5 mmol/1).

b) Fifteen days after Ly transfer: Ly from mice injected with diabetic Ly significantly inhibited hormonal response to glucose/theophylline when incubated with dispersed rat islets cells (uUI/5 x 10^3 cells/5 min, control Ly 32.6 ± 0.57, n = 15 vs diabetic Ly 18.08 ± 1.94, n = 7; p < 0.05).

Insulin response of perifused slices of pancreas from mice injected with diabetic Ly was diminished when stimulated by glucose (uU/area under the curve, 1st phase = control Ly 947 ± 42, n = 15 vs diabetic Ly 8958 ± 209, n = 5; p < 0.05). There was no difference in the I response by slices of pancreas from mice injected with Ly from controls or diabetics when arginine/glucose was used as stimulus.

c) Insulin response modulations: In another experimental group splenocytes from control and diabetic (m.l.d. STZ) mice were cultured in the presence of <u>Con A</u> for three days before transfer to syngeneic mice. Seven days after injection diabetic Con A treated Ly induced a significant inhibition of glucose-stimulated 1st phase insulin response by perifused pancreas slices (uU/area under the curve = 729 ± 19, n = 6, p < 0.01). Fifteen days after transfer, diabetic Con A treated Ly produced a greater impairment of 1st phase glucose under the curve: 549 ± 22, n = 4; p < 0.01). In this case, recipients mice also developed hyperglycemia (p < 0.001).

<u>Recipients mice pre-treatment with a single low dose of STZ</u>: Normal recipients mice were treated with a single injection of 40 mg STZ/kg body wt. before transfer of splenocytes. Fifteen days after transfer glycemia and hormonal secretion were evaluated. At this low dose, STZ did not cause, in itself or associated with control Ly transfer, neither hyperglycemia nor altered pancreas slices glucose stimulated I secretion.

STZ pretreated recipients transferred with diabetic Ly develop hyperglycemia (p < 0.001). Perifused pancreas slices showed a significant inhibition of first phase glucose-induced I secretion (uU/area under the curve): 504 ± 16, n = 5, p < 0.01). Insulin secretion was also lower than that obtained by recipients transferred with diabetic Ly (p < 0.02 for both I secretion phases).

<u>Repeated transfer of 5 x 10^7 cells</u> were performed at day 3 and 5 after first splenocytes injection. Hormonal response was evaluated at day 7 and 15. Recipients mice did not develop hyperglycemia at any of the times studied.

Perifused pancreas slices from diabetic by recipient mice showed, 7 days after first injection, a significant impairment of both phases of glucose-induced I secretion. (uU/area under the curve: 1st phase 691 ± 16, n = 5, p < 0.01; 2nd phase: 9395 ± 298, n = 5, p < 0.01). However, the I secretion pattern was normal when arginine/glucose was used as stimulus.

Fifteen days after first diabetic Ly transfer, perifused pancreas slices from recipient mice released diminished amounts of insulin in both phases when stimulated by glucose (uU/area under the curve, 1st phase: 625 ± 20, p < 0.01; 2nd phase 8502 ± 143, p < 0.01; n = 5 in both cases) or when stimulated by arginine/glucose (uU/area under the curve, 1st phase 631 ± 25, p < 0.01; 2nd phase 7552 ± 243, p < 0.01; n = 5 in both groups.

Comments

Ly transfer from diabetic (m.l.d.STZ) syngeneic did not produce any change in the blood glucose levels of recipients mice. However, splenic lymphoid cells from mice undergoing m.l.d. STZ diabetes were preferentially trapped in normal pancreas; in a similar way to those form Type I diabetics (10). This would suggest that Ly from m.l.d. STZ mice recognized a specific islet antigen(s) for population that was retained by the pancreas. Splenocytes not only were retained but also affected the beta cell function since they inhibited the stimulated release by dispersed rat islets cells "in vitro."

We studied in a temporal way some immunologic and hormonal response in the recipient mice. Seven days after diabetic splenocytes injection, anti-beta cell autoimmunity was present (indicated by recipients Ly-induced inhibition of I release from glucose/theophylline-stimulated dispersed islet cells). On the other hand, I response pattern from perifused pancreas slices was normal when stimulated by glucose or by arginine/glucose.

Fifteen days after transfer of diabetic Ly splenocytes anti-beta cell immunity still persists. Beta cell function was impaired when I release was induced by glucose, however the response was normal when arginine/glucose was employed as stimulus.

This temporal study allowed us to separate immune aggression from pancreatic I release and besides this showed that, also in this experimental model, impaired response to glucose was the most sensitive and earliest marker to detect loss of beta cell function.

Early pancreatic I response was modulated by 1) cultured diabetic Ly with Con A prior to transfer, 2) recipient mice pretreatment with a single low dose of STZ, 3) repeated splenocytes transfer.

Diabetic Ly-Con A culture before transfer not only produced an earlier but a greater impairment of beta cell function stimulated by glucose. Because Con A is a potent stimulator of IL_2 production by T-Ly the possibility of a Con A and IL_2-responsive cytotoxic cells (NK) was postulated (11).

Treatment of recipient mice with a single low dose of STZ also induced a greater impairment of glucose stimulated islet function and hyperglycemia also appeared. This result does not elucidate whether STZ treatment caused cytotoxic Ly from m.l.d. STZ to recognize STZ altered beta cells and then strongly react, or may simply reflect a reduction in beta cell mass or both.

It seems reasonable to speculate that many triggering events may initiate the autoimmune process and that multiple aggression may be necessary to destroy sufficient number of beta cells to produce IDDM (islets destruction versus cell regeneration). This seems to be supported by our data showing that repeated transfer of splenocytes made impairment of beta cell function to appear earlier and also increased their intensity.

Transfer of immunocytes seems to be one of the most useful methods for investigating cellular immunology and the pathogenesis of IDDM. Furthermore, it allows for "in vitro" manipulations of cells prior to transfer to determine, for instance, which cells types are related to a particular immune response. In addition Ly transfer offers an excellent model to test immuno-regulatory compounds to lead to effective and safe preventive and specific therapy.

REFERENCES

1. Eisenbarth, G.S.: Genes, generation of diversity, glycoconjugates and autoimmune beta cell insufficiency in Type I diabetes. Diabetes 1987; 36: 355-364.

2. Rossini, A.A., Mordes, J.P. and Like, A.A.: Immunology of insulin-dependent diabetes mellitus. Ann. Rev. Immunol. 1985; 3:289-320.

3. Ganda, O., Srikanta, S., Brink, S., Morris, M.A., Gleason, R., Soeldner, C.S., and Eisenbarth, G.S.: Differential sensitivity to beta cell secretatogues in "early" type I diabetes mellitus. Diabetes 1984; 33:516-521.

4.   Buschard K., Masbad, S., and Rygaard, J.: Passive transfer of diabetes mellitus from man to mouse.   Lancet 1978; 2:908-919.

5.   Rossini, A.A., Mordes, J.P., Williams, R., Pelletier, A., Like, A.: Failure to transfer insulitis to athymic recipients using BB/w rat lymphoid tissue transplant.   Metabolism 1983 (32, suppl. 1); 80-96.   (Sciences   1983; 220:727-733).

6.   Debray-Sachs, M., Sai, P., Boitard, C., Assan, R., and Hamburger, J.: Antipancreatic immunity in genetically diabetic mice.   Clin. Exptl. Immunol. 1983; 51: 1-7.

7.   Ono, J., Takabi, R., and Fukuma, M.: Preparation of single cells from pancreatic islets adult rat by the use of dispase.   Endocrinol. Jpn. 1987; 24:265-270.

8.   Burr, I.M., Stauffacher, W., Balant, L., Renold, A., and Grodsky, G.: Regulation of insulin release in perifused pancreatic tissue. Acta Diabet. Lat. 1969; 6:580-596.

9.   Herbert, V., Lau, K., Gottlieb, C., and Bleicher, S.J.:   Coated charcoal immuno-assay of insulin.   J. Clin. Endocrinol. Metab. 1965; 25:1375-1384.

10. Kaldany, A., Hill, T., Wentworth, W., Brink, J.A., D'Elia, M., Clouse, M., and Soeldner, J.S.:   Trapping of peripheral blood lymphocytes in the pancreas of oatients with acute-onset insulin-dependent diabetes mellitus. Diabetes 1982; 31:463-466.

LYMPHOCYTE SUBSETS IN PRE-DIABETES

¶W.J. Riley*, C.L. Hitchcock* and D.A. Schatz*

*Departments of Pathology and Pediatrics
University of Florida College of Medicine
Gainesville, Florida

Overwhelming evidence has accumulated in recent years that insulin dependent diabetes mellitus (IDD) is an autoimmune disease occurring in genetically susceptible individuals (1). Evidence for a possible role of humoral immunity in the autoimmunopathogenesis of IDD was initially suggested in the mid-1970's by the findings of 2 different autoantibodies reactive to either surface (islet cell surface antibodies) or cytoplasmic antigens (islet cell antibodies) (2). The presence of a mononuclear (predominantly lymphocytic) infiltration of the pancreatic islets had earlier provided evidence for involvement of the cellular arm of the immune system (3). More recently, "activated" T cells have been detected, both in these lymphocytic pancreatic islet infiltrates at the time of diagnosis as well as in recurrent insulitis following pancreatic transplantation (4-5). In addition, multiple defects in T cell mediated immunity (CMI) have been described in one of the prototypic animal model for human IDD, the biobreeding (BB) rat (6). These include severe lymphopenia, abnormal ratio of T lymphocyte subsets, an inability to reject skin grafts across major histocompatibility barriers, reduced proliferative response to T cell mitogens, and the ability to adaptively transfer diabetes.

These findings have prompted investigators to define more precisely the defects in CMI in human IDD. Previous studies in human IDD describing lymphocyte subset abnormalities have been contradictory (7). These studies, as well as functional lymphocyte assays, were hampered by the presence of the abnormal metabolic state in IDD (8). Islet cell autoantibodies (ICA) when present in the sera of nondiabetic individuals are now believed to reflect pre-clinical IDD associated with altered immunoregulation present long before the onset of symptoms (9). This ability to identify individuals prior to the onset of the abnormal metabolic state present once the diabetic state has already manifest has given us the opportunity to study cellular immunity without these confounding factors.

METHODS

Patients

The patients evaluated in these studies are part of an ongoing study attempting to define the natural history of IDD. ICA positive individuals

This work was supported by grants from the National Institutes of Health (1-RO-HD-19469-01 and RO-1-AM-36151-01) and the Clinical Research Center (RR-82). Dr. Riley is supported by a Research Career Development Award (K04-AM-01421-01).

are initially identified on sera obtained either as part of a screening
program of approximately 13000 high risk relatives of IDD probands (n =
7000) or from a general population of healthy school children from Pasco
County, Florida (n = 6000). These non-diabetic ICA positive persons and
matched ICA negative individuals are subsequently typed for human leukocyte antigens (HLA) A, B, C and DR and admitted to the Clinical Research
Center for intravenous glucose tolerance testing (IVGTT). Nine newly-
diagnosed IDD patients before insulin therapy was instituted were also
studied for comparison.

Laboratory Studies

ICA were determined by an indirect immunofluorescence assay as previously described (2). HLA typings were performed by an earlier reported two
color microcytotoxicity assay (8). After an appropriate 3 day preparative
high carbohydrate diet and overnight fasting, an IVGTT was carried out on
each patient using 0.5 gm./kg. of 25% glucose administered as a bolus over
2 to 4 minutes. Insulin concentrations were determined at -10, 1,3,5, 10,
30, and 60 minutes of the glucose bolus.

Lymphocyte subsets and activation studies

Peripheral blood was collected in heparinized tubes and leukocytes obtained by NH_4Cl lysis. The distribution of T lymphocyte populations were
then determined by direct immunofluorescence (IF) using flow cytometry. A
phycoerythrin (PE) conjugated Leu2a monoclonal antibody (MoAb) was used to
identify cytotoxic/suppressor (CD8+) T lymphocytes with Leu3a defining the
CD4+, helper T lymphocyte subset. Subsets of T helper lymphocytes (CD4+)
were enumerated by two color fluorescence using both PE conjugated Leu3a
and a fluorescein isothioscyanate (FITC) conjugated 4B4 MoAb to identify
the CD4+ 4B4+ helper-inducer T lymphocyte subpopulation and FITC conjugated
2H4 MoAb, the CD4+ 2H4+ suppressor-inducer T lymphocytes. These latter two
MoAbs have only recently been obtained and enumeration studies were performed on 10 ICA+ patients and 10 ICA- matched individuals. "Activated" T
lymphocytes were identified by a similar direct IF assay and flow cytometry
using FITC conjugated MoAbs to the interleukin 2 (IL-2) receptor (TAC) or
to a non-polymorphic DR antigen. B lymphocytes were used in the enumeration
of biotinylated B1 MoAb. Flow cytometry using the FACS Analyzer was used
for all enumeration studies. Four simultaneous parameters were determined
for each cell: electronic cell size, right angle (90°) scatter, green and
red fluorescence.

The relative antigen density of the DR antigen on lymphocytes, expressed as molecules per micrometers squared, was calculated from the following equations.

$$Fs = Fo \text{ x } Bs/Bo$$

$$RAD = Fs \text{ x } 1000/SA$$

$$SA = \pi D^2$$

Fs is the standardized mean channel number, either cell volume or green
fluorescence; Fo, the observed mean channel number, Bs, the standard mean
channel number from both the cell volume and the green fluorescence of the
#2 microbead on subsequent days; Bo the observed mean channel number for
the cell volume or the green fluorescence of the #2 microbead on subsequent
days: RAD, the relative antigen density; SA, the surface area; and D, the
cell diameter.

TABLE I

PERIPHERAL BLOOD T CELL POPULATIONS

PATIENT GROUP	n	TOTAL T CELLS	Th CELLS	T c/s CELLS	Th:Tc/s
Controls	16	68.0 ± 8.5	41.8 ± 9.2	20.6 ± 6.7	2.3 ± 0.9
New IDD	6	68.4 ± 8.7	43.1 ±18.6	22.0 ± 3.3	2.0 ± 1.2
ICA + Prediabetes	34	69.3 ± 6.8	45.3 ± 7.0	21.9 ± 4.5	2.1 ± 0.6

TABLE II

ENUMERATION OF LEU 3a SUBSETS
(HELPER T LYMPHOCYTES)

PATIENT GROUP	n	4B4+	2H4+
ICA+	10	25.3 ± 3	20.0 ± 4
ICA-	10	33.4 ± 4	18.0 ± 4

4B4+ Helper Inducer T Lymphocytes
2H4+ Helper Suppressor T Lymphocytes

RESULTS

The percentages of the various peripheral blood T lymphocytes between patients and controls are shown in Tables 1 and 2. No significant differences were detected in the percentage of total T lymphocytes or of the T cell subsets defined by Leu2a (CD8+. cytotoxic/suppressor) or Leu3a (CD4+, helper) monoclonal antibodies. However, the percentages of helper-inducer (CD4+ 4B4+) T lymphocytes were lower in ICA+ individuals compared to the ICA- individuals (matched for age, sex and relationship to a proband with IDD) (p < 0.05) (Table II).

No significant differences between controls and ICA+ individuals were seen in TAC antigen expression. However, the relative antigen density (RAD) of the DR antigen on T lymphocytes was significantly greater, (> 2 S.D. above the mean of the control), in 13 of 38 (34%) patients. Although this percentage was equivalent to the number of patients with increased percentages of DR staining T lymphocytes, only 7 patients had a concomitant significant increase in both the percentage of DR-positive T lymphocytes and the RAD DR antigen on T lymphocytes. In contrast, 11 of 13 with at least one value > 2 S.D. demonstrated increased RAD DR antigen on both Leu2a and Leu3a T lymphocytes; whereas, only 3 of 16 patients with at least one value > 2 S.D. had increased percentages of DR staining on both lymphocyte subsets.

The first phase insulin responses (sum of 1 & 3 minute insulin concentrations) to IV glucose were significantly different (p < 0.05) in those ICA+ patients with increased RAD of either helper or cytotoxic/suppressor T lymphocytes (Table III).

The relationship of RAD DR on T lymphocytes to the HlA DR phenotype

TABLE III

COMPARISON OF FIRST PHASE INSULIN RESPONSES AND RAD
IN ICA + PATIENTS

RELATIVE ANTIGEN OF DR	n	FIRST PHASE INSULIN RESPONSES	
		MEAN ± 1 S.D. μU/ML	RANGE μU/ML
> 2 S.D. of Normal * Population	13	126 ± 121	37 - 379
< 2 S.D. of Normal Population	21	247 ± 144	77 - 607

* Patients were included if either Leu 2a+ or Leu 3a+ positive lymphocytes had RAD DR > 2S.D. of the normal population as defined by Table 1.

TABLE IV

RELATIVE ANTIGEN DENSITY OF DR ON LYMPHOCYTES

PATIENT GROUP	n	LEU 2a+ CELLS	LEU 3a+ CELLS	B1 CELLS
All Patients	38	789 ± 412	575 ± 243	276 ± 93
DR X/X	4	684 ± 246	561 ± 203	167 ± 22
DR 3/X	11	695 ± 478	541 ± 263	287 ± 74
DR 4/X	12	685 ± 463	515 ± 261	258 ± 84
DR 3/4	11	887 ± 423	683 ± 212	275 ± 145

Leu 2a Cytotoxic/Suppressor T Lymphocytes
Leu 3a Helper T lymphocytes
X= Not HLA DR3 nor HLA DR4

of the patients was examined in all patients without respect to their ICA+ status (Table IV). This study demonstrated that the RAD DR on T lymphocytes was significantly higher in patients heterozygous for HLA DR3 and HLA DR4 than in patients with other DR phenotypes. A striking feature was the clear distinction the RAD DR on B1 staining lymphocytes compared to the T lymphocyte subsets.

DISCUSSION

The primary goal of this study was to determine whether peripheral blood lymphocytes may reflect the ongoing autoimmune process in the pancreatic islets during this pre-diabetic state. We did not find any significant imbalances of the total T lymphocyte subsets or the T helper/suppressor ratio or B lymphocytes in these pre-diabetic patients or in newly diagnosed patients. The reason for differences in our findings compared to other studies in the literature may be twofold. Firstly, our study made use of flow cytometry, only scantly used in the past for analysis of these lymphocyte subsets and, secondly, these studies performed in the prediabetic ICA+ patients eliminated the confounding metabolic abnormalities.

Interestingly however, we did find a significant decrease in a subset of the T cell lymphocyte helper (CD4+) population as defined by the helper-inducer (CD4+ 4B4+) phenotype. This sub-population of lymphocytes has been shown to play a pivotal role in T cells mediated immunoregulation. In vitro, these lymphocytes have been demonstrated to proliferate in response to soluble antigen and to provide help for B cell immunoglobulin synthesis in a pokeweed mitogen B and T cell coculture (10). The role of these cells in autoimmune disease has yet to be defined; however, the decrease in the number of these cells in pre-diabetic patients may reflect either the on-going autoimmune process and/or possibly the underlying immunoregulatory defect causing IDD. Functional studies need to be performed to define whether this numerical decrease is associated with detectable functional immunoregulatory defects.

We could not document increased number of T lymphocytes expressing the TAC antigen. This might be due to the fact that the IL-2 receptor appears to be present during the early stage of T lymphocyte activation and not later in the life of activated T lymphocytes. Thus, our findings of low percentage of IL-2 receptor positive T lymphocytes in the peripheral blood of prediabetic patients might reflect the chronic nature of this disease. However, we did find an increased percentage of the DR antigen on these patients both by the total percentage and by the increased relative anti-gen density. Relative antigen density appeared to be a more reliable and reproducible method probably because we were able to standardize the day to day variations in the instrumentation and reagents by using the fluor-esceinated microbeads. However, there were several ICA+ patients who had neither increased percentages of DR positive T cells nor increased RAD on their lymphocytes. Thus the destructive autoimmune process may be quies-cent at that point in time with the presence of ICA suggesting that the process was at one time active. The patients with the increased RAD of DR were, however, more likely to have impaired insulin response. Thus, these patients might have a more progressive disease. Fluctuation of disease activity has previously been reported in both multiple sclerosis and sys-temic lupus erythematosis (11). If longitudinal studies support these findings, the presence of these DR+ positive staining T cells in the peri-pheral blood of ICA+ individuals might have prognostic significance.

One of our findings suggested that the DR expression in these T lym-phocytes might be an expression of the underlying immunoregulatory defect in the predisposition to autoimmune disease. This was especially true in the DR3/4 heterozygote individuals who had significantly higher DR RAD on the surface of their T lymphocytes compared to other phenotypes. This was true regardless of the ICA state of the individual. More DR3/4 heter-ozygous patients without ICA, however, need to be evaluated to support this positive finding.

Our results represent only a single point along the continuum of the pre-diabetic state. The presence of activated lymphocytes as measured by the RAD of DR or the percent of DR+ staining cells correlated with the pre-sence of insulinopenia. Although the association with impaired insulin re-sponse suggest that the presence of increased numbers of "activated" T lym-phocytes in the peripheral blood may reflect the advanced activity of the immunological destructive process in the pancreatic islets, prospective longitudinal studies are needed to determine how predictive this test will be in predicting impending disease.

REFERENCES

1. Eisenbarth, G., 1986, Type I diabetes mellitus: A chronic auto-immune disease. N Eng J Med 314: 1360-1368.

2. Neufeld, M., Maclaren, N.K., Riley, W.J., Lezotte, D., McLaughlin, J.J., Silverstein, J., Rosenbloom, A.L., 1980, Islet cell and other organ-specific antibodies in U.S. Caucasians and Blacks with insulin-dependent diabetes mellitus. Diabetes 29: 589:92.

3. Gepts, W., 1965, Pathology anatomy of the pancreas in juvenile diabetes mellitus. Diabetes 14: 61-63.

4. Bottazzo, G.F., Dean, B.M., NcNally, J.M., Mackay, E.H., Swift, P.G.F., Gamble, D.R., 1985, In-situ characterization of autoimmune phenomena and expression of HLA molecules in the pancreas in diabetic insulitis. N Engl J Med 313: 353-360.

5. Sibley, R.K., Sutherland, D.E.R., Goetz, F., Michael, A.F., 1985, Recurrent diabetes mellitus in the pancreas iso- and allograft: A light and electron microscopic and immunohistochemical analysis of four cases. Lab Invest 53: 132-144.

6. Maclaren, N.K., Elder, M.E., Robbins, W.V., Riley, W.J., 1983, Autoimmune diathesis and T lymphocyte immunoincompetence in BB rats. Metabolism 32: 92-96.

7. Galluzzo, A., Giordano, C., Rubino, G., Bompiani, G.D., 1984, Immunoregulatory T-lymphocyte subset deficiency in newly diagnosed Type I (insulin-dependent) diabetes mellitus. Diabetologia 26: 426-430.

8. Gupta, S., 1984, Lymphocyte response to diabetes mellitus. In: Immunology of Clinical Experimental Diabetes, Gupta, S., Ed. Plenum Medical Book Company, New York & London 329-349.

9. Gorsuch, A.N., Lister, J., Dean, B.M., Spencer, K.M., McNally, J.M., Bottazzo, G.F., Cudworth, A.G., 1981, Evidence for a long prediabetic period in Type I (insulin-dependent) diabetes mellitus. Lancet 2: 1363-1365.

10. Reinherz, E.L., Kung, P.C., Goldstein, G., Schlossman, S.F., 1979, Separation of functional subsets of human T cells by a monoclonal antibody. Proc Natl Acad Sci (USA) 76: 4061-4065.

11. Morimoto, C., Hafler, D.A., Weiner, H.L., Letvin, N.L., Hagan, M., Daley, J., and Schlossman, S.F., 1987, Selective loss of the suppressor-inducer T-cell subset in progressive multiple sclerosis. N Eng J Med, 316: 67-72.

G. GRODSKY: Dr. Gleichmann, the really important question is how this development of antibodies against Streptozotocin has any effect? It's conceivable that immunizing with Streptozotocin by the technique you use is less effective as a diabetogenic agent.

H. GLEICHMANN: It's obvious that the schedule for inducing diabetes, according to the low dose Streptozotocin model, only occurs in T-cell positive mice in the majority of investigations. NUTE animals won't develop diabetes.

G. GRODSKY: NUTE animals will not develop diabetes against Streptozotocin?

H. GLEICHMANN: Not when you apply multiple low doses. If you go through the literature, few laboratories did that and in many of the laboratories they could inhibit diabetes initially by treatment of the recipients with monoclonal antibodies with specificity for T-cells. We know about the infiltration around the islets after Streptozotocin treatment and it's very obvious that this infiltration is T-cell dependent. I think that T-cells contribute to this. They do it via the specific reaction towards Streptozotocin as a hapten, and this inflammatory reaction or immunological reaction may contribute as an ischemic part to the islets where a subtoxic lesion has been set by Streptozotocin directly on the beta cells.

J. SCOTT: Dr. Riley, when you showed data that the DR3, DR4 patients had more intense density than the CD8 and CD4 antigens within your patient population, I didn't see data on your slide saying whether a 3, 4 heterozygote non-diabetic may also have increased antigen density. Did you look for that?

W. RILEY: The actual data was irrespective of the ICA positivity. All these people are non-diabetic. Every patient that we studied, that we showed the data on, were non-diabetic although there was ICA positivity. The data that I showed with the increased relative antigen density on those cells relate to the DR phenotype. This was irregardless of whether they had ICA or not. So, it was more a function of the DR phenotype.

J. SCOTT: Were they diabetic or non-diabetic at that point, on that slide?

W. RILEY: They were non-diabetic.

J. SCOTT: Relatives of diabetics?

W. RILEY; Relatives of somebody with diabetes.

J. SCOTT: Have you looked at this phenomenon in people who are not related to diabetics?

W. RILEY: We have done in a few people, but it's not very easy to find too many non DR3, DR4. We typed a lot of people and we only have 2 or 3% of that population that's related to somebody with diabetes that is a DR3, DR4 phenotype. So, we want to, but we don't have enough patients to really say anything.

D. KUMAR: Dr. Naji, if I understand your experiments correctly, it's very discouraging to physicians that if anybody thinks of pancreatic transplants the recipient is somehow going to destroy the graft.

A. NAJI: I think your impression is correct and I think we were one of the early ones, based again on BB rats, indicating that the recurrence of the auto-immune destruction of diabetes in a transplant is a real biologic threat for all of us who are interested in using the isolated islets for whole pancreas as a treatment for diabetes. You are very cautious in performing the experiments under circumstances where the immunologic rejection is completely excluded.

In 1984, the clinical experience of Dr. Sutherland from the University of Minnesota was virtually confirmed when he exchanged segmental pancreatic grafts between identical twins from a non-diabetic to a diabetic index. And, he noted a recurrence of insulitis and a selective loss of beta cells in segmental grafts. Fortunately, this biologic threat is amenable to control by immunosuppression. We do not know how much immunosuppression is needed to alleviate or to cool down this process, but from talking to Dr. Sutherland I know that in five patients that he has maintained on continuous immunosuppression he has not seen any loss of beta cells or recurrence of diabetes. And, interestingly enough, some of these patients require triple therapy. They need the prednisone, imuran and cyclosporine So, yes, in response to your question, Dr. Kumar. It's a real problem, but it appears that immunosuppression will take care of it.

D. PYKE: But, of course, if you're in that situation you lose advantage of being a twin, don't you, if in spite of receiving, say, pancreas graft from your identical co-twin you still need to have immunosuppression. You're no better off than the singleton diabetic.

A. NAJI: Yes, indeed. I think that these experiments are critical really to dissect how important or how vicious is, what I call this auto-immune threat to a normal mass of islets.

D. PYKE: Well, in the four cases you published, I think the longest one was 25 or 28 years, so it's clear that the immunological memory can persist for what is effectively a lifetime.

A. NAJI: Indeed.

G. GRODSKY: Do you think this will also apply to fetal islet transplants? Will they mature into rejectable islets?

A. NAJI: We really do not know what a pro-islet is. The so-called pro-islets need some time to mature and to become insulin secreting islets. What the evolution of phenotypes or markers are with this fetal islet no one knows. My suspicion is that it could occur with fetal islets, but we really don't have a clinical mass at the moment to assess that. That possibility may never be a testable one, because the experiments of identical twins could not be obviously done in that scenario. And, everyone who has so far been implanted with fetal islet has already been on immunosuppression for a loss of a kidney as a result of diabetic nephropathy, and those individuals are the ones who have been the potential recipients for fetal islet transplantation.

J. BARBOSA: In Denmark, by treating with insulin, pre-diabetic BB mice and presumably by suppressing the beta cell completely, the onset of diabetes was postponed. I think it would be fascinating if you did your transplants on rats receiving insulin to point out that those cells would not be at work and perhaps would be protected.

A. NAJI: I quite agree with you that this principle of putting the beta cell at rest has some merit. At what level it is operational, at the cell level, I really don't know. But, it is clearly established in BB rats, and also of course the human experiments indicate that individuals with intensive treatment of insulin may have a higher incidence of hormone. But, there is no doubt that a prophylactic use of insulin may put the machinery of the beta cell at rest and prolong the period of time that the individual is less dependent on insulin.

J. BARBOSA: Well, your experiment, does it suggest that immune attack is not MHC restrictive in the BB rat?

A. NAJI: Right. I think the way we had approached that in order to de-lineate the mechanisms of auto-immune recurrence, destruction of beta cell, we've got to come up with experimental scenarios that absolutely exclude the possibility of hematolytic rejection, because after all you're trans-planting foreign tissue. And, two laboratories, Dr. Lafferty and Dr. Like, have done this. Basically, what these investigators did was to use either an MHC compatible or MHC incompatible graft source along with a non pancreatic tissue like either adrenal or pituitary implanted in diabetes prone, or diabetic, BB rats. And, what they saw was evidence of lympho-cytic infiltration concordant with insulitis either MHC compatible or MHC incompatible. This type of analysis has merits, but we have to be cautious of our interpretation, whether the process is MHC restricted or not, based on just looking at the cellular infiltrate. In this type of experiment, we know that with every healthy graft, even if when we do transplant kidneys or liver, there is always some degree of lymphocytic infiltration in a normal functioning pancreas or kidney graft. So, having lymphocytic infiltration does not mean that the infiltration is insulitis. On a histologic level, insulitis and rejection are indistin-guishable.

We also tried to manipulate our islet tissue prior to transplantation by culturing. Everyone knows that the islets have a scattered population of antigen presenting cells that incite the immune rejection. And, if you delete those prior to transplantation you trick the immune system and you get away with rejection. And, when we did that in our experiments we found that there is clear destruction of MHC compatible grafts and the MHC incompatible grafts are involved indefinitely in the spontaneously diabetic graft. In our hand, the process appears to be MHC restrictive and interestingly in Sweden they analyzed the recurrence of disease in the MHC compatible as well as the twins and are seeing a preponderance of recurrence in HLA identical, but never in HLA mismatched category grafts. We are seeing some evidence, experimentally and clinically, that this very important T-cell function (i.e. MHC restriction) is not only operational, with respect to nominal antigen, but it appears that it is also operating for an auto-immune process.

J. BARBOSA: I may be wrong, but I thought Dr. Naji previously mentioned that in the BB rat the active T lymphocytes in the peripheral blood appear before insulitis. Did you mention that the appearance of active T lympho-cytes was earlier than insulitis? How do you explain where they come from?

DR. NAJI: The earliest that we have tested the BB rats in the prediabetic stage has been at age 35 days, and we don't have a simultaneous biopsy of pancreas to substantiate whether those animals, at that time, had any insulitis or not. But, I think a sequential biopsy from another group of BB rats would show that insulitis could appear 16-20 days before the onset of hyperglycemia.

R. MC EVOY: Do you have any direct evidence that the IA positive cells are in fact reactive to any islet antigen, or is it just the association with the presence of the positive cells in animals who eventually develop diabetes that leads you to that implication?

A. NAJI: I only tried to refer that these animals do, indeed, have some status of immune activation as presented by RA positive cells. Under no circumstances could I claim, or can anybody else, that every single one of these effector cells have anti-beta cell activity.

W. RILEY: I have to agree. I think the next step really is to try to get some antigen specificity in the assay and that's not an easy test to do.

D. PYKE: Dr. Riley, can I ask you a question? I think you said in your talk that you weren't clear whether the increased antigen density was a genetic feature or an acquired one. You showed the grafts before and as they became diabetic. What happens if you follow the animals thereafter?

W. RILEY: We've only followed a handful of people over time and I don't know what's going to happen with all of them. The ones that have had relatively high antigen density stayed there, but we had some variation in others, so that I'm not sure if it's reflecting that there is increased activity or what kind of noise in the background there is over time.

THE IN VIVO VISUALIZATION OF INSULITIS

A NEW MARKER OF PREDIABETES

A. Signore, P. Pozzilli, ¶G. Tamburrano and D. Andreani

Endocrinologia (I), Clinica Medica (II), Policlinico Umberto I
Universita di Roma "La Sapienza"

Type 1 (insulin-dependent) diabetes is a disease characterized by a prodromal period with beta-cell destruction mediated by mononuclear white blood cells and their products. Several markers have been identifyed to characterize the prodromal phase of the disease. During this phase alterations involving lymphocyte activation are present; an increased percentage of circulating activated lymphocytes is detectable and these cells show a decreased interlukin (IL2) production (1) together with an increased release of IL2 receptors (IL2R) which can be detected in serum (2).

The alterations observed in the peripheral blood, may be the expression of insulitis and beta-cell destruction occurring gradually in the pancreas. Insulitis has been studied particularly in diabetes prone animal models (3,4) but it has also been described in newly diagnosed diabetic patients who died soon after diagnosis (5).

We have studied a nuclear medicine approach to visualize in vivo the insulitis in diabetes prone animals. This technique is based on the intravenous administration of 123I-labelled IL2 which binds to activated, IL2R+ve, lymphocytes present in the pancreas with insulitis. Radioactivity is detected externally by sequential gamma camera imaging.

MATERIALS & METHODS

Labelling of IL2: Human recombinant IL2 (Glaxo) was labelled with 123Iodine (Harwell) using a modified chloramine-T method as previously described (6). After labelling, unbound iodine was eliminated by gel filtration chromatography on Sephadex G10 column.

In Vivo Studies: Labelled IL2 was injected i.v. in 6 anaesthetized NOD mice and 6 BB/W rats. NOD mice were kindly provided by Dr. E. Simpson (Transplantation Biology Center, Nortwick Park Hospital, London) and BB/W rats by Dr. A. Parman (Bramtan Hospital, London). For control experiments normal Balb/c mice and Wistar rats were used. Mice were injected at the age of 15 weeks and rats at the age of 14 weeks. All animals were not diabetic at the time of study.

This work was supported by grants from CNR International project n. 87.00 20204 and Ministero P.I. n. 2.12.1.2. A.S. is recipient of a fellowship from the Juvenile Diabetes Foundation.

The anaesthetic mixture (5 ml/Kg body weight) consisted of Diazepam (1 mg/ml) and Hypnorm (Yanssen) diluted 1:10 in saline and was injected i.p. 15 minutes before the injection of the tracer. Also 6 mg/Kg body weight of $KClO_4$ were injected with the anaesthetic in order to avoid thyroid and stomach uptake of free iodine.

Labelled IL2 was injected i.v. in a vein of the tail: 50 μCi/100 μl saline, in each mouse and 200 μCi/400 μl saline, in each rat. Gamma camera images were collected every minute for 45 minutes using a pinhole collimator and time-activity curves were generated by computer analysis in different organs.

In Vitro Studies: These studies were performed in 9 BB/W and 9 Wistar rats. Animals were injected i.v. with $2x10$ c.p.m. of labelled IL2 and sacrificed after 5, 30 or 60 minutes. Liver, spleen, pancreas and kidneys were immediately removed, counted for radioactivity and frozen in liquid nitrogen for subsequent histological examination and autoradiography as previously described (6).

RESULTS

Gamma camera images of normal animals after the in vivo injection of 123I-IL2 showed a distribution of radioactivity in the heart, liver, kidneys and bladder (figure 1).

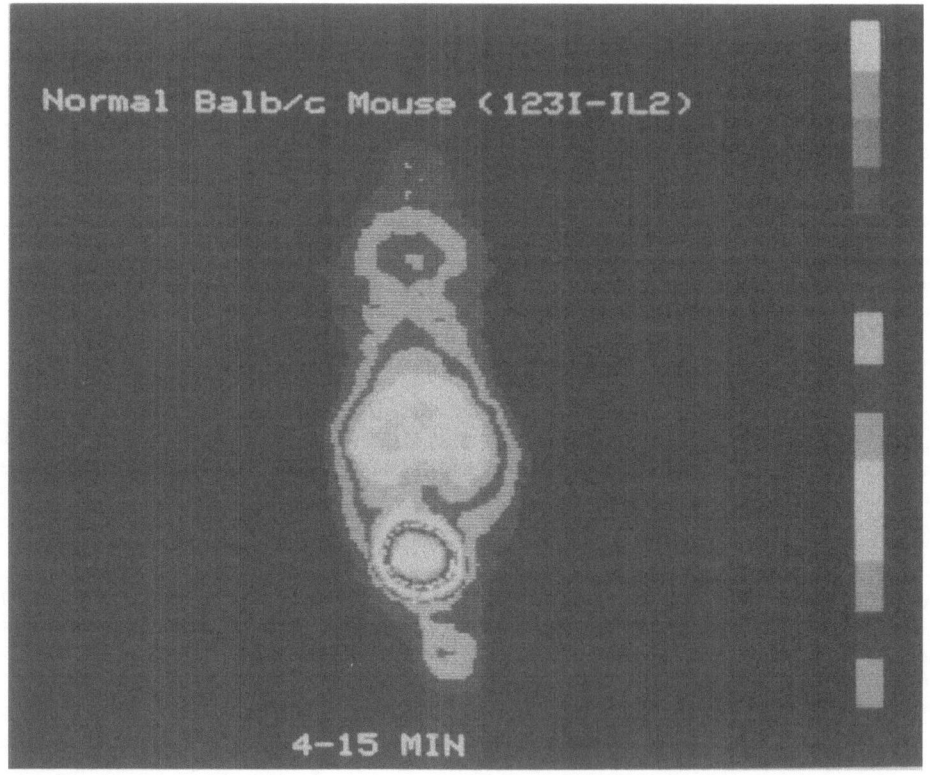

Figure 1. Gamma camera image of a normal Balb/c mouce of 15 weeks of age

120

In diabetes prone NOD mice (figure 2) and BB/W rats (figure 3) we found a different distribution of radioactivity. This was concentrated in the pancreatic region suggesting a high binding to lymphocytes infiltrating the pancreas. Kidneys and bladder were also visible due to renal metabolization of IL2.

Time-activity curves generated by computer analysis also showed a higher radioactivity in the pancreatic region of diabetes prone animals compared to normal controls (data not shown).

The in vitro count of radioactivity in organs of animals sacrificed at different time points showed that liver radioactivity fell rapidly in both normal and BB/W rats. Thus, in animals sacrificed at 60 minutes, we found only 14% of the radioactivity found in animals sacrificed at 5 minutes. By contrast spleen radioactivity was still high after 60 minutes in both normal and BB/W rats (about 60% compared to 5 minutes). The decrease of radioactivity in the pancreas of normal rats was similar to that observed in the liver whereas in BB/W rats it was similar to that of spleen indicating a high binding into the organ and a substantial retention of the tracer.

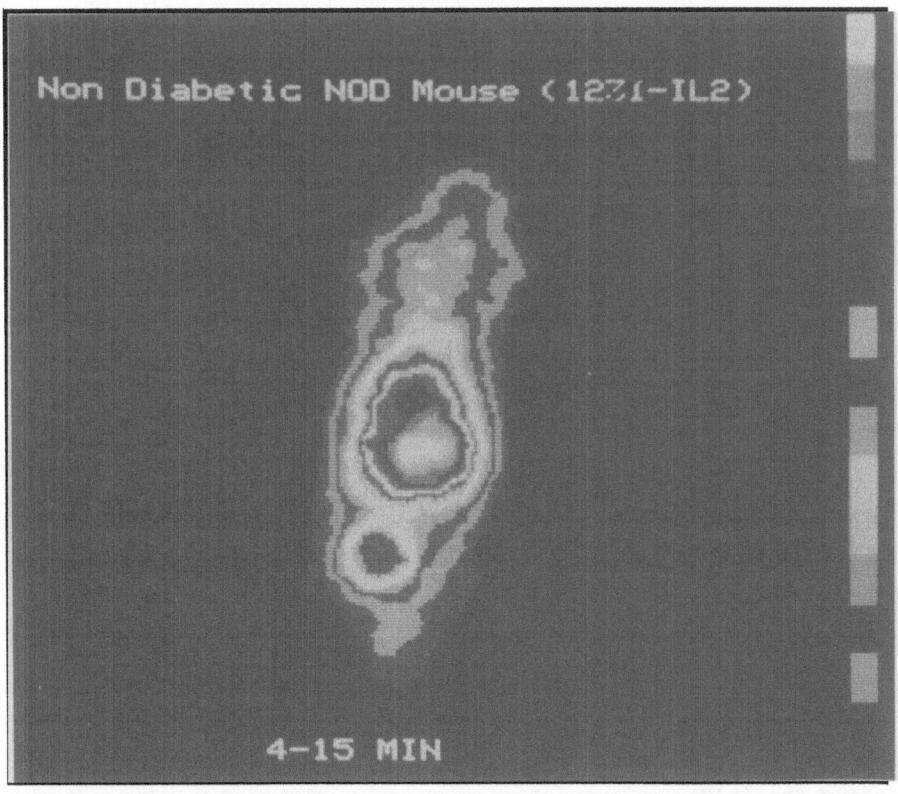

Figure 2. Gamma camera image of diabetes prone NOD female mouse of 15 weeks of age after the i.v. injection of 123I-labelled IL2. The picture is the sum of images acquired from minute 4 to 15. The radioactivity is accumulated in the pancreatic reagion.

By autoradiography and combined immunoperoxidase staining of pancreas sections with an anti-IL2R monoclonal antibody (OX39), we found that the radioactivity was specifically associated to IL2R+ve lymphocytes infiltrating the islets (figure 5). Moreover, we found that most of the brown staining

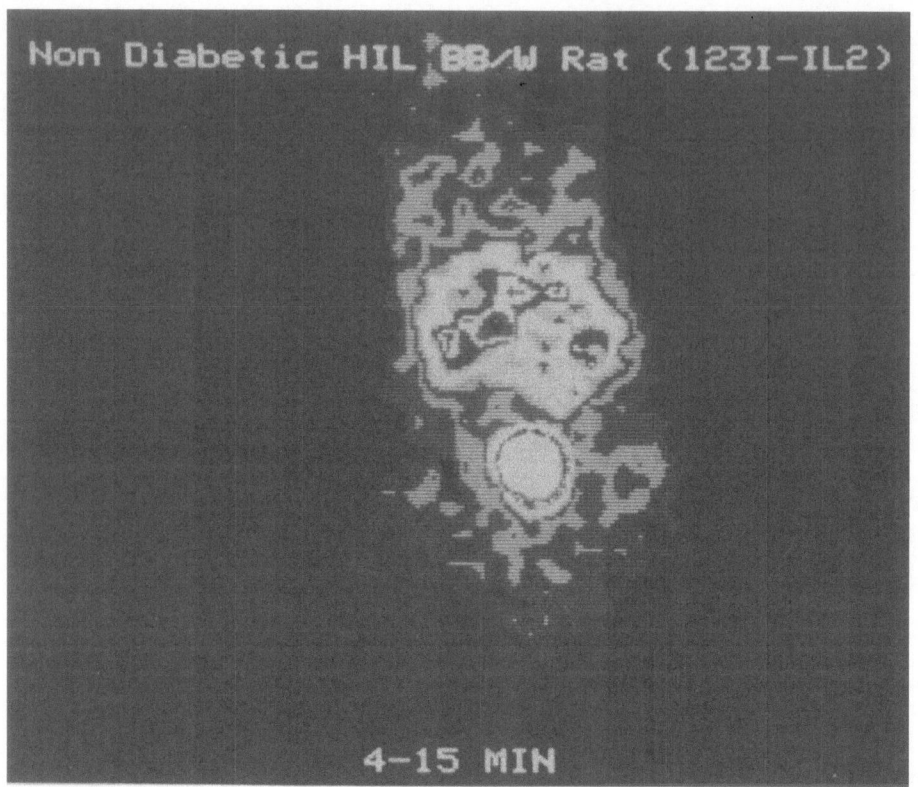

Figure 3. Gamma camera image of a diabetes prone BB/W male rat of 14 weeks of age after the i.v. injection of 123I-labelled IL2. The picture is the sum of images acquired from minute 4 to 15. The bladder and the two kidneys are visible and the pancreas between them.

(representing the IL2R) was not cell associated and this may represent the presence of cell-free receptors released by activated lymphocytes. The association of this staining with radioactivity, revealed by autoradiography, suggests that also soluble IL2R may efficiently bind IL2 in the pancreas (figure 5).

122

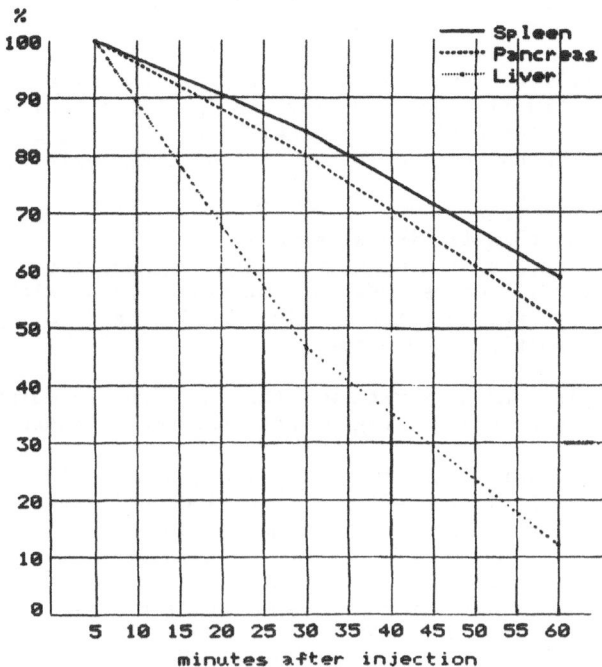

% decrease of radioactivity
in BB/Wistar HIL rats

Figure 4: Percentage decrease of radioactivity in organs of BB/W rats of the high incidence line (HIL) for diabetes. Radioactivity at minute 5 was calculated as 100%. Each time point is mean of three rats.

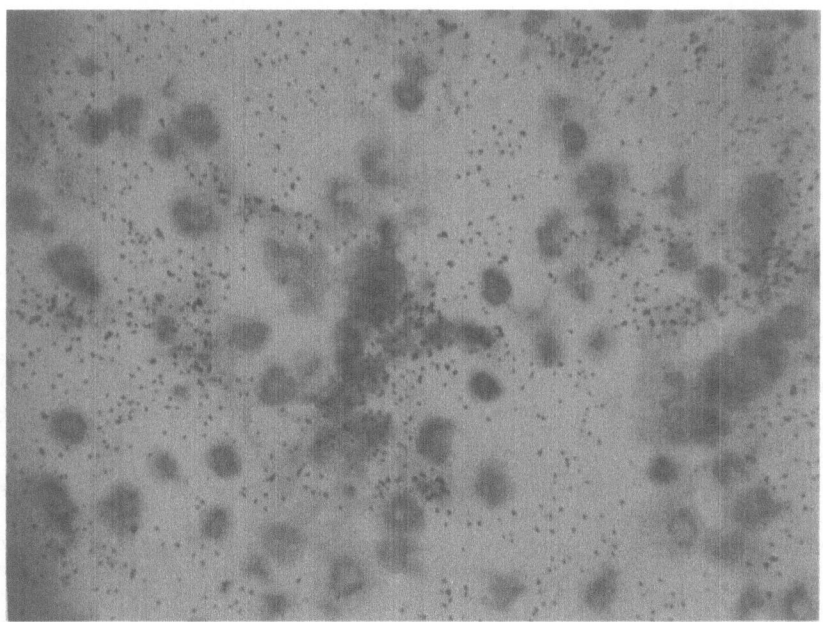

Figure 5. Combined autoradiography and immunoperoxidase staining with an anti-IL2R monoclonal antibody of a cryostat section of pancreas of a BB/W rat sacrificed 5 minutes after the i.v. injection of labelled IL2.

DISCUSSION

The lymphocytic infiltration of the endocrine pancreas is an early sign of type 1 diabetes and may be considered as the histopathological marker of this disease.

We have recently reported, in diabetes prone NOD mice, that insulitis starts as early as the fifth week of life and persists until diabetes becomes clinically evident (7). Among cells infiltrating the pancreas, a large percentage is constituted by activated, IL2R positive, lymphocytes (7).

On the basis of this finding we studied a non invasive technique for the in vivo visualization of lymphocytic infiltration in the pancreas. We labelled IL2 with 123Iodine, a x-ray emitting isotope with a very short half life (13 hours), suitable for in vivo studies, and we injected it intravenously in diabetes prone animals.

In both NOD mice and BB/W rats was found a high accumulation of radioactivity in the pancreatic region not observed in control animals.

IL2 has a very short plasmatic half life (about 7 minutes) and therefore from 5 to 15 minutes after the in vivo administration it is bound to target cells or degraded by kidney metabolism.

In vitro organ counting, after the animals were sacrificed, showed a retention of radioactivity into the pancreas of BB/W rats. This suggests a specific binding of labelled IL2 into the organ. By contrast, no retention of radioactivity was found in the liver of either BB/W or normal rats and therefore the radioactivity observed in vivo in this organ during the first minutes after injection is mainly due to blood flow activity. In the spleen of both BB/W and normal rats we found a decrease of the radioactivity with time similar to that observed in the pancreas of BB/W rats suggesting the presence of activated IL2R+ve lymphocytes which was confirmed histologically in this organ.

However, the radioactivity observed in vivo by gamma camera imaging was much higher in the pancreas than the spleen and both these organs, in diabetes prone animals, are infiltrated by activated lymphocytes. This finding was difficult to interpret and an autoradiography of pancreas and spleen sections combined with a staining to evidentiate IL2R was performed. Thus, in the spleen the radioactivity was associated only to IL2R+ve lymphocytes whereas in the pancreas it was also associated with cell-free IL2 receptors likely released by activated lymphocytes infiltrating the organ.

The presence of high levels of soluble IL2R in the serum of type 1 diabetics was previously reported and these receptors may be released by the cells infiltrating the pancreas. Soluble IL2R may play an important local immunoregulatory role and their presence in the pancreas may help in visualizing the insulitis at a very early stage of prediabetes as labelled IL2 could also bind to them locally.

Previous approaches for the in vivo visualization of insulitis, such as the labelling of peripheral white blood cells with 111 Indium, had failed so far (8), probably because only a small percentage of circulating lymphocytes are labelled with this technique and only a portion of these migrate into the pancreas.

In conclusion, our technique has proven to be successful in detecting, in diabetes prone animals, the insulitis which is the histopathological marker of type 1 diabetes.

· This technique is non invasive and the amount of IL2 and 123I injected are clinically insignificant and therefore it may be applied in humans for the early diagnosis of type 1 diabetes, particularly in genetically suscep- tible subjects.

REFERENCES

1. Kaye, W.A., Adri, M.N., Soeldner, J.B., Rabinowa, B.L., Kaldany, A., Kahn, C.R., Bristrain, B., Srikanta, S., Ganda, O.P., and Eisenbarth, G.S., 1986, Acquired defect of interleukin-2 production in patients with type 1 diabetes mellitus. N Engl J Med 315: 920-24.

2. Galluzzo, A., Caruso, C., Giordano, C., Modica, M.A., Marco, A., and Zambito, P.M., 1987, High release of soluble interleukin-2 receptors by peripheral mononuclear cells in Type 1 (insulin-dependent) diabetes. Diabetologia 30: 521A.

3. Marliss, E.B., Nakhooda, A.F., Poussier, P., and Sima, A.A.F., 1982, The diabetic syndrome of the BB Wistar rat: possible relevance to Type 1 (insulin-dependent) diabetes in man. Diabetologia 22: 225-32.

4. Miyazaki, A., Hanafusa, T., Yamada, K., Miyagawa, J., Fujino- Kurihara, H., Nakajima, H., Nonaka, K., and Tarui, S., 1985, Predominance of the lymphocytes in pancreatic islets and spleen of prediabetic non-obese diabetic (NOD) mice: a longitudinal study. Clin Exp Immunol 60: 622-30.

5. Foulis, A.K., Liddle, C.N., Farquharson, M.A., Richmond, J.A., and Weir, R.S., 1986, The histopathology of the pancreas of type 1 (insulin- dependent) diabetes mellitus: a 25 year review of deaths in patients under twenty years of age in United Kingdom. Diabetologia 29: 267-74.

6. Signore, A., Parman, A., Pozzilli, P., Andreani, D., and Beverley, P.C.L.: Detection of activated lymphocytes in endocrine pancreas of BB/W rats by injection of 123I-interleukin-2: an early sign of type 1 diabetes. Lancet 2: 537-40.

7. Signore, A., Cooke, A., Pozzilli, P., Butcher, G., Simpson, E., and Beverley, P.C.L., 1986, Class-II and IL2 receptor positive cells in the pancreas of NOD mice. Diabetologia 30: 902-5.

8. Gallina, D.L., Pelletier, D., Doherty, P., Koevary, S.B., Williams, R.M., Like, A.A., Chick, W.L., and Rossini, A.A., 1985, 111-Indium-labelle lymphocytes do not image or label the pancreas of BB/W rat. Diabetologia 28: 143-7.

GENETIC RELATIONSHIPS BETWEEN TYPE I AND TYPE II

DIABETES MELLITUS

¶Jose Barbosa, Miriam Segall, and Stephen Rich

Division of Endocrinology and Metabolism, Department of Medicine
and Department of Laboratory Medicine and Pathology
University of Minnesota, Minneapolis, Minnesota

Both Type I and Type II diabetes mellitus are phenotypically heterogeneous. These two diseases are clearly dependent on genetic susceptibility which is also quite likely heterogeneous (1). During the last decade, findings of several HLA antigen associations in humans with Type I diabetes and clear evidence of autoimmunity in both animal models of Type I diabetes and in humans with Type I diabetes, coupled with the apparent absence of such attributes in Type II diabetes, have led to the belief that these two disorders are unrelated. This conclusion, however, may have been premature. We present in this report epidemiologic and genetic evidence suggesting that at least a subset of Type II diabetes shares genetic susceptibility with Type I diabetes.

METHODS

The methods and clinical material used for the epidemiologic studies have been reported before in detail (2).

HLA (3) and haptoglobin determinations were performed by methods described previously.

RESULTS

A. Epidemiologic studies. 493 diabetic families were classified according to diabetic status as described previously (2) and then analyzed for cumulative risk up to age 40 in the sibs of the proband as a function of the parental diabetic phenotype.

Table 1 shows that when the joint effects of the probands age at diagnosis and parental diabetes are taken into consideration, the risk in the subgroup of families with probands who developed diabetes before age 10 is highest when one parent had Type II diabetes. Thus, the risk curve is significantly higher when one parent had Type II diabetes ($x^2 = 12.8$, $p < 0.0005$) as compared with the group having neither parent diabetic.

This work is supported by NIH Grant AM20729, U.S.-Spain Joint Committee for Technological Cooperation - Grant NO. CCA 84/105, Eli Lilly and Company, Indianapolis, Indiana, and Clinical Research Center GRant #RR-400.

B. <u>Genetic studies</u>. Twenty diabetic families with at least one Type II diabetic parent and a Type I diabetic child proband, typed for HLA and haptoglobin, have been studied. Type I diabetic probands showed increased frequencies of the haptoglobin 2 allele (0.69) as compared to frequencies recorded in the literature (0.61) and in unaffected sibs (0.52). HLA studies revealed that there was a significant increase in the frequency of HLA DR4 (0.63), (with relative risk = 15.7, p < .01) as compared with the frequency in controls (0.10) or in affected sibs (Type I diabetes) without a Type II diabetic parent (.42).

Analysis of sharing of HLA and haptoglobin haplotypes in affected pairs of Type I diabetic siblings in families with Type II diabetic parent showed a deviation from expectation, with an excess of sharing of both haplotypes.

TABLE I

RELATIONSHIPS BETWEEN SIB'S EMPIRICAL RISK (%) FOR IDD AND COMBINATIONS OF PARENTAL DIABETIC STATUS AND PROBAND'S AGE AT DIAGNOSIS.

Proband's age at diagnosis	Diabetes in parents	Number of probands	Number of Sibs		Crude risk $\pm$ SE	$CR_{40} \pm$ SE
			Total	with IDD		
<10 *	None	111	310	16	5.2 $\pm$ 1.3	7.5 $\pm$ 2.0
	One with IDD	6	17	1	5.9 $\pm$ 5.7	12.5 $\pm$ 11.7 **
	One with NIDD	7	18	4	22.2 $\pm$ 9.8	24.7 $\pm$ 10.7
	None	305	917	34	3.7 $\pm$ 0.6	4.7 $\pm$ 0.8
	One with IDD	24	68	3	4.4 $\pm$ 2.5	4.6 $\pm$ 2.6
	One with NIDD	36	93	4	4.3 $\pm$ 2.1	3.8 $\pm$ 2.2
Total	None	416	1227	50	4.1 $\pm$ 0.6	5.3 $\pm$ 0.8
	One with IDD	30	85	4	4.7 $\pm$ 2.3	5.3 $\pm$ 2.6
	One with NIDD	43	111	8	7.2 $\pm$ 2.5	7.1 $\pm$ 2.6

* When the age of diagnosis is <10, the three risk curves for sibs in the parental diabetic status groups are significantly different from one another (x^2 = 13.1, P = 0.0001). The only significant pair-wise comparison is that between the "None" and the "One with NIDD" groups (x^2 = 12.8, P <0.0005).

** CR_{30} is given since no sibs in this group were older than 30.

TABLE II

B44 haplotype of IDD patient

	B44-DR4	B44-non-DR4
NIDD parent	6	0
IDD parent	1	6

p<0.005

The HLA haplotype B44-DR4 seems to be of pariticular interest. B44 tends to be decreased in frequency in the general Type I diabetic population and the B44-DR4 haplotype is a "non-susceptibility" or perhaps even a "resistance" (decreased frequency) haplotype. Interestingly, B44-DR4 seems to be increased among Type I diabetic probands with a Type II diabetic parent as shown in Table II.

DISCUSSION

The concept of entirely different pathogenesis for the two identifiable types of diabetes has prevailed for the last decade, in spite of frequently observed families including both types of the disease. However, evidence against the complete seperation of the two diseases is emerging. Since both Type I and Type II diabetes are believed to be heterogeneous, it could be argued that at least a subset of one of them may be related to the other.

For instance, some cases of Type II diabetes with onset in the 4th decade of life and later could be milder forms of Type I diabetes. Indeed, Groop et al. (4) have reported that a fraction of Type II diabetics who require treatment with insulin display immunologic and genetic characteristics which are often seen in Type I diabetics. Thus, the insulin requiring Type II diabetic patients had significantly higher prevalence of islet cell and thyroid antibodies than the milder Type II diabetics and showed associations with HLA antigens different from those seen in either Type I diabetics or milder Type II diabetics.

The finding of higher risk for siblings of Type I diabetics when one of their parents has Type II diabetes suggests that at least some of the genetic susceptibility to one disease is shared by the other. These results, however, are compatible with bias, since parents of two diabetic children may be more aware of their medical status than other parents, including those with only one diabetic child.

Genetic studies, however, strongly suggest a genetic connection between these two disorders. Stern et al. (5) have reported an association between the haptoglobin 1-1 genotype and Type II diabetes in a population study. This finding was of particular interest because no genetic markers have been available to study this most common disease. In view of our interest in searching for genetic common denominators between the two forms of identifiable diabetes, we studied haptoglobin in HLA typed diabetic probands and also the segregation of haptoglobin in HLA typed diabetic multiplex families. Since HLA provides strong genetic susceptibility to Type I diabetics it is important to study new genetic markers in patients and families also HLA typed. Like Stern et al. (5) we also found an association between haptoglobin and diabetes (6). Type I diabetic probands with Type II diabetic parents have an excess of the haptoglobin genotype 2-2. In addition, in multiplex families (one Type II diabetic parent and two or more Type I diabetic children) both haptoglobin and HLA haplotypes were more often shared in affected sib pairs than expected (6). This latter finding, in particular, suggests that one of the genetic factors providing susceptibility to both diseases seems to be in linkage disequilibrium with haptoglobin.

We find a slightly higher relative risk (RR) for HLA DR4 in probands with a Type II diabetic parent as compared with probands with unaffected parents (RR - 2.4, p = .06), although this is not significant (probably because of the small sample size). It may be that DR4 or DR4-linked genes provide susceptibility shared by subsets of the two diseases. Type I diabetes is associated with DQw3.2 but not DQw3.1 patterns as analyzed by Southern blotting with cDNA probes for the DQ beta gene (7). The B44-DR4 haplotype, which is not a susceptibility haplotype in Type I diabetes (8), frequently carries DQw3.1 in normal individuals, and susceptibility in Type I diabetics with a Type II parent may thus be associated with HLA markers not associated with susceptibility in other Type I diabetics. Cellular typing, Southern blotting analysis and DNA sequence studies of B44-DR4 cells may elucidate this question.

These findings on haptoglobin and HLA are compatible and supportive of the theory that at least two genes, one in the HLA D region, and the other in chromosome 16 in linkage with haploglobin, are involved in susceptibility to both disorders in these doubly affected families.

SUMMARY

We propose that at least certain subsets of Type I and Type II diabetes share factor(s) responsible for genetic susceptibility. The data presented here to support this contention include:

1. A significantly increased cumulative risk (CR40) to age 40 for Type I diabetes in sibs of probands in families with a Type II diabetic parent (Type II diabetic parent: CR40-24.7 ± 10.7%; normal parent: CR40 = 7.5 ± 2.0%, x^2 = 12.8, $p < 0.0005$).

2. The relative risk (RR) for HLA DR4 in Type I diabetic probands with a Type II diabetic parent is higher than in probands with normal parents (RR = 2.4).

3. The haptoglobin genotype 2-2 is increased in Type I diabetics with Type II parents and the sharing of both HLA and haptoglobin haplotypes in affected sib pairs is distorted with an excess sharing of both haplotypes.

REFERENCES

1. Rossini, A.A., Mordes, J.P., Handler, E.S., 1988, Speculation on etiology of diabetes mellitus. Diabetes 37: 257-261.

2. Chern, M.M., Anderson, V.E., Barbosa. J., 1982, Empirical risk for insulin-dependent diabetes (IDD) in sibs. Diabetes 31: 1115-1118.

3. Barbosa, J. Bach, Fritz H., Rich, S.S., 1981, Clinical Genetics 20: 1-7.

4. Groop, L., Miettinen, A., Groop, P., Meri, S., Koskimies, S., Bottazzo, G.F., 1988, Organ-specific autoimmunity and HLA-DR antigens as markers for beta-cell destruction in patients wth Type II diabetes. Diabetes 37: 99-103.

5. Stern, M., Ferrell, R., Rosenthal, M., Haffner, S., Hazuda, H., 1986, Association betwenn NIDD, RH blood group, and haptoglobin phenotype: results from the San Antonio Heart Study. Diabetes 35: 387.

6. Rich, S.S., Panter, S.S., Reusch, J., Barbosa, J.J., Joint susceptibility of IDD and NIDD: The role of a non-HLA linked susceptibility factor. Submitted for publication.

7. Nepom, G., 1986, HLA Class II variants: Structural Studies and Disease Associations. In Autoimmunity, Schwartz, R. and Rose, N., Eds., New York Acad of Sci, 475.

8. Segall, M., Barbosa, J., 1988, HLA markers in insulin dependent diabetic (IDD) children of a non-insulin dependent diabetic (NIDD) parent: A distinct subset of IDD? American Diabetes Association Meeting, New Orleans, LA.

DISCUSSION

A. ROLLA: Dr. Tamburrano, is it possible that the IL2 receptors are present in cells that are not lymphocytes?

G. TAMBURRANO: It's possible that they are not lymphocytes, but I think we demonstrate that they are lymphocytes.

A. ROLLA: The reason for my question is that there are very strong possibilities that IL2 have effects outside of lymphocytes as well.

G. TAMBURRANO: Yes, maybe.

D. PYKE: Dr. Tamburrano, in your studies of activated insulitis, as it were, do you ever see spontaneous remission?

G. TAMBURRANO: Yes, we have observed in a few animals a spontaneous remission.

D. PYKE: You mean it remits, but it comes back? You don't ever see a complete remission?

G. TAMBURRANO: No, there's not complete remission. We have animals without insulitis. Twenty percent of the animals do not show any insulitis, but 8% of these animals show diabetes and insulitis.

J. BARBOSA: Is there some evidence that salivary glands also undergo some inflammation?

G. TAMBURRANO: I don't really know, but I'm sure that is true.

A. REDDI: Dr. Tamburrano, can you prevent this insulitis by cyclosporine treatment?

G. TAMBURRANO: We didn't perform those experiments.

F. PUCHULU: Dr. Barbosa, what is your idea of the role of the short allele in the 11th chromosome, that is the flanking region, and the connection of that allele with insulin dependent diabetes?

J. BARBOSA: My impression right now is that the earlier reports have not been confirmed and general consensus is that there is no association at all between that polymorphism and type 1 diabetes; or, perhaps even type 2. I think it's very shaky. Perhaps someone else will know more about it. There has been a suggestion that it's possibly related to atherosclerosis.

S. EFENDIC: Our studies would support your notion that there is no relation between the polymorphism and the diabetes, but there seems to be some relation between insulin response and this flanking region which is interesting, because then you can envisage that you have a lower insulin gene stimulating secretion.

J. BARBOSA: Unfortunately, there have been several false starts on genetic markers of type 2 diabetes. For example, the famous flush which was a British phenomenon. We even had an NIH meeting on the flush and perhaps Dr. Pyke can tell us what happened to the flush.

D. PYKE: It's not a British phenomenon. Regardless of whether it's important or not, it happened everywhere for patients taking chlorpropamide. And, in the East, in Japan and in China, it happens very frequently. What its etiological or genetic significance is, I don't know, but that is happens I do not doubt. And, those who don't think it happens often are people who don't ask their patients questions or come from countries where they don't drink alcohol.

D. KUMAR: A comment on interleukin-2, because it has become interesting in the immune relationship and immune functions of type 1 diabetes. We have been looking into the polymorphics of the interleukin-2 gene itself in type 1 patients. In a very limited forum, we have found the polymorphil of interleukin-2 gene in type 1 Caucasian patients which we did not find in our control population. The information is very primitive and I can't say anything more than that at this time. Interleukin-2 doesn't have alpha and beta. It's supposed to be non-polymorphic.

F. PUCHULU: Is our belief that insulin dependent diabetes follows a very long period of the non-insulin dependent type? Is that a pre-diabetes type 1 period?

J. BARBOSA: I think there are pre-type 1 diabetic stages that are defined by genetic means, especially HLA and auto-immune means, such as islet cell antibodies. Also, the progressively decreasing acute phase insulin secretion which can be measured and has been reported. The implications of this are far reaching and gives us a chance to be at the scene of the crime while the crime is happening, so to speak, rather than after it is accomplished. That is when blood sugar goes up. Ideally, any intervention should be done at this stage. We are trying nicotinamide, but I don't think cyclosporine or imuran can be tried at the stage where the child is still normal. But, we also need to better characterize this pre-diabetic stage. We are far from being able to predict in how many weeks or months the child will develop diabetes. I don't know if these considerations are pertinent to your question.

M. RUIZ: Yes. I agree with Dr. Barbosa. I think this is a heterogeneous group, some of them are pre-type 1 diabetics, slow IDDM, the others are non-insulin dependent diabetics without the genetic marker or genetic pattern.

P. BENNET: I think this morning we've seen two phenomena mentioned that seriously challenge our conventional classification as the synonymous use of type 1 and IDDM. I think this is coming from two directions. Firstly, we have heard that islets have antibodies that can be detected quite fre- quently in NIDDM and secondly, Dr. Barbosa, you suggested that IDDM, or type 1 diabetes, occurs more frequently in the offspring of NIDDM parents. The specific question I would like to ask is do you have any evidence about the frequency of islet cell antibodies in the offspring of the NIDDM parents manifesting IDDM? And, secondly, do you have any comments or suggestions to adjust or amend our current classification?

J. BARBOSA: We are now trying to get some data on the prevalence of antibodies in these families, but we cannot yet report on them. Classi- fications are difficult to make when our knowledge is so limited.

IV.   PATHOLOGY OF PREDIABETES

KIDNEY DISEASE IN KK MICE: STRUCTURAL, BIOCHEMICAL AND FUNCTIONAL RELATIONSHIPS

¶A.S. Reddi[+], H. Wehner[*], M.Y. Khan[+],
and R.A. Camerini-Davalos[++]

[+]Department of Medicine, UMDNJ-New Jersey Medical School, Newark, N.J.
[*]Institute of Pathology, University of Freiberg, West Germany
[++]Department of Medicine, New York Medical College
Metropolitan Hospital Research Center, New York, New York

Renal disease in diabetic patients causes increased morbidity and mortality. About 30 to 40% of insulin-dependent diabetic patients develop end stage renal disease and require either dialysis or transplantation for survival. Several animal models of diabetes have been developed to understand the renal disease with regard to structural, biochemical and functional changes that occur in the diabetic kidney. Our interest has been to delineate these relationships in diabetic nephropathy using the KK mouse as an animal model. Therefore, we evaluated the kidney disease in KK mice from three perspectives. The first one is to demonstrate glomerulosclerosis in a reasonable number of animals. The second perspective is to establish the biochemical basis of diabetic glomerulosclerosis, and finally to correlate these structural and biochemical abnormalities with the functional defect, namely, proteinuria. This correlation has clinical relevance because of possible prevention of diabetic proteinuria through improvement in structural or biochemical abnormalities.

STRUCTURAL CHANGES

Diabetic glomerulosclerosis, which involves an excessive deposition of mesangial matrix is demonstrable in KK mice as early as 40 days of age. This deposition continues to increase with duration of diabetes (Fig. 1 and 2).

Electron microscopic studies revealed an increase in mesangial matrix with widening of mesangial space (Fig. 3). As the mesangium widens, it grows into the capillary wall and tends to become inserted between the basement membrane and the endothelium. In advanced cases, the capillary lumen was partly occluded by the mass of mesangium. Electron-dense deposits were also seen in the mesangium beneath the endothelium. There was focal loss of foot processes in many of these glomeruli.

This work was supported in part by the Diabetes Research Fund, New York, New York and the Michael J. Bilotto Research Fund of Hope for Diabetics Foundation, New York, New York.

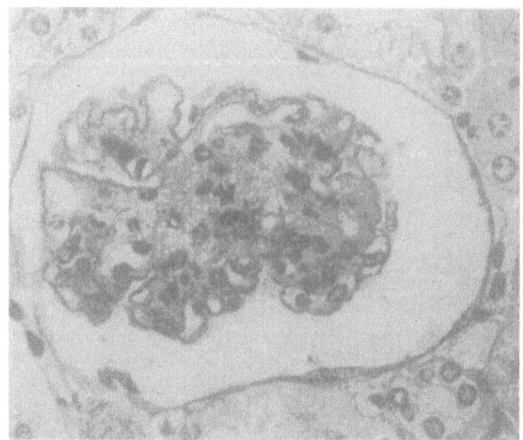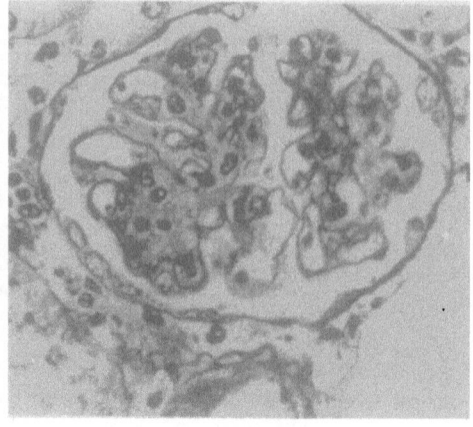

Figure 1. Almost complete nodule of intercapillary glomerulosclerosis.
Marked thickening of capillary walls by superimposition of
mesangial matrix. 12 mth. animal C-SM stain 800 X. Spec.
glom. lesions in spont. Diab. Mice of KK strain.

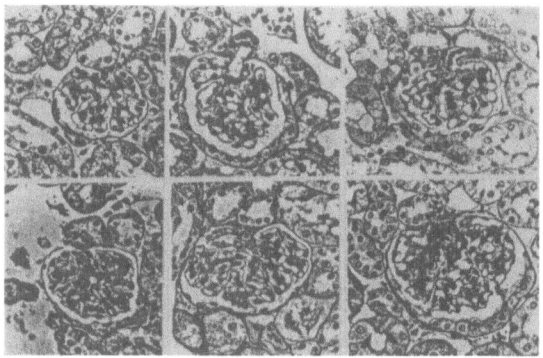

Figure 2. Increase in severity of glomerulosclerosis within 2 months
in 3 KK mice. Upper panel: 1st biopsy at 4 months of age;
lower panel: 2nd biopsy at 6 months of age.

Thickening of the glomerular basement membrane (GBM) was observed
in some KK mice. Mean GBM width of KK and control Swiss albino mice,
according to the methods of WIlliamson and Siperstein, are summarized
in Table 1. Although the mean GBM width was found to be higher in
KK than in control mice when measured by both methods, these differences
were not statistically significant. SD_1 and SD_2 (Table 1) reflect the
segmental variation in mean GBM width per capillary loop. They were calculated by averaging the standard deviations of GBM width obtained by the
Williamson and Siperstein methods, respectively. These values were also
found to be higher in KK than in control mice; however, these were not
statistically significant.

Standard deviations of GBM width per capillary loop were averaged
in order to obtain the focal variation (SD_3) in GBM width around the
circumference of the loop. Although the difference for SD_3 between KK
and control mice was greater than those in segmental variation (Table 1),
it is not statistically significant. This observation indicates that
variation in GBM width around the circumference of glomerular capillaries
is greater than variation in mean GBM width from vessel to vessel.

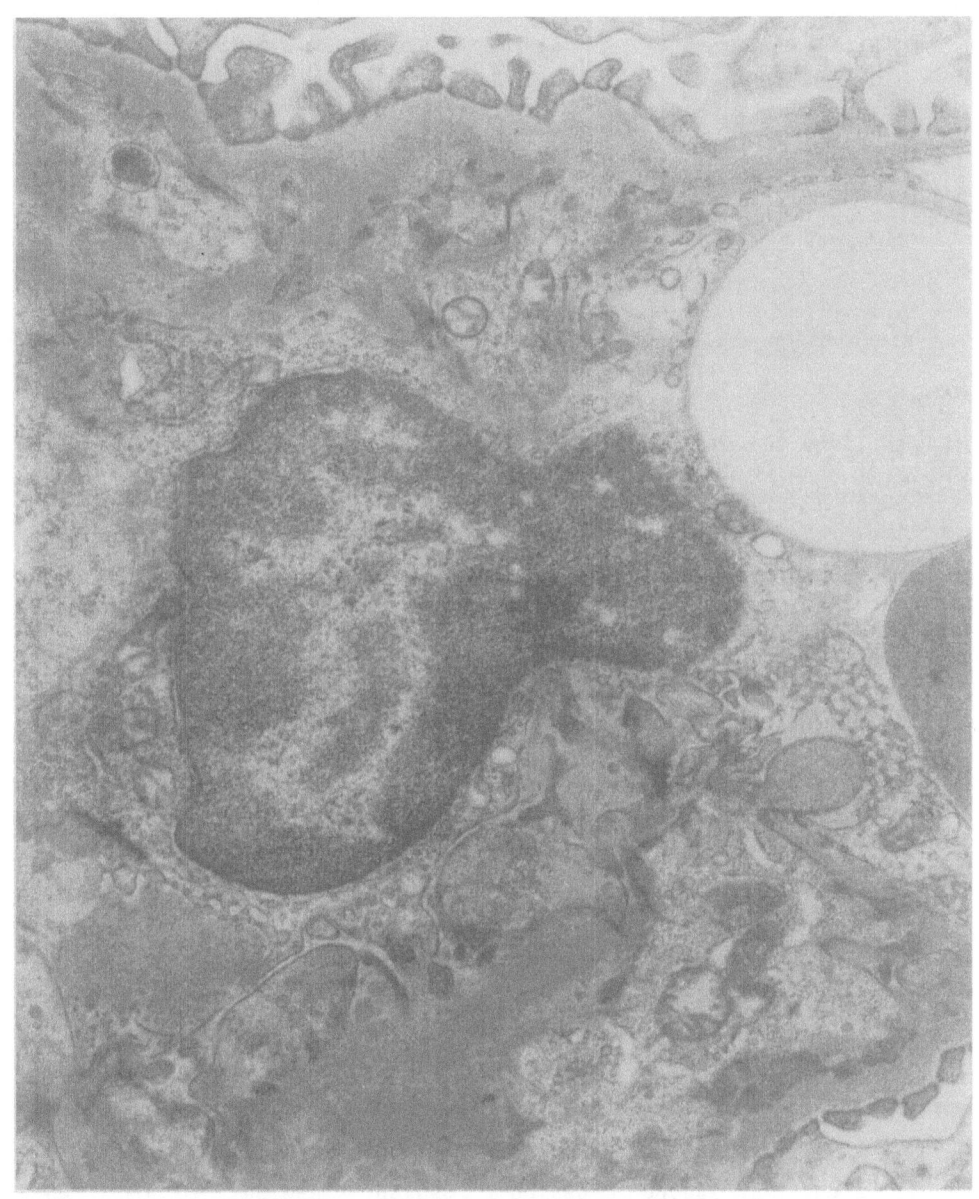

Figure 3.   Mouse 161 Mesangial X 28,700.

TABLE I

EVIDENCE OF SEGMENTAL AND FOCAL GLOMERULAR BASEMENT MEMBRANE (GBM) width
IN CONTROL SWISS ALBINO I AND KK MICE (1 DAY TO 21 MONTHS OF AGE).*

	Swiss albino I (Å) (N = 16)	KK (Å) (N = 19)
Mean GBM width		
Williamson method	1,810 ± 610	2,310 ± 1,660
Siperstein method	2,390 ± 820	2,960 ± 1,980
Segmental variation in GBM width		
Williamson method (SD_1)	442 ± 300	507 ± 556
Siperstein method (SD_2)	533 ± 316	609 ± 489
Focal variation in GBM width		
Siperstein method (SD_3)	680 ± 538	803 ± 591

*Values shown are means ± SD.

Both light and electron microscopy studies indicate that the
majority of KK mice demonstrate significant increase in the mesangium,
resulting in widening of the mesangial area or volume. We were able
to confirm this by morphometric studies. As shown in Table 2, both the
total and percent mesangial areas either in 40- or 70 day-old KK mice
were found to be greater than age-matched control mice. Furthermore,
an increase in mesangial area is evident with an increase in age in both
groups of mice. However, no difference in glomerular area was found
between the two groups of mice.

TABLE II

TOTAL GLOMERULAR AND MESANGIAL AREAS (μ^2) AND PERCENTAGE OF MESANGIAL
AREA IN GLOMERULI OF SWISS ALBINO (SA) AND KK MICE AT 40 and 70 DAYS OF AGE.*

	Age in days				Significance (SA vs. KK)	
	40		70		40	70
	SA	KK	SA	KK		
Glomerular area	3671.00 ± 122.98	3554.80 ± 160.99	4441.40 ± 145.98	4151.40 ± 130.14	NS	NS
Mesangial area	342.00 ± 18.36	465.00 ± 19.68	490.60 ± 42.48	650.50 ± 35.23	<0.005	<0.02
% of Mesangial area	9.54 ± 0.64	13.18 ± 0.89	10.98 ± 0.66	14.24 ± 1.31	<0.02	<0.005

*Each value is the mean ± SEM of 5 animals.

Although the presence of diabetic glomerulosclerosis has been reported in these KK mice (1-4), one study (5) demonstrated amyloidosis and concluded that this pathologic feature is misinterpreted as diabetic glomerulosclerosis. In an analysis of 395 KK mice of different age groups, using both Congo red staining and EM studies of the mesangium at high magnification, 247 mice (63%) showed glomerulosclerosis, 33 (8%) amyloidosis and 4 (1%) pyelonephritis (Fig. 4). These studies showed that the majority of our KK mice demonstrate diabetic glomerulosclerosis.

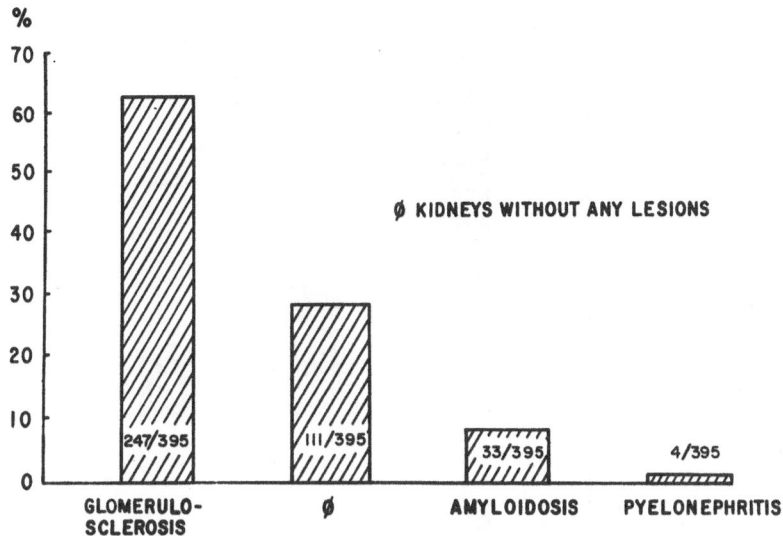

Fig. 4. Prevalence of glomerulosclerosis, amyloidosis and pyelonephritis in KK mice 2-18 months of age.

BIOCHEMICAL CHANGES

Several studies have shown that the diabetic glomerulosclerosis involves not only an increase in GBM width and accumulation of mesangial matrix, but changes in their chemistry and metabolism as well (6,7). It has now been established that the GBM is composed of collagenous, noncollagenous and carbohydrate moieties. The collagen of the GBM is termed type IV collagen which is genetically and biochemically distinct from types I, II and III; the latter being present in interstitial collagens. The collagen molecule is composed of three polypeptide chains called alpha-chains. Type IV alpha-chains of the GBM contain substantial amounts of proline, hydroxyproline, hydroxylysine and glycine. The noncollagenous component of the GBM contains glycosaminoglycan (GAG) proteoglycans, laminin, fibronectin, nidogen and entactin.

The carbohydrate portion of the GBM glycoprotein accounts for 10-11% of the dry weight. It is present in the form of glucose, galactose, sialic acid, fucose, mannose, glucosamine, glucuronic acid and iduronic acid. These sugars are distributed in three distinct units. They are disaccharide, heteropolysaccharide and GAG units. Disaccharide units consist of glucose and galactose; the latter is linked to the hydroxyl group of hydroxylysine in the peptide chain. The heteropolysaccharide unit contains sialic acid, fucose, mannose, glactose and glucosamine. This unit is linked to the protein chain through asparagine by glycosylamine bonds. The GAG unit comprises galactose, glucose, glucosamine,

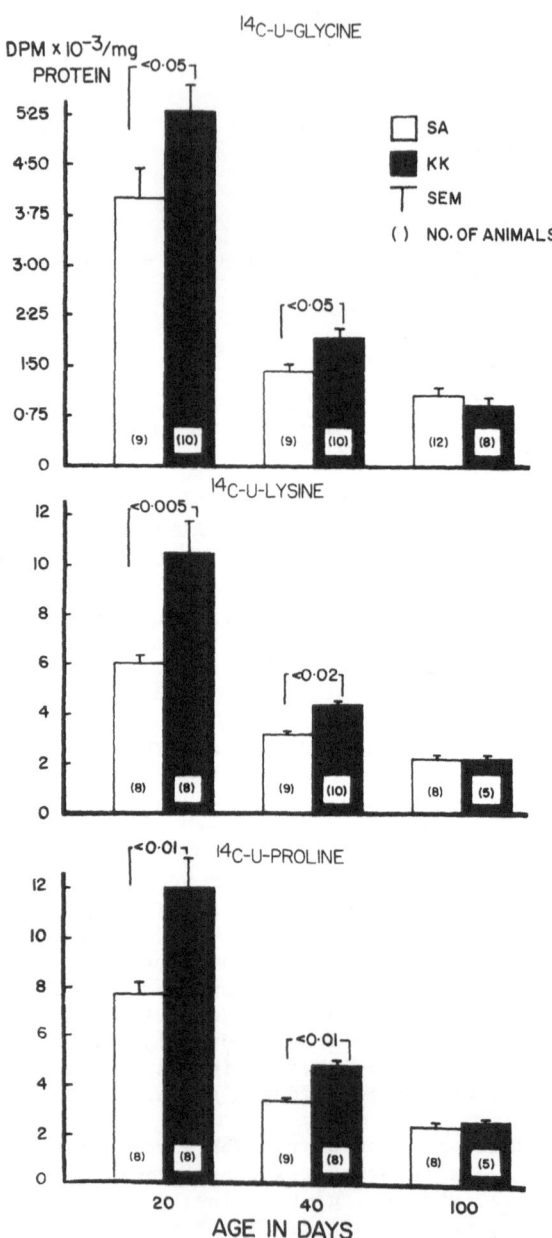

Figure 5. Incorporation of ^{14}C-U-labeled glycine, lysine and proline into protein by the renal cortex in vitro in 20, 40 and 100 day-old Swiss albino (SA) and KK mice.

glucuronic acid and iduronic acid. Sulfate comprises about 35% of the unit. The GAG unit is linked to the peptide through serine by disulfide bonds.

The synthesis of the GBM glycoprotein is analogous to the synthesis of other glycoproteins and involves many steps. These include: 1) assembly of amino acids to form polypeptide chains on polysomes; 2) hydroxylation of appropriate prolyl and lysyl residues to hydroxyproline and hydroxylysine, respectively; 3) glycosylation of the hydroxyl residues to galactosylhydroxylysine and glucosylgalactosylhydroxylysine; and 4) the formation of cross-links to form an insoluble product.

The assembly of amino acids and the formation of polypeptide chains occur by the well-established mechanisms of protein synthesis. Subsequently, hydroxylations of proline and lysine take place. These reactions are catalyzed by prolyl and lysyl hydroxylases, respectively. Both enzymes require molecular oxygen, ferrous iron, alpha-ketoglutarate and ascorbic acid as cofactors.

The attachment of carbohydrate to the peptide portion (glycation) occurs by both enzymatic and nonenzymatic reactions. The enzymatic reaction involves highly specific uridine diphosphoglycosyltransferases. There are two enzymes which require manganese as a cofactor. One enzyme is galactosyltransferase. It transfers galactose from uridine diphosphogalactose to hydroxylysine on the peptide chain to form a high molecular weight galactosylhydroxylysine residue. The other enzyme is a glucosyltransferase. This enzyme facilitate the attachment of glucose from uridine diphosphoglucose to hydroxylysine-linked galactose to form glucosylgalactosylhydroxylysine residue.

We investigated the various steps involved in the biosynthesis of the collagenous glycoprotein in the kidneys of KK mice before and after the development of significant glomerulosclerosis, and these results were compared with age-matched control Swiss albino mice. The studies include; 1) determination of protein synthesis; 2) measurement of prolylhydroxylase activity, and 3) measurement of glucosyltransferase activity.

As evident from Figure 5, the in vitro incorporation of 14C-U-labeled glycine, lysine and proline into protein by the renal cortex was found to be higher in KK at 20 and 40 days of age. No difference in protein synthesis was found at 100 days of age. The increase in protein synthesis seems to be localized in the microsomal and cytosol fractions of the cell (Figure 6). Prolyl hydroxylase activity in renal cortical homogenates of KK mice was found to be significantly increased at 40 days of age (Figure 7). A similar increase was found in glomeruli from KK mice suggesting that changes in renal cortical homogenates reflect changes in glomeruli in these KK mice.

Glucosyltransferase activity in renal cortical homogenates of KK and control mice showed no difference up to 20 days of age. However, significantly higher activity was found in KK mice from 25th to 55th days of life compared to age-matched controls. Later on, no difference in enzyme activity was observed between the two groups of mice (Figure 8).

In order to ascertain whether the observed transient increase in glucosyltransferase activity in KK mice is specific or due to species variation, the enzyme activity was determined in two other strains of control mice at 40 and 70 days of age (Table 3). The glycosyltransferase activity was found significantly increased in 40 day-old KK, when compared to that of normal control Swiss Webster or C57BL/6J mice. At 70 days of age, no difference in enzyme activity was observed between KK and the two groups of control mice.

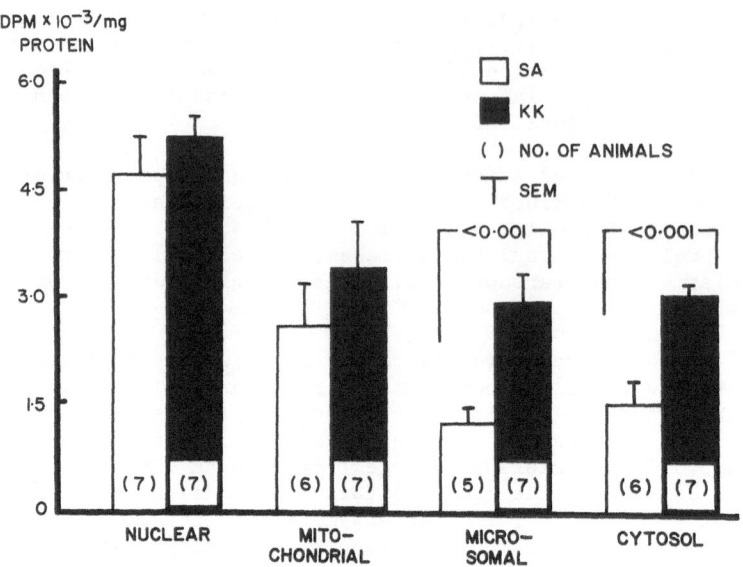

Figure 6. Incorporation of ^{14}C-U-proline into protein by various subcellular fractions of the renal cortex from 20 day-old Swiss albino (SA) and KK mice.

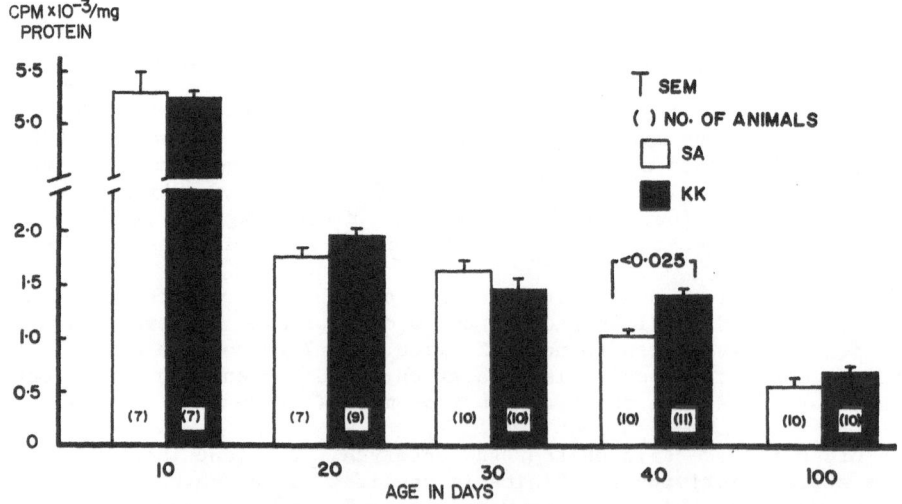

Figure 7. Prolyl hydroxylase activity in renal cortical homogenates of Swiss albino (SA) and KK mice at different age periods.

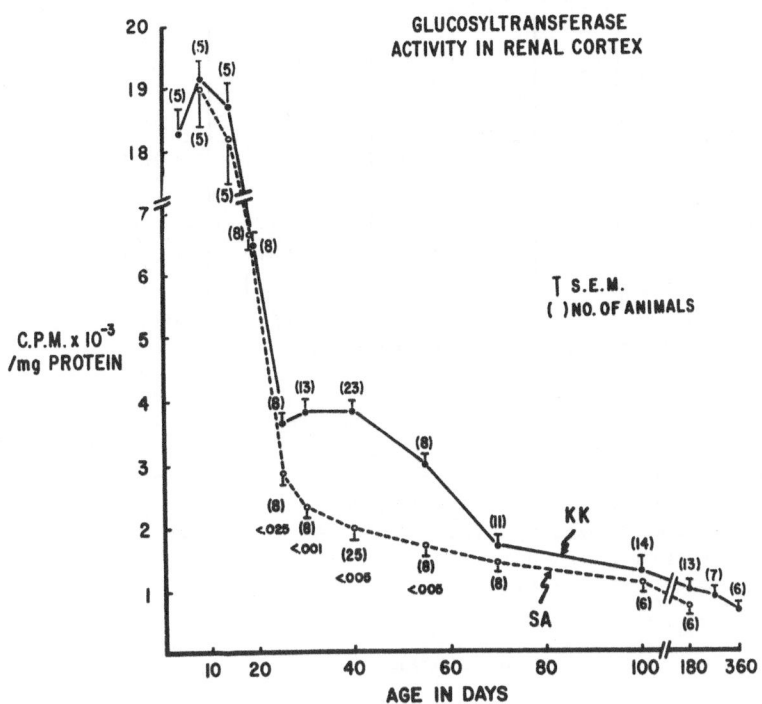

Figure 8. Glucosyl transferase activity in renal cortical homogenates of Swiss albino (SA) and KK mice at different age periods.

TABLE III

COMPARISON OF KIDNEY GLUCOSYLTRANSFERASE ACTIVITY BETWEEN SWISS ALBINO (SA), C57BL/6J, SWISS WEBSTER (SW) and KK MICE AT 40 AND 70 DAYS OF AGE. NUMBERS IN PARENTHESES INDICATE NUMBER OF ANIMALS. ENZYME ACTIVITY IS EXPRESSED AS CPM/MG PROTEIN.

Mice	Age in days	
	40	70
SA	$2207 \pm 123^{*}$ (6)	1575 ± 107 (5)
CBL	$1922 \pm 164^{**}$ (7)	1456 ± 54 (7)
SW	$2086 \pm 78^{***}$ (8)	1790 ± 162 (8)
KK	4217 ± 110 (6)	1743 ± 157 (5)

*SA vs. KK: $P < 0.001$; **CBL vs. KK: $P < 0.001$; ***SW vs. KK: $P < 0.001$

Age	1 Month		2 Months		4 Months		6 Months		9 Months		12 Months	
	Prot.	#An.	Prot.	#An.	Prot.	#An.	Prot.	#An.	Prot.	#An.	Prot.	#An.
Swiss Albino I+II	Trace +	1 3	+	31	0 Trace + ++	1 2 4 1	Trace + ++ +++	3 26 1 1	++	6 1		
	Prot.	#An.	Prot.	#An.	Prot.	#An.	Prot.	#An.	Prot.	#An.	Prot.	#An.
KK Mice	Trace + +++	1 5 1	+ ++ +++	1 2 1	+ +++ ++++	1 2 1	+ ++ +++	1 4 9	+ ++ +++ ++++	10 7 10 3	+ ++ +++ ++++	3 1 2 2

Figure 9. Dipstick (qualitative) proteinuria in Swiss albino and KK mice at different age periods.

All of these studies suggest that increased collagen-like glycoprotein is synthesized in KK mice and these biochemical changes precede significant development of glomerulosclerosis. Increases in kidney protein synthesis, prolyl hydroxylase and glucosyltransferase activity have been reported in other animal models of diabetes (6,7).

FUNCTIONAL CHANGES

The clinical hallmark of diabetic nephropathy is proteinuria. Compared to control mice, KK mice demonstrate significant proteinuria, which progresses with duration of diabetes (Figure 9). This suggests that progressive structural changes, particularly increases in mesangial matrix and volume, are causally related to functional changes of the kidney in KK mice.

In summary and conclusion, our data in KK mice demonstrate: 1) human diabetic-like glomerulosclerosis as early as 40 days of age. Diffuse increase in mesangial matrix and volume are consistently demonstrable pathologic lesions in these KK mice and the severity of these lesions progresses with age and duration of diabetes. Amyloidosis is seen only in less than 4% of our KK mice, 2) increases in protein synthesis and glucosyltransferase activity in renal corical homogenates precede structural abnormalities, and 3) these structural and biochemical changes seem to be responsible for enhanced proteinuria. Thus the KK mouse appears to be an ideal animal model for the study of the natural history and treatment of diabetic glomerulopathy.

REFERENCES

1. Camerini-Davalos, R.A., Oppermann, W., Mittl, R., and Ehrenreich, T., 1970, Studies of vascular and other lesions in KK mice. Diabetologia 6: 324-329.

2. Wehner, H., Hohn, D., Faix-Schade, U., Huber, H., and Walzer, P., 1972, Glomerular changes in mice with spontaneous hereditary diabetes. Lab Inverst 27: 331-340.

3. Duhault, J., Lebon, F., Boulanger, M., and DuBoistesselin, R., 1973, KK mice as a model of microangiopathic lesions in diabetes. Bibl. Anat. 11: 453-458.

4. Volkmann, H.P., and Wehner, H., 1986, Renal vessel cahnges in diabetic KK-mice. Virchows Archs. Pathol Anat 409: 669-678.

5. Soret, M.G., Peterson, T., Wyse, B., Block, E.M., and Dulin, W.F., 1977, Renal amyloidosdis in KK mice that may be interpreted as diabetic glomerulosclerosis. Archs Pathol Lab Med 101: 464-468.

6. Reddi, A.S., 1978, Diabetic microangiopathy. I. Current status of the chemistry and metabolism of the glomerular basement membrane. Metabolism 27: 107-124.

7. Reddi, A.S., and Camerini-Davalos, R.A., 1983, Metabolism of glomerular basement membrane in diabetes mellitus. In Diabetes 1982, Mngola, E.N., Ed., Amsterdam, Excerpta Medica, 449-57.

SEQUENCE OF CHANGES IN KK MOUSE NEPHROPATHY

¶Herbert Wehner

Institute of Pathology
General Hospital, West Germany

The KK mouse is suitable for investigations of diabetic kidney changes (1) because it develops spontaneous diabetes mellitus with a genetic pre-diabetic phase. In addition, it develops the known vascular and neurogenic lesions which are comparable to those in human diabetics. It survives without therapy. Long-term observations are hence possible without interfering side effects of medication.

The development of nephropathy is comparable to that of human diabetes, in which all structures of the kidneys (renal glomeruli, vessels, tubules, and interstitium) are finally altered. Corresponding lesions also developed in KK mice in the course of time. These can be demonstrated with suitable methods (morphometry) in very young animals, with blood sugar values and the glucose tolerance test within the normal ranges (2).

This animal model thus permits a study of the development of the diabetic lesions in very early stages which are characterized by "silent pathology." Early functional abnormalities such as glomerular hyperfiltration and intensified tubular glucose reabsorption are also known in diabetic mice so that a "non-silent physiology" is present which is possibly not without consequences for structural alterations and for the pathogenesis of diabetic nephropathy (3).

After the first communications on this species (4,5), we investigated the early stages of the glomerular alterations in these animals (2) and their therapy (6). Investigations on the immunological transmission of the glomerulosclerotic changes (7) and intrarenal vascular lesions in these animals (3) as well as on the proximal tubules of the kidney have been published recently. In this paper, the sequence of glomerular, vascular and tubular alterations of KK mouse nephropathy will be described.

MATERIALS AND METHODS

Animals

The investigations described were carried out on more than 100 KK mice (Central Institute for Laboratory Animals, Tokyo, Japan). Since a nondiabetic KK variant does not exist, we used more than 50 nondiabetic NMRI mice (Ivanovas, Kisslegg, Germany) as controls. The age of the diabetic animals was between two months and two years, and the control animals were aged between two and 18 months. The morphometric investigations of the glomeruli, vessels and tubules were performed in two, five and 12 month-old KK mice and age-correlated NMRI control mice. All animals were male. The body weight of the KK mice was between 20.9 ± 0.6 g (two months) and 0.3503 ± 0.011 g (12 months). The body and kidney weight of the control mice were similar. Five animals were investigated in each age group. All animals received Ssniff mixed mouse food (Internast GmbH, Bockum-Hovel, Germany) and had free access to water.

Blood glucose

We investigated the fasting blood glucose levels in the serum using the enzymatic ultraviolet test with hexokinase (Boehringer, Mannheim, Germany).

Light microscopy

The light microscopic investigations were performed on the kidneys of 60 KK mice and corresponding NMRI mice. The kidneys were fixed in buffered formalin. Half a kidney was embedded in paraffin and stained as follows: PAS reaction, van Gieson, Masson-Goldner, HE and Congo red. After fixation in buffered osmic acid, the other kidney half was embedded in roughly $1mm^3$ dices in Plexiglas and worked up into 1μ thick sections on the ultra microtome. The sections were silver-stained according to Movat. In these preparations, we have investigated 50 different glomeruli in each animal and determined the percentage incidence of the various alterations which could be demonstrated by light microscopy.

Morphometry

The morphometric investigations were generally performed in accordance with the methods of renal morphometry (8). The evaluation was carried out on 1μ thick sections which were silver-stained according to Movat. All sections were coded. The measurements were carried out blind, i.e., the histological preparations and the pertinent measurement values were assigned to the various age groups only after completion of the analysis. The following methods were applied for the various renal structures:

Glomerular morphometry. In each of the animals specified above, 80 different glomeruli were evaluated. The following values were determined:

1. The mean percentage mesangium content (mesangial volume) of the glomeruli by means of the point counting method on the Visopan Reichert (scale 800:1, point interval 3.75μ).

2. The mean total glomerular surface and the mesangial area on the Visopan Reichert.

3. The total number of glomerular cells, the number of individual glomerular cells (mesangial, endothelial and epithelial cells) as well as their percentage distribution by direct counting in the microscopic picture (oil immersion, 1,000 times).

4. The glomerular cell density, i.e. the total cell count in 1,000 μ^2 glomerular surface.

5. The mesangial cell density, i.e. the number of mesangial cells in 100 μ^2 mesangial surface.

Vessel morphometry

In the kidneys of the animal groups specified above, we investigated
1. small intrarenal arteries (ART), 2. arterioles (ALE) and 3. preglomerular afferent arterioles (PAA). The morphometric investigations were carried out on unequivocal perpendicular sections with the point counting
method on the Visopan Reichert (scale 800:1, point interval 3.75 μ). The
following parameters were determined:

1. vessel cross-sectional area
2. vessel lumen area and
3. vessel wall area

Altogether, 408 ART, 5,140 ALE and 518 PAA were evaluated.

Tubular morphometry

In the kidneys of the animal groups specified above, we investigated
the main sections of the proximal tubules. The morphometric investigations
on silver-stained 1 μ sections by means of the point counting method on
the Visopan Reichert. Per animal, 30 different cross-sections of the proximal tubules were investigated. Only tubule sections were evaluated which
displayed an unequivocal structure and a largely circular cross-section.
We determined the following parameters:

1. mean area of the cross-section of the proximal tubules
2. mean lumen area
3. mean epithelial area and
4. mean nuclear area

Statistics

Results are expressed as mean ± SEM. The significance of differences
was assessed using Student's t test. The limit for the probability of
error was 2 p less than 0.05.

RESULTS

Blood Sugar

The mean fasting blood glucose was 141.2 ± 25.2 mg/100 (SEM) ml in
the KK mice at two to five months, 164.2 ± 20.1 mg/100 ml in six to eight
month, 143.5 ± 9.9 mg/100 ml in nine to 11 month, and 202.1 ± 10.2 mg/100
ml in KK mice 12 to 14 months old. The NMRI mice displayed a value of
125.2 ± 3.3 mg/100 ml at an age of two to five months and of 95.8 ± 14.6
mg/100 ml at an age of 12 to 14 months.

Light microscopy

Diffuse glomerular sclerosis

Diffuse glomerular sclerosis of the mesangium is the most frequent
alteration in the glomeruli. By light microscopy, it can already be detected in 10% of glomeruli in two to four month-old KK mice. With increasing age, the alteration is more frequent and can be demonstrated in more
than 60% of the glomeruli in 19 to 22 month-old animals (Table I, Figure 1).

Nodular glomerular sclerosis

Typical glomerular sclerosis such as has been described in human

TABLE I

FREQUENCY OF THE MOST IMPORTANT GLOMERULAR ALTERATIONS
IN KK MICE OF VARIOUS AGES

Glomerular Change	Percentage at age (months)						
	2 - 4 (n = 15)	5 - 8 (n = 10)	11 - 12 (n = 6)	13 - 14 (n = 9)	15 - 16 (n = 3)	17 - 18 (n = 14)	19 - 22 (n = 3)
Diffuse Glomerulo-sclerosis	.10	14	16	12	30	60	61
Nodular mesangial enlargement	2	7	3	6	13	28	43
Hypercellularity	15	11	7	4	2	2	4
Exudative lesions		2	4	6	11	7	4

diabetics does not develop in the mice. On the other hand, a nodular mesangial thickening occurs in the course of time which increases from 2% to
43% in 19 to 22 month-old animals at the time specified above (Tab.1, Fig.
2).

Hypercellularity

GLomerular cell proliferation visible in light micrograms can be detected in 15% of the glomeruli in the young KK mice. With increasing sclerosis, the cell proliferation decreases, and only 2% to 4% of the glomeruli
are altered in this way in old KK mice (Tab. 1, Fig.3).

Exudative lesions

This lesion which is relatively characteristic for human diabetes also

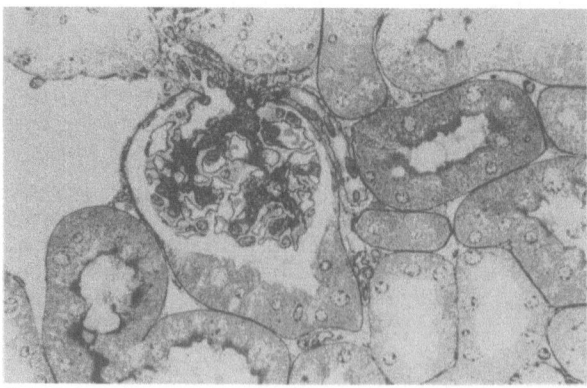

Figure 1. Diffuse glomerular sclerosis (KK mouse, two month-old,
silver staining according to Movat, 400:1).

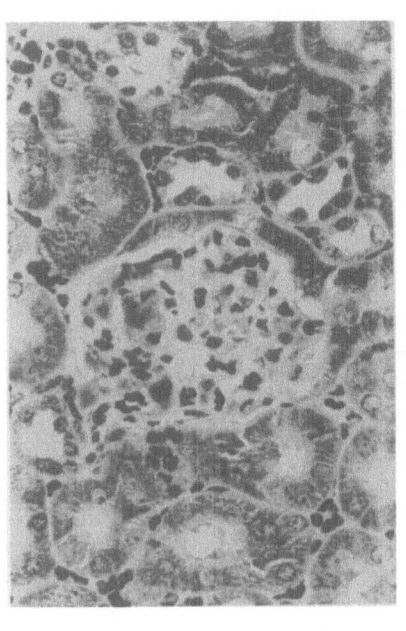

Figure 2. Nodular mesangial thickening in the lower part of the glomerulus (KK mouse, eight months old, silver staining according to Movat, 400:1).

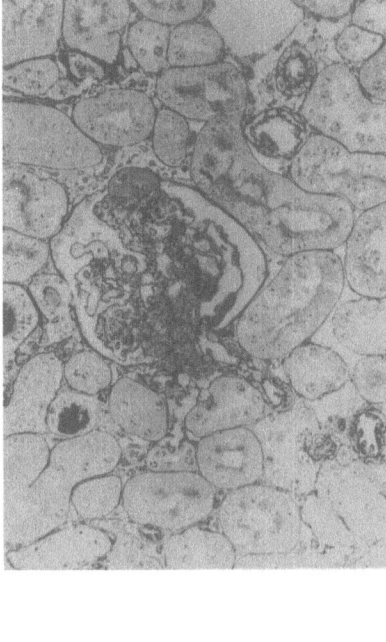

Figure 3. Glomerular cell proliferation and small fibrinoid necroses in the upper part of the glomerulus (KK mouse, five months old, Masson-Goldner staining, 512:1)

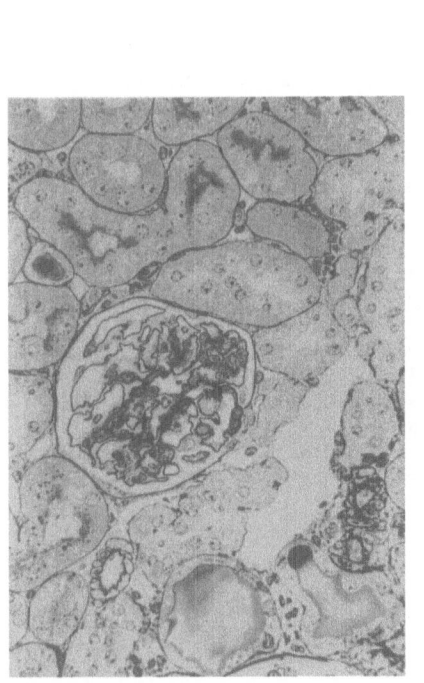

Figure 4. Fibrinoid caps near to the vascular pole (KK mouse, 12 months old, silver staining according to Movat, 400:1).

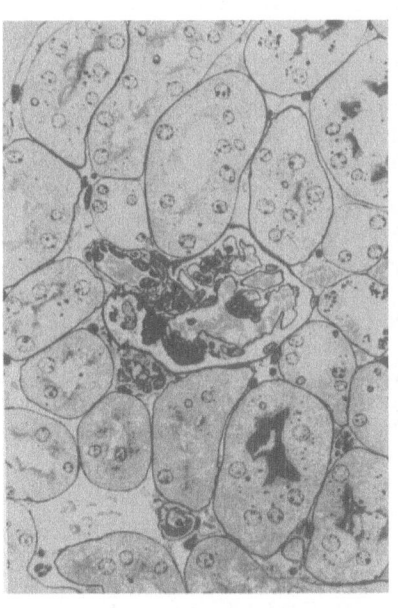

Figure 5. Aneurysm in the peripheral glomerular loop convolution (KK mouse, ten months old, silver staining according to Movat, 512:1).

occurs in the glomeruli of KK mice. We found fibrinoid caps, especially in the 13 to 16 month-old animals at an incidence of 6% to 11% (Tab. 1, Fig. 4).

Further rare glomerular alterations

The rare alterations in the glomeruli of the older KK mice include: homogenous thickening of the basement membrane, membranous changes of the basement membrane, splintering of the basement membrane (as in membranoproliferative glomerulonephritis) aneurysms (Fig. 5), adhesions (synechias) and a complete hyalinization of glomeruli which are visible in the light microgram.

Glomerular morphometry

The most important morphometric parameters in connection with diabetic nephropathy are the mesangial area and the glomerular cell density. The normal two to five month-old NMRI mice display a mean mesangial area of 7.5% on the overall glomerular surface. This value is significantly higher (9.5%) in KK mice of the same age and decreases to 11.7% with increasing age (Table II). The normal glomerular cell density is 3.9 cells in 1,000 μ^2 glomerular area. In the young KK mice, there is glomerular cell proliferation which is manifested in a raised glomerular cell density of 6.5. With increasing age (and/or progressive sclerosis), the cell density decreases (Table 2).

Vascular morphometry

The most important result of our investigation concerns the vessel lumen area. At the age of two months, the diabetic arteries and arterioles are significantly narrower than the nondiabetic arteries and arterioles (360 vs 515 μ^2 and 70.9 vs 94.3 μ^2). In the preglomerular afferent arterioles, no difference is shown. With increasing age, all vessels show an increase in lumen. However, this enlargement is very much more pronounced in diabetic mice. At the age of 12 months, the diabetic arteries and arterioles have a significantly larger lumen than that of the NMRI mice (1,057 vs 616 μ^2 and 176 vs 115 μ^2). The same applies to the preglomerular afferent arterioles (Table III). Expressed in percentage terms, this entails an enlargement of the lumen with increasing age (two to 12 months) between 92% and 194% in the diabetic vessels in contrast to 20% to 38% in the nondiabetic vessels (Table IV). A similar situation is shown in the determination of the vessel wall area. The 12 month-old diabetic animals display a larger vessel wall area (however, this is not statistically significant) than the non-diabetic 12 month-old animals (for the ART 1.83 vs 1.52 mm^2, for the ALE 344 vs 331 μ^2, for PAA at five months 835 vs 810 μ^2). This can also be discerned in the percentage alteration which is between 15% and 51% in the KK mice and is 14% in the NMRI mice. With the exception of the arteries of nondiabetic mice, all vessels of all animals show an increase in area of the overall cross-section with increasing age. However, at an age of 12 months, the cross-section of all vascular reegions investigated is greater in the diabetic animals (ART 2.89 vs 2.13 mm^2, ALE 520 vs 447 μ^2, PAA (five months) 970 vs 905 μ^2).

Tubular morphometry

We could observe the following as the most important morphometric alterations of the tubules:

The mean luminal area, the mean tubular cross-section and the mean epithelial area increase significantly with age from two to 12 months in diabetic animals. There was no increase in the course of these ten months of life in the NMRI mice: the areas remain the same (Table 5). The mean

TABLE II

PERCENTAGE MESANGIAL AREA AND GLOMERULAR CELL DENSITY IN NORMAL AND DIABETIC MICE OF VARIOUS AGES (MEAN ± SEM)

Group (age in months)	Mesangial area (%)	Glomerular cell density
Normal 2 - 5 (n = 10)	7.5 ± 0.3	3.9 ± 0.6
KK 2 (n = 5)	9.5 ± 0.4	6.5 ± 0.5
KK 5 (n = 5)	10.8 ± 0.7	4.8 ± 0.3
KK 12 (n = 6)	11.7 ± 0.6	4.3 ± 0.4

TABLE III

VESSEL LUMEN AREA (SQ. μ) OF ARTERIES (ART), ARTERIOLES (ALE) AND PREGLOMERULAR AFFERENT ARTERIOLES (PAA) IN NON-DIABETIC NMRI-MICE AND DIABETIC KK-MICE

* = A SUFFICIENT NUMBER OF PAA COULD NOT BE FOUND IN THIS GROUP

Vessel Group	Age (months)	NMRI	KK	
ART	2	515.52 ± 69.29	360.00 ± 34.48	S
	5	594.72 ± 49.42	462.96 ± 36.80	
	12	616.68 ± 72.99	$1.057.68 \pm 142.46$	S
ALE	2	94.32 ± 2.80	70.92 ± 1.78	S
	5	113.76 ± 3.75	102.34 ± 2.29	S
	12	115.56 ± 4.55	176.04 ± 7.36	S
PAA	2	68.76 ± 4.01	68.76 ± 6.23	
	5	95.04 ± 7.31	131.76 ± 8.53	S
	12	91.44 ± 9.48	-*	

TABLE IV

MEAN PERCENTAGE CHANGES IN LUMEN AREA IN DIFFERENT VESSELS
COMPARED TO THE 2-MONTHS VALUES

Vessel group	NMRI	KK
ART (at 12 months)	+ 20 %	+ 194 %
ALE (at 12 months)	+ 23 %	+ 148 %
PAA (at 5 months)	+ 38 %	+ 92 %

TABLE V

DIFFERENT CROSS-SECTIONAL AREAS OF PROXIMAL TUBULES IN NMRI AND KK MICE
OF VARYING AGE (MEAN ± SEM)

Area	Age	NMRI	KK	
Lumen area (sq.µ)	2	181 ± 95	245 ± 99	n.s.
	5	180 ± 75 n.s.	180 ± 80 s.	n.s.
	12	206 ± 98	395 ± 130	s. !!
Cross sectional area (sq.µ)	2	2603 ± 300	2470 ± 500	n.s.
	5	2640 ± 320 n.s.	2565 ± 485 s.	n.s.
	12	2700 ± 400	3250 ± 490	n.s.
Epithelial area (sq.µ)	2	2422 ± 300	2200 ± 420	n.s.
	5	2464 ± 420 n.s.	2390 ± 410 s.	n.s.
	12	2510 ± 380	2863 ± 380	n.s.

luminal area is significantly increased ($395 \mu^2$ vs $206 \mu^2$) in 12 month-old KK mice compared to normal mice, i.e. there is an unequivocal dilation of the proximal tubules in 12 month-old KK mice (as compared to normal and two month-old diabetic mice) (Table V). A significant alteration of the nuclear area of the tubular epithelia can be demonstrated neither in the KK mice nor in the NMRI mice at the age of two, five and 12 months.

DISCUSSION

The sequence of glomerular alterations in the context of diabetic nephropathy in the KK mouse is characterized by progressive glomerular sclerosis which can be demonstrated in two month-old animals (prediabetics) and by glomerular cell proliferation which can be demonstrated in young animals. The latter regresses within increasing glomerulosclerotic alterations. This development is also shown in the course of the morphometric parameters with the increase of mesangial volume and the decrease of glomerular cell density with the increasing age of the animals. In addition, in the course of the first years of life of the KK mouse, intrarenal vascular lesions develop in the small arteries, the arterioles and the preglomerular afferent arterioles: these are characterized morphometrically by a progressive and excessive dilation of the vascular lumen which amounts to 194% in the small arteries of the 12 month-old animals compared to those with an age of two months. At the same time, the proximal tubule system of the diabetic animals also shows morphometrically demonstrable alterations which consist of a marked enlargement of tubular lumina compared to nondiabetic animals and a progressive increase of the lumen area and the epithelial area in the diabetic animals in the first year of life. The diabetic tubules evidently show a very much more intensive growth than normal tubules. We did not find the tubule mineralizations (calcium deposits) demonstrated in spontaneously diabetic rabbits (9). We were also unable to detect a marked storage of glycogen in the tubular epithelia (Armani-Ebstein cells) or tubule atrophy with thickening of the tubule basement membrane.

From a pathogenic point of view, our results indicate on the one hand a major influence of the hyperglycemia (2). On the other hand, the renal vasodilation described is accompanied by intraglomerular hypertension with consequent glomerular hyperfiltration. This is associated with the mesangial thickening (3, 10). These alterations which can still be demonstrated in the stage of the nonmanifest diabetes and the increase with age finally allows the conclusion that in addition to a specific genetic predisposition environmental factors are also necessary for the development of nephropathy (1,11). The alterations of the proximal tubules are possibly secondary phenomena of the glomerular and vascular functional disorders. The findings may also be based on a true growth in terms of hypertrophy of the nephron regions concerned. This is supported in particular by the fact of the excessive growth of diabetic tubules compared to normal tubules. The alteration of glomerular hemodynamics with subsequent morphological lesions thus appears to initiate the alterations and be at the center of the pathogenesis of diabetic nephropathy of KK mice.

As the KK mice of our laboratory are still normoglycemic at the age of 2 months the following alterations can definitely be attributed to the period before hyperglycemia: Diffuse glomerulosclerosis with morphometrically demonstrable enlargement of the mesangial area; glomerular hypercellularity with morphometrically demonstrable increase in glomerular cell density and finally a narrowing in lumen of intrarenal arteries and arterioles.

REFERENCES

1. Camerini-Davalos, R.A., Reddi, A.S., Velasco, C.A., Oppermann, W., Wehner, H., Bloodworth, J.M.B., 1979, Microangiopathy in genetic prediabetes. Front Matrix Biol 7: 281-295.

2. Wehner, H., Hohn, D., Faix-Schade, U., Huber, H., Walzer, P, 1972, Glomerular changes in mice with spontaneous hereditary diabetes. Lab Invest 27: 331-340.

3.   Volkmann, H.P., Wehner, H., 1986, Renal vessel changes in diabetic KK mice. Virchows Archiv (Pathol Anat) 409: 669-678.

4.   Kondo, K., Nozawa, K., Tomita, T., Ezaki, K, 1957, Inbred strains resulting from Japanese mice. Bull Exp Anim 6: 107-112.

5.   Treser, G., Oppermann, W., Ehrenreich, T., Lange, K., Levine, R., Camerini-Davalos, R.A., 1968, Glomerular lesions in a strain of genetically diabetic mice. Proc Soc Exp Biol Med. 129: 820-823.

6.   Wehner, H., Wagner, H., Podmaniczky, A., Heidbrink, V., Kiessling, B., 1978, Influence of short-term insulin therapy on th mesangial structure in young KK-mice. Nephron 22: 460-472.

7.   Wehner, H., Konig, I., 1982, Immunological transmission of glomer-ulosclerotic changes in KK-mice with spontaneous diabetes. 1. Transplantation of spleen cells. Virchows Archiv (Pathol Anat) 396: 61-71.

8.   Wehner, H., 1983, Kidney morphometry, 1983, In J.P.A. Baak and J. Oort: Manual of morphometry in diagnostic pathology. Springer, Heidelberg: 124-126, 174-175.

9.   Roth, S.I., Conaway, H.H., Sanders, L.L., Casali, R.E., Boyd, A.E., 1980, Spontaneous diabetes mellitus in the New Zealand white rabbit. Preliminary morphologic characterization. Lab Invest 42: 571-579.

10.   Cohen, A.J., McGill, P.D., Rossetti, R.G., Gubersi, D.L., Like, A.A., 1987, Glomerulopathy in spontaneously diabetic rat. Impact of glycemic control. Diabetes 36: 944-951.

11.   Oppermann, W., Ehrenreich, T., Patel, D., Espinoza, T., Camerini-Davalos, R.A., 1973, Related factors in the progression of microangiopathy in KK mice. In R.A. Camerini-Davalos and H. Cole, Eds., Early Diabetes, Adv Metab Dis; Suppl. 2: 281-290.

DISCUSSION

H. LAUBE: Dr. Reddi, I wonder if you have any information to what extent the biochemical changes in the kidney of your mice are reversible after islet transplantation?

A. REDDI: We have not used islet transplantation, but we have data. Dr. Camerini is going to discuss the effect of insulin on these biochemical abnormalities. If we improve the blood glucose levels, the activity of one of the enzymes responsible for basement membrane degradation increases and then we can ameliorate the glomerular deposition.

R. RODRIGUEZ: In our rats we found after 6-8 months of diabetes an increase in the size of the kidney of about 30% and also a mixture of nephrosis and nephritis so there was an infection usually in the animals. Also, we find a deposition of glycogen in the tubules.

C. HOWARD: Dr. Reddi, there have been some attempts to find circulating markers to indicate potential glomerulosclerosis. Isn't glucosyl-transferase one of those enzymes? So, my question here would be two-fold actually. First of all, have you examined the level of the enzyme in the kidneys as they progress towards the nephropathy? And, secondly, have you examined for circulating levels of the enzyme and does it mean anything?

A. REDDI: Yes. I have shown the glucosyl-transferase activity in one of the slides here in relation to age. When compared to Swiss Albino mice the enzyme activity in the KK mouse is increased only from 25th to 55th days of life. It is a transient increase, then the enzyme levels decrease in the renal cortex. We did determine the glucosyl-transferase activity in the plasma, but the data are inconclusive.

C. HOWARD: What I really had in mind was enzyme levels. You measured the enzyme activity. I wonder about the actual levels.

A. REDDI: No, we did not. When we examined the kidneys of 700 animals, we found amyloidosis in only 33 animals. But, when we did the E.M. studies on the remaining kidneys, we could not show the presence of amyloid fibrins. The amyloid fibrins measure about 100 nanometers, and we were unable to detect any amyloid fibrin in the majority of our KK mice either with a congo red staining or under high magnification using electron microscopy. Since you mentioned amyloidosis, I think I should refer to a paper published by Dulin from UpJohn and he is the only one that reported amyloidosis in his colony of obese KK mice. Usually we send the specimens to various nephropathologists and one of them is Dr. Wehner. We specifically request looking for presence of amyloidosis because we are interested in this animal model for diabetic glomerulosclerosis. And, nobody so far reports amyloidosis other than in those 33 animals out of 700.

R. CAMERINI-DAVALOS: I think that it is important to point out Dulin's strain of KK mice is completely different from Dr. Wehner's and ours in the sense that these animals are markedly obese and they have a really tremendous amount of insulin in the fasting state, something like 5000 microunits. In those animals, in his colony, they published a paper where they found amyloidosis.

If glycosyl-transferase is a marker or not, we don't know, but we measure in tears and in muscle and we also found that in those two locations there is an increase during the prediabetic period of the KK mouse. So, there is something in that particular enzyme that may be a marker.

H. LAUBE: Dr. Wehner, did you ever observe a case of papillary necrosis in the kidneys of your mice?

H. WEHNER: No.

H. LAUBE: How come? This is a typical lesion which was frequently, or is frequently, described in diabetes.

A. REDDI: Can I answer that question, please? We evaluated for the presence of pyelonephritis and papillary necrosis in relation to amyloidosis in our KK mice. Again, 700 kidneys is a large study and only four animals out of 700 animals had pyelonephritis, but only one mouse showed papillary necrosis. And, when we went back and reviewed the morphologic characteristics of these mice, these were the mice that had some skin lesions. So, the majority of the animals do not show a pyelonephritis or amyloidosis or papillary necrosis.

J. HOET: Regarding the amyloidosis, it might very well be that certain strains of animals cannot make local amyloidosis. For instance, in the pancreas of rodents, I do not know of any amyloisis description. It could be strain specific. It could also be sex determined. In these 33 KK mice, were these male or female animals?

A. REDDI: We used both males and females.

J. HOET: Well, but in the ones where you showed some amyloidosis in the kidney. Were these both males and females or only males showing it or only females showing it?

A. REDDI: It is a very interesting observation. We had one group of female mice, they were mated consecutively four times, and after the 4th pregnancy, we sacrificed them and looked into the kidneys and the majority of them had amyloidosis. I do not know how to interpret this, whether pregnancy stimulated the production of amyloid formation, but these are the animals that fell into those 33 animals which showed amyloidosis. The majority are the females and the males seem to have no amyloidosis.

ABNORMAL RESPONSE TO GLUCOSE IN THE PREHYPERGLYCEMIC STAGE

¶R.A. Camerini-Davalos[+], A.S. Reddi[*], H.S. Cole[++] and C.A. Velasco[+]

[+]Department of Medicine, New York Medical College
Metropolitan Hospital Research Center, New York, New York
[*]Department of Medicine, UMDNJ-New Jersey Medical School, Newark, N.J.
[++]Department of Community & Preventive Medicine, New York Medical College
Bronx Developmental Center, OMRDD

If conception marks "the beginning" of the disease, how early in life is the disease trend manifest? Even in those highly predisposed to diabetes on a genetic basis there is a period in life when the "dynamic resistance" is so effective that no abnormalities can be detected with our present capabilities and where diabetes can only be suspected. Jackson (1) called this first stage without abnormalities "suspected prediabetes." The second with detectable abnormalities (but normal carbohydrate metabolism) we recognize as prediabetes.

Can the art of predictive medicine anticipate the development of diabetes? If disease in a person is testimony of failure, we need to use the concept of predispostion to heed the signs of incipient failure. But, in those predisposed to hyperglycemia, what are the abnormalities inherited with the diabetic predisposition that will allow us to attempt to delay the progression of the disease? How early is early enough to intervene?

We published our first retrospective study on prediabetes in 1951 (2) and the first prospective ones in 1961 and 1963 with Marble (3-4). In a previous publication (5) we listed 16 abnormalities recognized, at that time, at the prediabetic stage. Today the list is constantly increasing. In this presentation we will discuss some hormonal-metabolic deviations from "normal" in prediabetics.

MATERIAL AND METHODS

From our large group of an ongoing study on early diabetes, Caucasian, identical nondiabetic twins of diabetic patients, offspring with normal glucose tolerance of proven conjugal diabetic parents: genetic prediabetics (GP) and, nondiabetic controls (C) who have no history of any type of diabetes in a first or second degree relative; and within 15% of ideal body weight (according to the table of Average Weights of Adults from the Society of Actuaries. Build and Blood Pressure Study, Vol. II, Chicago, IL.) were included.

This work was supported in part by General Research Support Grant RR05398 from the General Research Support Branch, Division of Research Resources NIH. Health Research Council of the City of New York. Diabetes Research Fund, New York. The Michael J. Bilotto Research Fund of HOPE for Diabetics Foundation, New York.

Blood glucose values were considered abnormal during the morning test if they exceeded the upper tolerance limits for the patients' sex and age group as determined from our previous studies on 117 control subjects for the intravenous and 249 for the oral glucose tolerance test (6-7). Our criteria is different from those accepted by the American Diabetes Association in that they are more stringent (lower upper limit of normal) and also, any deviation from "normal" will exclude the subject from the study of prediabetics. Fasting blood glucose for our 366 non-diabetic control subjects between 15 to 44 years of age were 88 ± 7 mg/dl. (mean + 2SD = 102 mg/dl).

Tolerance to glucose was performed in the morning after 3 days on at least 300 g carbohydrate diet by oral administration of 100 g glucose in a cold cola-flavored preparation (Koladex) after an overnight 14-hr. fast. (OGTT). Three milliliters of blood were drawn for blood glucose determinations via an indwelling catheter (Longdwel no. 18) in the antecubital vein at zero time and after the glucose load at 30, 60, 120, and 180 min. Blood glucose was determined in whole blood in the Autoanalyzer by Hoffman's ferricyanide method (n-2A). Serum immunoreactive insulin was determined by mixing the samples with the tracer and a Sephadex anti-insulin complex. After 3 h incubation at room temperature, the precipitate was settled by centrifugation, washed with saline and counted. The concentration of immunoreactive insulin was read directly in microunits/ml from a Standard curve (8).

Glucose or insulin area (glucose or insulin area under the curve) was determined according to the formula area = $[t_0 + 2(t_{30} + t_{60} + t_{90} + t_{180}) + 3t_{120}]/4$ where t_j = blood sugar in milligrams per dl at j min., and t_0 = fasting blood glucose.

In order to determine the rate of disappearance of glucose from the blood following an acute glucose load and to compare the results in different subjects and in a given subject at different times, rapid intravenous glucose tolerance tests were performed after three days on the preparatory diet (IVTT). Glucose in a dosage of 0.5 gm. per kilogram of actual body weight was mixed as a 50 per cent solution with an equal amount of a 0.9 per cent solution of sodium chloride (sodium and chloride each 154 mEq. per liter) and injected intravenously in two to four minutes. Blood samples were collected at ten-minute intervals after the end of the infusion. Determination of the glucose assimilation coefficient (K) was effected by transcription on semi-logarithmic graph paper (concentration in logarithmic scale in ordinates, time in abscissas of the blood glucose values observed). The slope of the line connecting the points shows the rate of disappearance of glucose. Value of the mean less 2 S.D. in normal control subjects was 1.17 (S.D.:.574). Values below this were considered to indicate diabetes.

RESULTS

Baseline

From 1965 to 1970 we studied 114 genetic prediabetics. Among them there were 11 twin siblings not affected with diabetes:

A: No statistically significant difference and no uniform pattern of difference was found between the mean blood glucose or insulin levels of C and GP during the OGTT. When the glucose area, 1- and 2-h, and 1-, 2- and 3-h blood glucose values, and Δ glucose or the mean serum insulin levels, insulin area, 1- and 2-h, 1-, 2- and 3-h blood glucose values, and Δ glucose or the mean serum insulin levels, insulin area, 1- and 2-h, 1-, 2- and 3-h serum insulin values, and insulin to glucose area ratio of that day were compared. When the IRI increments at 30' were determined a significant

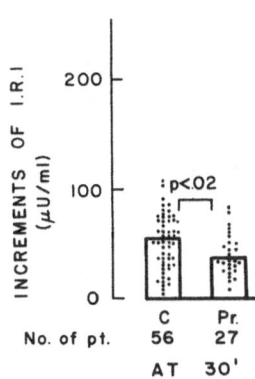

Figure 1. Increments above fasting, at 30 minutes, of immunoreactive insulin (IRI).

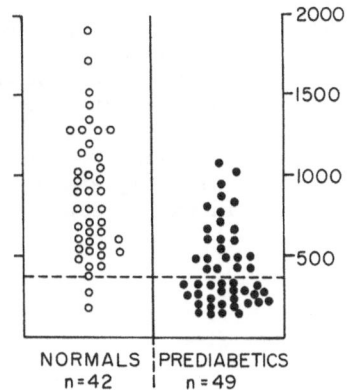

Figure 2. Insulin area above baseline for the first 10 minutes of the IVTT. Milliunits per liter x minutes after glucose.

(p < 0.02) lower mean was found in the GP (Figure 1). Fifteen of them (55%) had values velow the mean.

B: During the rapid I.V. test the rate of disappearance of glucose from blood (glucose disposal) was slow in the GP when compared to C: K = 169 ± 6 to 226 ± 9, p < 0.01. Thirty nine of them (57%) had the glucose assimilation coefficient (K) values below the mean less 1 SD of C.

Immunoreactive insulin levels during the IVTT were significantly lower (p < 0.05) at 3,5, and 10 minutes. The abnormal insulin response to glucose was normalized after glucagon (7), arginine and tolbutamide. When the early-phase insulin response in these patients (with very similar blood glucose concentrations: GP and C) was expressed as the insulin area above baseline for the first 10 minutes of the I.V. test at the fifth percentile, only 2 of 42 controls showed a deficit in the insulin response, but 26 of the 49 GP (53%). (Figure 2).

C: In a pilot investigation (with J. Tobin, unpublished data) we studied C and GP under continuous IV glucose sufficient to keep the arterial blood glucose at a 300 mg/dl plateau (constant, equal hyperglycemia) measuring the arterial IRI trying to determine the biological activity of "effectiveness" of the IRI in these patients using the formula:

$$\frac{M}{IRI} = \frac{mg/Kg/Min}{U/ml}$$

M = glucose metabolized is equal to I - S - U
I = infusion rate   (mg/Kg/min)
S = glucose necessary to fill the glucose space
U = urinary glucose loss

When the final analysis of each case was tabulated no significant difference was found between the two groups (GP and C).

After 15 years

Excluding 7 patients that developed overt diabetes with abnormal fasting BG and symptoms (OD), 83 patients of the original group when retested in 1985 had normal fasting BG. Twenty nine GP developed abnormal OGTT and

10 abnormal IVTT (chemical diabetes: CD). Four patients had abnormal IVTT with normal OGTT. When all those with abnormal fasting (and syptoms) or tolerance to glucose were excluded we were left with 50 GP. Five of them were twin siblings not affected with diabetes.

Early-phase insulin response was abnormal in 12 of 29 GP or 41%. The slope of the linear regression of serum insulin with regard to blood glucose concentration in the GP can be seen in Figure 3.

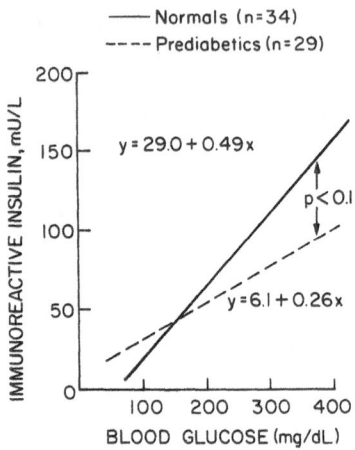

Figure 3. Regression line for insulin versus blood glucose.

Markers of Progression

At the end of this study period, 33 patients were found with CD and 7 with OD. In trying to find the major factor predicting the risk for the progression from prediabetes, we analyzed blood glucose and IRI response to glucose and the glucose disposal during the IVTT test.

Sixty three patients from the original groups with OGTT (with BG and IRI determinations) were reviewed and divided arbitrarily according to their blood glucose response into average, low or high responders. As may be seen in Figure 4, progression to CD was frequent in those older than 29 years of age regardless of their response to the glucose load.

As may be seen in Table I, the percentage of genetic prediabetics who progressing to diabetes (CD or OD) is remarkably high in those with low first phase IRI response during the IVTT, low IRI increments at 30 minutes during the OGTT, slow glucose disposal and/or more than 29 years of age.

When the IRI area of GP, CD, and OD was compared, it was found higher at the stage of CD (Figure 5).

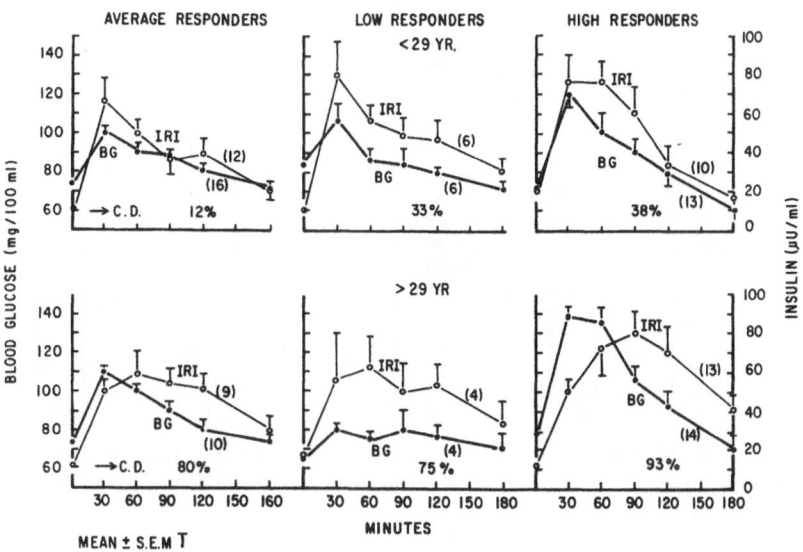

Figure 4. Percent progression to asymptomatic chemical diabetes (CD) according to their blood glucose response during the OGTT.

TABLE I: SOME MARKERS OF PROGRESSION
N = NUMBER OF PATIENTS; * = TOTAL PERCENTAGE, BASED ON NUMBER
OF PREDIABETICS PROGRESSING TO CD OR OD.

	Prediabetics	Chemical Diabetics		Overt Diabetics		Total*
	N	N	%	N	%	%
Immunoreactive Insulin						
IVTT: Low first phase IRI response	26	20	76	3	11	88
OGTT: Low increment at 30'	15	12	81	1	7	87
Glucose Disposal						
Low K	37	33	89	2	5	94
Age of Patients						
Older than 29 Y	28	23	83	3	11	93

Immunoreactive Insulin						
IVTT: Normal	23	7	30	2	9	39
OGTT: Increments at 30' above the mean	12	5	12	2	17	58
Glucose Disposal						
Normal K	30	9	30	3	10	40
Age of Patients						
Younger than 29 Y	35	10	28	1	3	31

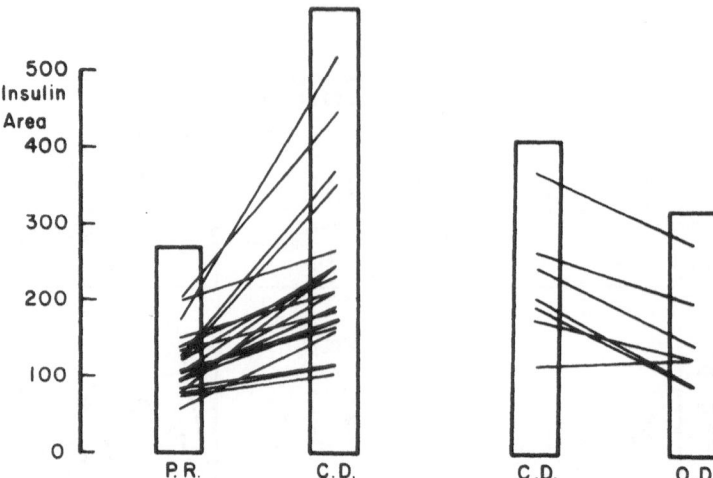

Figure 5. Insulin area, of the same patients, according to their progression of the disease. PR: Prediabetics, CD: Chemical diabetics, OD: Overt diabetics.

DISCUSSION

The probability that a person is genetically liable to diabetes as a function of the relationship to a diabetic patient is well accepted today. During the last 30 years, it has become clear even to clinicians, that a barely significant abnormality in the glucose tolerance curve is a late event in the development of diabetes. But what happens before? What happens at the stage of prediabetes?

In this presentation we reviewed some hormonal-metabolic deviations from "normal" during the phase of dynamic resistance to diabetes, that period of life (up to the first abnormal tolerance to glucose) that in subjects highly predisposed to diabetes on genetic bases, is recognized as prediabetes.

In reviewing the "markers of progression" we were surprised to find that age was such a significant factor (Table I). Nevertheless, in a previous investigation on the prevalence of macrosomia in relation to age (9) we found a highly significant increase in those patients older than 25 years. What is the common denominator (if any) of these two findings is not clear at the present time.

Clearly (Table I) a subnormal insulin response to oral or IV glucose load is strongly predictive of progression from prediabetes. If the impaired insulin secretion, is more predictive than the slow glucose disposal cannot be answered from our study, since the total percentage (Table I) is very similar.

But, why this impaired insulin secretion in prediabetics when their blood glucose levels are normal and very similar to the ones of normal control subjects? Insulin secretion is regulated by a complex interaction of nutrient, hormonal, and neural factors. Which one is altered in prediabetes? Is that the "beginning?" Is that what is inherited with diabetes? The fact that the diminished insulin response to glucose can be normalized by insulinogogues suggests that what is inherited is a decreased sensitivity of the recognition of the B cell for glucose. Studies have now identified a high affinity receptor on the plasma membrane of the B-cell specific for sulfonylureas (8)., suggesting that the "normalization" of the insulin response by tolbutamide in GP is due to the fact that the signal to the pancreas is transmitted through a different "channel." But what "channel" is deranged in GP? A glucose receptor in the B cell as recently suggested again? (10).

Another question to be answered is why the apparent improvement of the insulin response to glucose (Figure 5) with the progression of GP to CD. Is it that the threshold for glucose, to elicit release of insulin, is higher in those highly predisposed to diabetes?

REFERENCES

1. Jackson, W.P.U., 1962, That expression "Prediabetes." Diabetes 11: 334.

2. Camerini-Davalos, R.A., Landabure, P., Serantes, N., 1951, Obstetric reference of pregnant diabetics in the prediabetic period. Rev. Med. de Cordoba 39: 187.

3. Camerini-Davalos, R.A., Marble, A., Dhamdhere, M., Rees, S.B., Lawrence, D.G., and Freedlender, A., 1961, Development of methods for early detection of prediabetes, Proc IVth Intern Diabetes Federation, Geneva: 212.

4. Camerini-Davalos, R.A., Caulfield, J., Rees, S., Lozano-Castaneda, O., Naldjian, S., Marble, A., 1963, Preliminary observations on subjects with prediabetes. Diabetes 12: 508.

5. Camerini-Davalos, R.A., 1978, Early Diabetes. Concept. Terminology. In: Camerini-Davalos, R.A, Hanover, B., Eds., Treatment of Early Diabetes. New York and London, Plenum Press 119: 1-6.

6. Szabo, O., Oppermann, W., Victor, C., Camerini-Davalos, R.A., 1974, A new concept for the evaluation of the blood glucose and insulin responses of healthy subjects following an oral glucose load. Acta Diabetol Lat 11: 265-275.

7. Camerini-Davalos, R.A., Oppermann, W., Rebagliati, H., Glasser, M., Bloodworth, J.M.B., 1979, Muscle capillary basement membrane width in genetic prediabetes. J Clin Endocrinol Metab 48: 251-9.

8. Velasco, C.A., Oppermann, W., Camerini-Davalos, R.A., 1973, Critical variables in the radioimmunological technique for measuring immunoreactive insulin with use of immunosorbents. Clin Chem 19: 201-4.

9. Oppermann, W., Gugliucci, C., O'Sullivan, M.J., Hanover, B., Camerini-Davalos, R.A., 1974, Gestational Diabetes and Macrosomia. In: Camerini-Davalos, R.A., Cole, H.S., Eds, Early Diabetes in Early Life. New York, Academic Press Inc.: 455-68.

10. Zollner, N., 1980, Stoffwechselkrankheiten, Kohlenhydratstoffwechsel. In: Forth, W., Henschler, D., Rummel, W., eds., Pharmakologie und Toxikologie. Mannheim, Wissenschaftsverlag: 295.

LOW INSULIN RESPONSE: A MARKER OF PREDIABETES

¶Suad Efendic, Valdemar Grill, Rolf Luft and
Alexandre Wajngot

Department of Endocrinology, Karolinska Hospital
Stockholm, Sweden

It is generally accepted that genetic factors play a decisive role in
the development of non-insulin dependent diabetes (NIDDM). Accordingly,
the manifest disease develops gradually from a genetically determined initial
stage, prediabetes, over a stage characterized by a decrease in glucose
tolerance only. This process might be slow or rapid, possibly dependent on
the type and 'weight' of the genetic trait as well as on factors precipitat-
ing the disease.

Insulin responsiveness was best characterized by i.v. administration
of glucose (square wave or constant stimulus) known to induce a biphasic
insulin response. The first phase lasts about 10 min with the peak at 3-5
min. The second phase persists as long as glucose is given. It appeared
that in subjects with decreased intravenous glucose tolerance (IVGTT) only,
as well as in mild manifest diabetes, the first-phase insulin response to a
glucose infusion test (GIT) was diminished and often virtually abolished,
while the second phase could be preserved in patients with mild hyperglycemia
(1). In contrast, studies with other insulinogogues, such as tolbutamide,
glucagon and isoproterenal, showed that many mild NIDDM's responded normally
to these stimuli (2). These findings suggested that a deranged transmission
of the hyperglycemic signal to the cellular machinery controlling insulin
release (stimulus-secretion coupling) constitutes an early and possibly
the primary defect in NIDDM.

In the above studies Cerasi and Luft (1) included a large number of
healthy subjects and observed that 15-20% demonstrated a delayed and sluggish insulin response to glucose. They proposed that these subjects with
low insulin response and normal IVGTT - low insulin responders - are genetic
prediabetics. This presumption led in 1967 to the following hypothesis
regarding the pathogenesis of maturity onset diabetes (3): 1)a prerequisite
for the disease is a genetically determined condition, prediabetes, characterized by delayed and decreased insulin secretion; 2)additional diabetogenic factors may induce glucose intolerance in prediabetics by increasing
the demand for insulin, a condition which, when not delt with, leads to
decompensation of the metabolic equilibrium, with latent or manifest diabetes as a consequence; 3)a prediabetic subject is protected from the full
consequences of insulin deficiency by compensatory mechanisms which maintain
glycolysis and hepatic glucose output within normal limits.

Since the first presentation of the above hypothesis we have tried to elucidate a series of questions developing from the hypothesis. In the following we shall consider some important aspects of low insulin response:
- comparison of insulin and C-peptide responses in low insulin responders,
- insulin release and sensitivity as predictive factors for the development of NIDDM,
- impact of hereditary factors on insulin release,
- mechanisms responsible for low insulin response

KINETICS OF INSULIN RELEASE AND INSULIN SENSITIVITY

A quantitative analysis of the time dynamics of glucose-induced insulin secretion is complicated by the variation in glucose levels that occur during GIT. Another point of concern when comparing insulin responses among individuals relates to the extraction of insulin that takes place in the liver. Differences in hepatic extraction of insulin could thus, in theory, account for differences in peripheral insulin levels between individuals. Therefore we have evaluated, in two groups of low insulin responders (LIR) and in high insulin responders (HIR), insulin and C-peptide responses under constant hyperglycemia as achieved by the hyperglycemic clamp technique (Fig 1) (4). A second stimulation with glucose served to assess a priming effect of glucose. In order to put the findings in the perspective of pre-diabetes, the study also included a group of subjects with a high propensity to develop diabetes, namely, women with a history of gestational diabetes with a low insulin response to glucose and with a normal oral glucose tolerance (OGTT) after pregnancy.

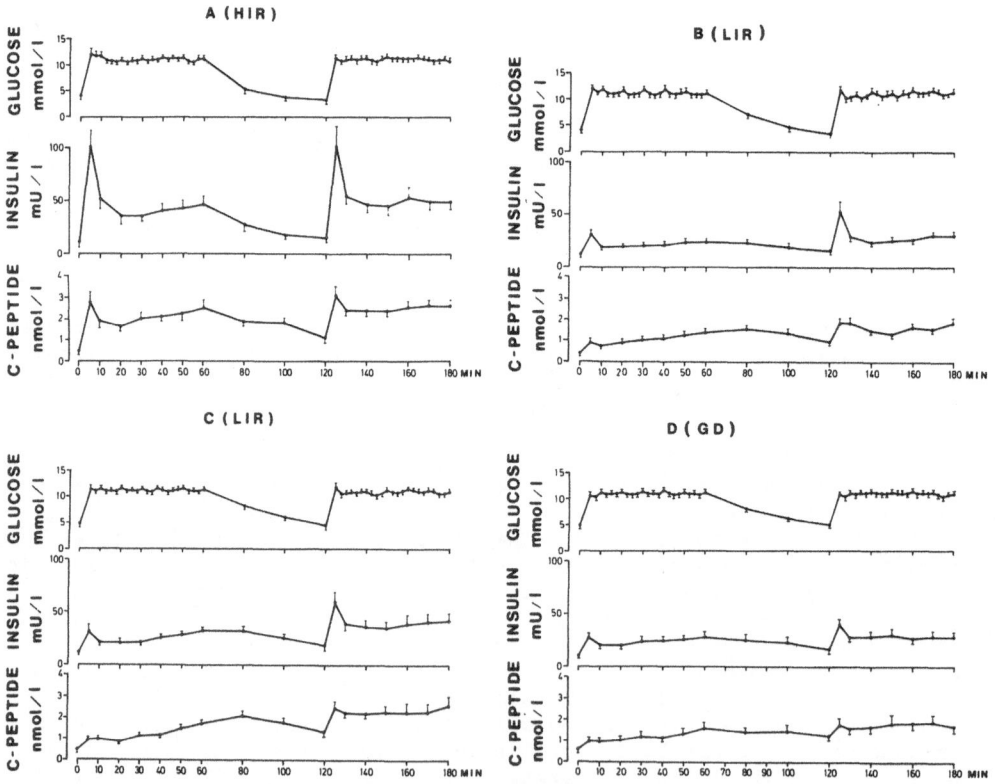

Figure 1. Effect of two sequential hyperglycemic clamps on glucose and insulin levels. Mean± SEM. A (HIR), high insulin responders; B (LIR), low insulin responders; C (LIR), low insulin responders; D (GD), previously gestational diabetes (4).

The hyperglycemic clamp used was modification of that introduced by DeFronzo et al (5). The procedure aimed to raise and maintain the level of blood glucose at 11 mmol/L. To this end, a bolus injection of glucose was injected and followed by a variable infusion of 15% solution of glucose during a 60 minute clamp period. Sixty minutes after the end of the first clamp, a second clamp was initiated. The level of hyperglycemia was similar during the first and the second clamp in all groups.

The elevated blood glucose induced a diphasic insulin release in all four groups of subjects. In comparison with other groups, HIR (group A) demonstrated higher insulin as well as C-peptide responses. No differences in insulin responses were observed between groups B, C and D with regard to the total or to the first or second phase of insulin and C-peptide secretion. After five minutes of hyperglycemic clamping ratios between incremental insulin and C-peptide levels were not significantly different between groups, which suggests a similar liver extraction of insulin. The second clamp raised insulin to levels that were significantly higher than during the first clamp with regard to first phase and mean 60 min levels in groups B and C, and with regard to first phase in group D. Neither first phase nor mean levels of insulin were significantly different between the two clamps in group A. Due to the long half-life of C-peptide, it was difficult to quantify a priming response from determinations of this peptide; however, the initial response seemed higher during the second than during the first clamp in groups B and C.

We concluded that a low insulin response in healthy subjects with a normal OGTT reflects a decreased endogenous insulin secretion and not an altered insulin extraction in the liver. This study confirmed previous observation that LIR were more sensitive than HIR to induction of a priming effect of glucose (6). The reason for this seemingly paradoxical observation is not clear. Although the LIR studied had, by definition, a normal glucose tolerance, it has been suggested that they may still have experienced somewhat larger glycemic excursions after meals than HIR. A mild and intermittent stimulation by glucose could then have increased the potential for inducing a priming effect. A different possibility could, however, also be envisioned. Thus, if lower demands on insulin secretion exist in some LIR, that condition could leave room for a larger priming effect because of a larger reserve capacity of the B-cell to respond.

FOLLOW UP STUDIES OF SUBJECTS WITH DIFFERENT GLUCOSE TOLERANCE

The subject material comprised 226 volunteers (7-9). They had normal fasting blood glucose (<5.2 mmol/1) and normal IVGTT (K-value > 1.0). In some of these subjects OGTT was borderline or decreased. A group of 10 subjects had decreased IVGTT.

Insulin response to GIT was evaluated by a mathematical model previously described in detail (10). The model assumes that glucose initiates insulin release, first, by an immediate action (parameter KI) and, second, by a time-dependent potentiating mechanism (parameter KP) which amplifies the former action. The sensitivity of tissues to insulin is measured by a further parameter, KG. Low insulin responders were arbitrarily defined as those with KI $\leqslant$ 0.30 and high responders or controls as those KI $>$ 0.30. From the above 236 subjects 111 were available and willing to submit themselves to a new OGTT 5-8 years after the first one. This group included the following subjects listed according to their original OGTT: 83 normal; 26 borderline OGTT; eight decreased OGTT and normal IVGTT; six decreased OGTT and IVGTT.

As shown in Fig 2, 11 normal subjects developed decreased OGTT or diabetes mellitus over a 7-year follow-up period. Nine of these originally demonstrated either low insulin response, KI<0.30, in combination with KG less than 80, or marked insulin resistance, KG<20. The one patient who developed diabetes had severely decreased insulin sensitivity as well as low insulin response.

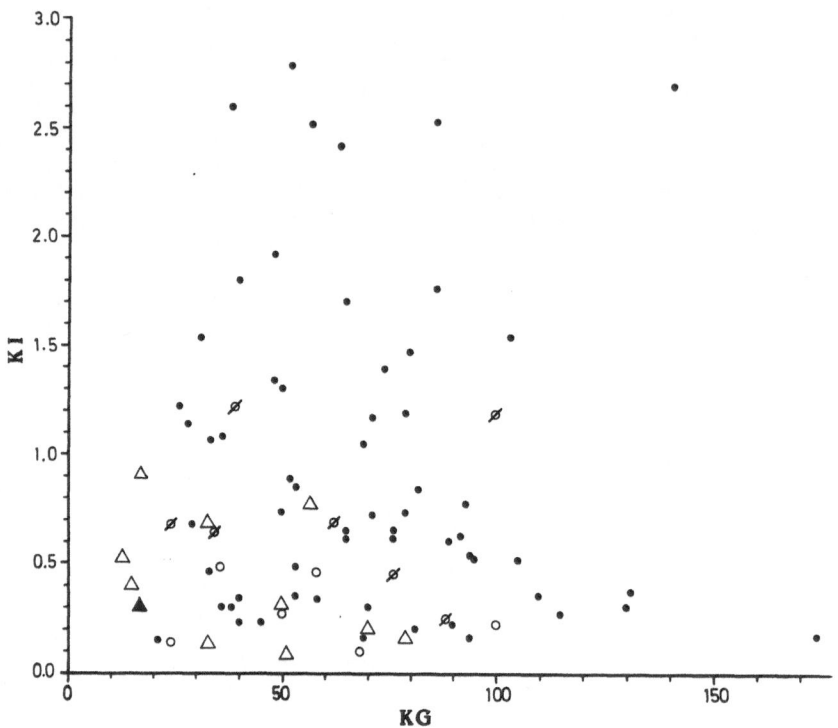

Figure 2. Impact of KG and KI on the development of type 2-diabetes. KG and KI were determined on the basis of GIT. All 83 subjects had normal OGTT at the initial investigation which was performed close to GIT. After a follow-up of 5-8 years they demonstrated a variety of glucose tolerances: normal (●); borderline-1 (0); borderline 2 (∅); decreased OGTT (△); and manifest diabetes (▲) (9).

Among the 26 subjects who initially showed borderline OGTT, 3 who were originally low insulin responders with decreased KG developed manifest diabetes or decreased OGTT only (Fig 3). Out of 8 subjects with initially decreased OGTT, 3 developed manifest diabetes (Fig 4). At the beginning of the study GIT showed severely impaired insulin release in all three. Three subjects in this group originally had a decreased OGTT with high insulin response during GIT, and none of these developed diabetes. Four out of 6 subjects with decreased IVGTT and low insulin response developed diabetes. Hence among subjects with decreased glucose tolerance those with a low insulin response run a risk to develop NIDDM during a follow-up period of 5-8 years.

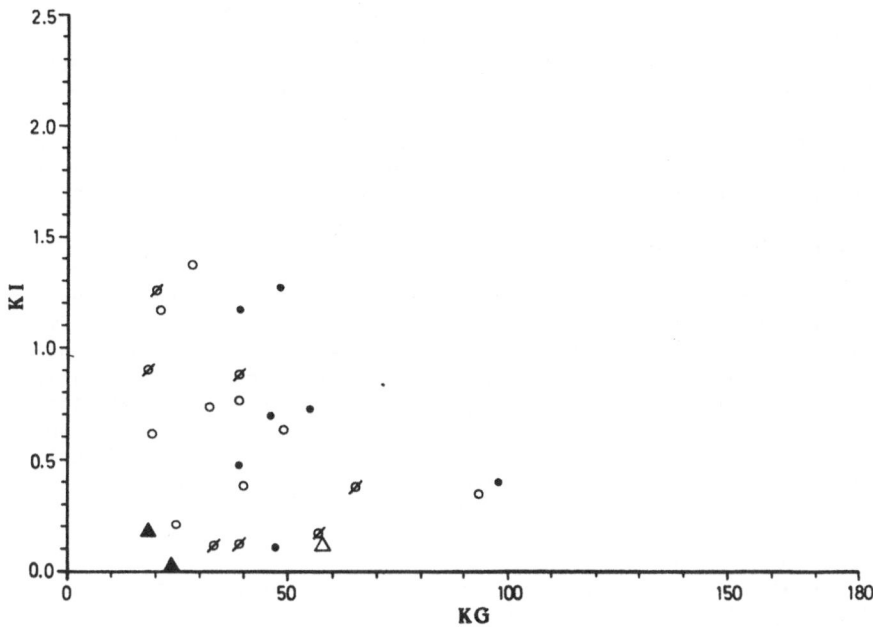

Figure 3. Follow-up of 26 subjects who demonstrated borderline glucose tolerance at the initial OGTT (see legend Fig 2) (9).

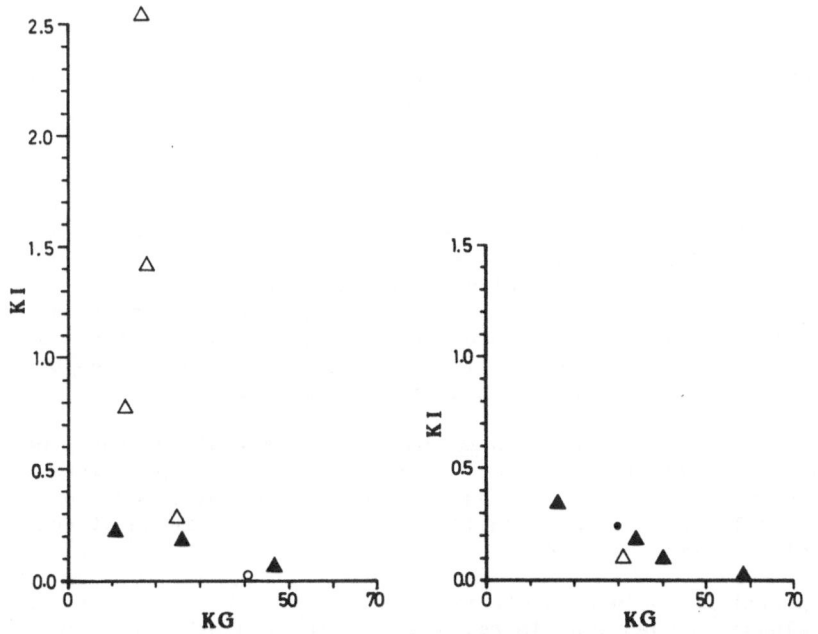

Figure 4. Follow-up of subjects with decreased OGTT and mormal IVGTT (left panel, n=8) and with impaired OGTT and decreased IVGTT (right panel, n=6) at the initial investigation (see legend to Fig 2) (9).

Studies of Kosaka et al (11) have also emphasized the importance of low insulin response for the development of NIDDM. In 39 out of 330 subjects, equivocal diabetes progressed to overt diabetes during a mean follow up period of 3.3 years. In all these 39 subjects, insulin response was subnormal at the initial glucose tolerance test and remained low throughout the follow-up period, during which glucose tolerance varied, being normal, borderline or decreased at different times. The later study as well as the present one indicates, firstly, that low insulin response is either a primary event or at least an early marker in most instances of NIDDM. Secondly, they demonstrate that a substantial number of subjects with decreased glucose tolerance and decreased insulin response develop manifest diabetes although the exact percentage may vary depending on a number of factors.

IMPACT OF HEREDITARY FACTORS ON INSULIN RELEASE

Plasma insulin response to glucose infusion was measured in 52 non-diabetic family units consisting of the proband, his parents, children and sibs. In addition, 24 monozygous and 29 dizygous like-sexed twin pairs were studied. The blood glucose and plasma insulin curves of each individual were used for analysis of the principal eigen-values, which were then used for the selection of compound variables, characterizing the relationship between the glucose and insulin curves. After correction for changes of sex, age, and body weight, and standardization with regard to mean and variance, the heritability of the compound variables was evaluated. When the hypothesis of heritability alone was fitted to the data, the chi-square values for the residual variance were non-significant. In contrast, when the hypothesis of the common environmental component alone was tested, highly significant residual chi-squares were obtained. Therefore, these findings indicate that insulin response to glucose is indeed genetically regulated. In this study, the magnitude of the familiar correlation for some of the variables was 0.32-0.72, the highest figure reflecting early insulin response.

Thus, genetic factors are of major significance for the responsiveness of the beta-cell to glucose, in spite of the fact that a number of environmental factors - such as nutritional state, stress, physical training, etc - influence insulin response in a significant manner.

MECHANISMS RESPONSIBLE FOR LOW INSULIN RESPONSE

In subjects with low insulin response and even in some maturity-onset diabetics the maximal response of the pancreas to glucose, expecially the late response, may look normal but the threshold glucose concentrations - needed to elicit release of insulin - are higher than in controls. Thus, for diabetics the glucose-insulin dose-response curve is displaced towards the right of the control curve in a parallel manner in diabetics during intravenous and during oral glucose loading. The situation in the LIR is intermediate, between responses in diabetics and normals.

Although it may be hazardous to draw firm conclusions from studies in man in whom, for example, a maximal insulin response can practically never be achieved, we believe that the basic defect in the mild forms of diabetes manifests itself as decreased sensitivity of the recognition of the beta-cell for glucose (increased Km).

The prevailing opinion about the molecular basis of glucose initiated insulin release is that insulin release is triggered by glucose metabolism in the beta-cell. Accordingly the increased K_m for glucose in prediabetics and diabetics could be ascribed to impairment of glucose metabolism of the beta-cells.

DISCUSSION

It is well known that some healthy subjects run an increased risk to develop diabetes. They have been termed potential diabetics. Recognizing this, the WHO Expert Committee on Diabetes Mellitus in 1964 stated that the period of time from onset to the diagnosis of an episode of diabetes of any defined severity should be termed prediabetes. The term should be used retrospectively. Already in 1967, Cerasi and Luft defined the prediabetic state in NIDDM on the basis of measureable criteria, and proposed low insulin response to glucose in the presence of normal IVGTT to be a characteristic feature of this state. This approach was based on the assumption that the insulin response to glucose is mainly genetically determined.

Over the years, evidence has accumulated which is compatible with the above hypothesis. First of all, it has been established that a low insulin response could be accounted for by a defective insulin secretion and is not related to hepatic insulin extraction. Secondly, the similarity of insulin response in monozygotic twin pairs, where one sibling was non-diabetic and the other had NIDDM, has been demonstrated at length. Thirdly, a follow-up of a large group of volunteers with normal IVGTT showed that low insulin responders run a higher risk of developing glucose intolerance. Finally it has been established that insulin response to glucose is mainly controlled by heredity, while other factors play a secondary role in this connection.

The molecular basis of diabetic heredity is not clarified. The biochemical background of the deranged insulin responsiveness in NIDDM is not fully characterized either. We believe that the latter defect resides in impaired glucose metabolism in the beta-cell, resulting in a deranged transmission of the hyperglycemic signal to the cellular machinery controlling insulin release.

REFERENCES

1. Cerasi, E., Luft, R., 1967, The plasma insulin response to glucose infusion in healthy subjects and in diabetes mellitus. Acta Endocrinol (Copenh) 55: 278-304.

2. Luft, R., Efendic, S., 1979, Low insulin response - genetic aspects and implications. Horm Metab Res 11: 415-454.

3. Cerasi, E., Luft, R., 1967, 'What is inherited - what is added'; hypothesis for the pathogenesis of diabetes mellitus. Diabetes 16: 615-627.

4. Grill, V., Efendic, S., 1987, Studies of high and low insulin responders with the hyperglycemic clamp technique. Metabolism 36: 1125-1131.

5. De Fronzo, R.A., Tobin, J.D., Andres, R., 1979, Glucose clamp technique: A method for quantifying insulin secretion and resistance. AM J Physiol 237: E214-E223.

6. Cerasi, E., 1975, Potentiation of insulin release by glucose in man. III. Normal recognition of glucose as a potentiator in subjects with low insulin response and in mild diabetes. Acta Endocrinol (Copenh) 79: 511-534.

7. Efendic S., Cerasi, E., Elander, I., 1980, Studies on low insulin responders. Acta Endocrinol (Copenh) 90: 1-32.

8. Efendic, S., Wajngot, A., Cerasi, E., Luft, R., 1980, Insulin release, insulin sensitivity, and glucose intolerance. Proc Natl Acad Sci USA 77: 7425-7429.

9. Efendic, S., Luft, R., Wajngot, A., 1984, Aspects of the patho-genesis of type 2 diabetes. Endocrine Rev 5: 395-410.

10. Cerasi, E., Fick, G., Rudemo, M., 1974, A mathematical model for the glucose induced insulin release in man. Eur J Clin Invest 4: 267-278.

11. Kosaka, K., Hagura, R., Kuzuya, T., 1977, Insulin responses in equivocal and definite diabetes, with special reference to subjects who had mild glucose intolerance but later developed definite diabetes. Diabetes 26: 944-952.

STUDY OF GLUCOSE REMOVAL RATE AND FIRST PHASE INSULIN SECRETION
IN THE OFFSPRING OF TWO PARENTS WITH NON-INSULIN-DEPENDENT DIABETES

¶James H. Warram*, Blaise C. Martin*, J. Stuart Soeldner+
and Andrzej S. Krolewski*

*Joslin Diabetes Center, Boston, Mass.
+University of California at Davis Medical Center, Sacramento, Calif.

Is non-insulin-dependent diabetes (NIDDM) a disease of insulin deficiency, a disease of insulin resistance, or both? This problem has con-
fronted diabetologists and researchers for years.

Perhaps, this question would not have remained unanswered so long if
individuals who are going to develop diabetes were marked or labeled in
some way that could be detected readily. If that were the case, it would
have been possible to follow these individuals in order to observe successive steps of the pathogenesis of diabetes. However, we are unable to
recognize them until many metabolic disturbances are already present; therefore, we have not been able to witness the temporal sequence of appearance
of insulin resistance and insulin deficiency. If there is a distinct order
to their appearance, this would be strong evidence that the first to appear
is the more basic defect.

While a specific marker does not exist, it has long been recognized
that NIDDM diabetes is more common in relatives of cases than in the
general population; therefore, a family history of diabetes can be thought
of as a marker (1). Presumably the evidence in this type of marker would
be strongest in the children of cases since parent-child pairs share more
genes than any other type of pairs of relatives except identical twins.
Moreover, this marker would be even better if both parents have NIDDM. In
fact, this approach was undertaken by investigators at the Joslin Diabetes
Center who began a follow-up study of the offspring of two diabetic parents.
At that time, there was no way to know what the incidence rate of diabetes
would be in the offspring. However, about 200 families were identified
through the patients of the Joslin Clinic and information on their 606 offspring gathered by questionnaire and telephone interviews.

Recently, we at the Joslin Diabetes Center have reviewed the accumulated data on the men and women in this cohort of offspring. The supposition
of the investigators who started this project has been born out: individuals who have both a mother and a father with NIDDM, have a very high probability of developing diabetes sometime during their lifetime. This is
clearly seen in Figure 1. In the study population of offspring of two
parents with NIDDM, the cumulative risk of diabetes by age 65 is 44%. This
is five times the risk at that age in the general population, represented
here by the Framingham Heart Study Population (2). Moreover, median age
at onset was a few years younger than in the general population. This

demonstrates very effectively that the population of offspring of diabetic parents is highly enriched with individuals who are predisposed to NIDDM, although the specific nature of the predisposition remains unknown.

By studying such populations, it is possible to examine some aspects of the predisposition in order to shape hypotheses about it. For example, when this population was stratified according to the age at onset of diabetes in the parents, the results suggested that the predisposition included the age at which diabetes would manifest itself. If both parents had the onset of diabetes before age 50, the offspring had their onset about 15 years earlier than if both parents had their onset after age 50 (Figure 2). If only one parent had the onset of diabetes before age 50 and the other had the onset after age 50, the onsets in the offspring were intermediate between the other two groups.

Tracking of the age at onset from one generation to another could be the result of a genetic mechanism or familial environment or behavioral pattern. This could be the basis for an hypotheses about the failure of a genetically determined metabolic process which is triggered by some maturation process. Alternative hypotheses could be developed about the role of environment in families with an early onset versus those with late onsets. For example, obesity is conceded to be an important risk factor for NIDDM diabetes (2). This association is clearly demonstrated in the offspring of two parents with NIDDM diabetes, where the risk of developing NIDDM diabetes was 29% by age 50 in those who were obese (ideal body weight greater than 125%) but only 2% in those who were lean (ideal body weight less than 110%). One could undertake a study in this population of offspring to investigate a hypothesis that the familial clustering of the age at onset of diabetes can be explained by familial clustering of obesity, or more precisely, the age at onset of obesity.

The results presented so far demonstrate the value of a population of offspring of two parents with NIDDM diabetes for conducting studies of the prediabetic stages that precede the clinical onset of diabetes mellitus. Because these individuals are at high risk, it is possible to observe the onset of diabetes in enough cases to test a variety of hypotheses. More-

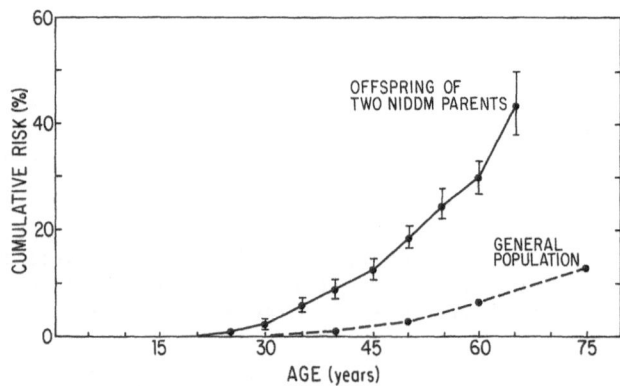

Figure 1. Cumulative risk of diabetes in offspring of two parents with non-insulin-dependent diabetes. The parents (158 families) were ascertained from among the patients of the Joslin Clinic. Data for the general population were derived from incidence rates of diabetes in the Framingham Heart Study (2). Cumulative incidence of diabetes according to attained age is the net cumulative risk obtained using life table techniques.

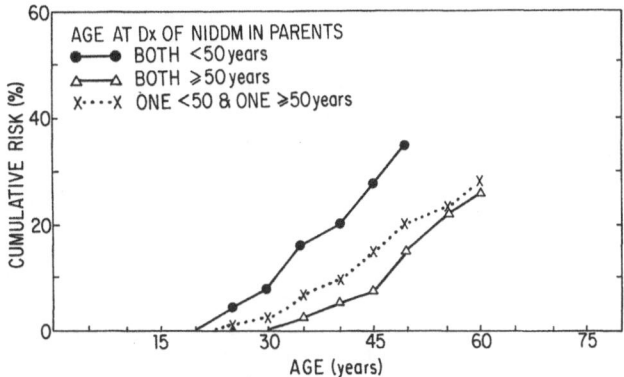

Figure 2. Cumulative risk of diabetes in offspring of two parents
with non-insulin-dependent diabetes according to age at
onset of diabetes in the parents. The population of offspring is the same as that shown in Figure 1.

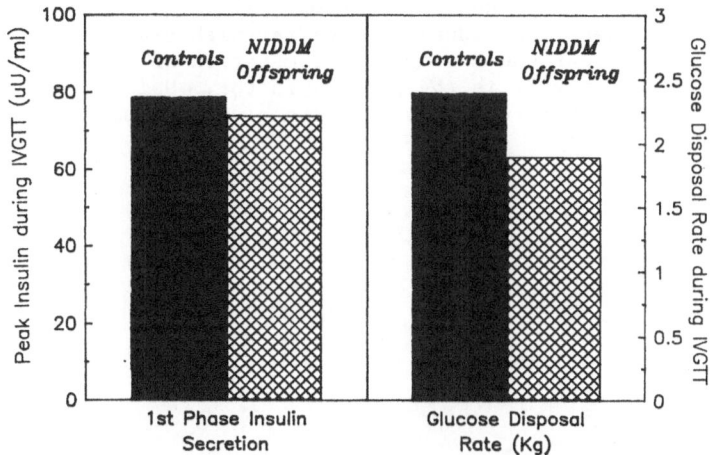

Figure 3. Comparison of insulin secretion and glucose disposal during intravenous glucose tolerance test in a group of normoglycemic offspring (n = 165) of two parents with non-
insulin-dependent diabetes and in normoglycemic individuals
(n = 203) without a family history of diabetes.

over, it is important to emphasize that the studies do not have to be as
general as the examples that have been given. More interesting than the
number of offspring with NIDDM diabetes are the physiologic data that it
was possible to obtain on them before the disease developed.

For this analysis, we selected only the offspring with normal glucose
tolerance by NDDG criteria when they were first seen for follow-up. Average
age was 32 years and average weight was 114 of ideal body weight. All had
normal fasting glucose, range 56 to 98 mg/dl with a mean of 70 mg/dl, and
normal 2-hour glucose, range 43 to 139 mg/dl with a mean of 97 mg/dl. There
were two questions that were posed in studying this population: (1) Does
this group differ from the general population with regard to insulin sensitivity and insulin secretion, and (2) if so, does that characteristic which

is different from the general population also predict those individuals who eventually develop diabetes?

From an intravenous glucose tolerance test one can obtain a measure of insulin secretory capacity, i.e. first phase insulin response, and a measure of insulin sensitivity, i.e. the insulin stimulated glucose disposal rate of K_g. First phase insulin response was defined here as the peak rise in serum insulin above basal during the first five minutes of the IVGTT, and K_g was estimated from the linear portion of the exponential fall in blood glucose after the first five minutes of the IVGTT. When compared to non-diabetic controls, who have no history of any type of diabetes in a first or second degree relative, the offspring of two NIDDM patents and controls had very similar measures of insulin secretion (Figure 3). By contrast, slow glucose removal rates were significantly more common in the offspring population. Thus in answer to the first question, these individuals with a high risk of developing NIDDM have relatively normal insulin secretion but an excess of individuals with low glucose disposal rates even when they have normal glucose tolerance.

Turning to the second question, we looked to see whether the glucose removal rate also predicted which individuals progressed to diabetes during follow-up. Of course, many subtleties complicate a comparison of these two populations since these individuals may differ with regard to age and body weight in ways that confound a simple determination of whether insulin secretion or insulin sensitivity is the primary factor. Using a multivariate analysis of all risk factors we found that the glucose removal rate K_g at the

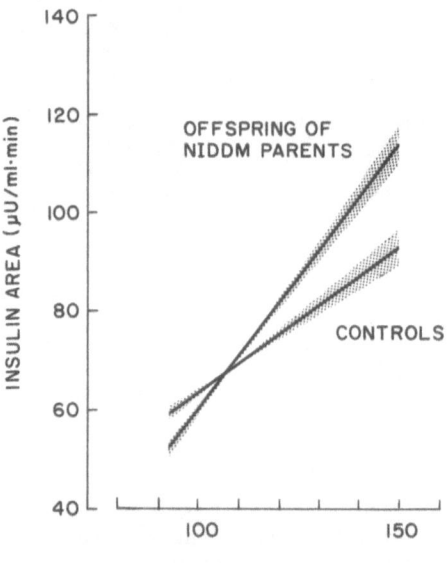

PERCENT OF IDEAL BODY WEIGHT

Figure 4. Stimulated insulin levels during oral glucose tolerance test as a function of ideal body weight in offspring of two parents with non-insulin-dependent diabetes and controls. Stimulated insulin level is represented as the insulin area above baseline during a three hour oral glucose tolerance test. Each line represents the regression slope of the insulin response on percent ideal body weight. The shaded area around each line represents one standard error of the slope. The difference between the slopes is significant at the 0.05 level.

first examination was the single most important predictor of the development of diabetes during the subsequent 13 years of observation. For example, an individual at the 25th percentile of the distribution of K_g had an 8.5 fold higher risk of developing Type II diabetes than an individual at the 75th percentile. On the other hand, an individual at the 25th percentile of the distribution of first phase insulin response had only a 1.3 fold higher risk than an individual at the 75th percentile. Furthermore, in the multivariate analysis, 2-hour post challenge blood glucose, ideal body weight, and age at the time of study all had less than a doubling effect on the risk of developing NIDDM. Therefore, it appears that the major factor predicting the risk of diabetes is not impaired insulin secretion but is slow glucose disposal, and this we believe to be evidence of underlying insulin resistance.

Given the evidence presented previously that obesity is an important risk factor for NIDDM, the findings in the multivariate analysis regarding the roles of obesity and glucose removal rate are surprising. When the two factors were examined simultaneously, we found that the risk of development of NIDDM was mainly related to a low K_g and only weakly related to obesity. This find can be explained if one postulates that obesity is associated with insulin resistance in some individuals but not in others, and that obesity has its effect on the risk of diabetes mainly in those with slow glucose removal. This interesting hypothesis requires additional study.

Some support for the hypothesis that obesity assumes an important role only in individuals with a predisposition to diabetes comes from a comparison of the offspring of two parents with NIDDM with the control population of individuals with no first or second degree relatives with diabetes. When we measured stimulated insulin levels during an oral glucose tolerance test as a function of ideal body weight, the insulin level rose in heavier individuals, presumably as a result of increasing insulin resistance (Figure 4). However, this linear relation between insulin levels and obesity in the offspring of two diabetic parents differed markedly from that in the control population. For each increment in obesity, individuals who have a genetic predisposition to diabetes increased their insulin resistance twice as much as controls. Thus obesity is not an additive factor in determining the risk of NIDDM, but interacts synergistically with whatever gene or genes there are for diabetes or insulin resistance.

In summary, the offspring of two parents with NIDDM constitute a rich population for studying the pathophysiology of prediabetic states. Preliminary data from a follow-up study of such a population suggest that a state of insulin resistance precedes the development of a relative insulin deficiency and the subsequent emergence of clinical diabetes.

REFERENCES

1. Simpson, N.E., 1969, Heritabilities of liability to diabetes when sex and age at onset are considered. Ann Hum Gen 32: 283-303.

2. Krolewski, A.S. and Warram, J.H., 1985, Epidemiology of Diabetes Mellitus. In: Marble, A., Krall, L.P., Bradley, R.F., Christlieb. A.R., Soeldner, J.S., eds., Joslin's Diabetes Mellitus. Philadelphia, Lea & Febiger: 12-42.

DISCUSSION

H. LAUBE: Dr. Camerini, in your studies how often did patients with an impaired glucose tolerance eventually become overt diabetics?

R. CAMERINI-DAVALOS: After 10-15 years of the first abnormality in the OGTT, around 30% of our subjects would be overt diabetics, or around 2-3% per year.

B. WAJCHENBERG: Dr. Efendic, you mentioned that in those with impaired glucose tolerance there is a question of the glucagon secretion rate. As in diabetes, you have an increase glucagon secretion.

S. EFENDIC: You mean it's decreased suppression?

B. WAJCHENBERG: Decreased suppression and the basal level of glucagon was quite increased from a normal of around 20 picograms. Four times more the basal values. Dr. Warram, you know the data of the value of the IVGTT that Richard Bergman has postulated in his model. Did you compare the KG with the sensitivity index, because we found very significant discrepancies between the KG and the sensitivity in the index. If the KG would be a good marker of peripheral resistance in well known cases, you should have a parallel change in both and we, as Bergman, could not find that. Therefore, did you recalculate your data?

J. WARRAM: You're just a little faster than we are. Now, I have Bergman's model operating in our laboratory with 1000 IVGTT's. The preliminary work we've done so far is looking at a difference between the controls and the offspring in two diabetic parents and we find differences in the insulin sensitivity between the offspring and the controls. Now, I haven't gone to the next step of seeing if that is the predictor of who goes on to diabetes.

S. EFENDIC: Just a comment. The statement which I've made is based on the computer elevation of insulin response and insulin sensitivity, and I think that's very essential to evaluate an insulin response in relation to the prevailing blood glucose levels. Otherwise, it's very difficult to evaluate insulin responses.

G. GRODSKY: I think the question was already handled and this is an old debate we hear and nothing seems to change, and the old question of obesity still comes in. When you discussed, Dr. Warram, that your studies were preliminary, the last studies that you showed us which put the resistance primary, are you sure that study was also controlled for obesity and that you got the same data with it?

J. WARRAM: Well, we've approached obesity in several different ways. As you noticed, in the first slide, you get a very pronounced separation of the risk in the offspring according to the level of obesity. And, so it's a little surprising that when you start a file by obesity and K rate, K rate dominates and in the multivariant model the effect of obesity is still there a little bit, bit it is overwhelmed by the effect of the K rate. And, this is readily explained. I can show you some data, later perhaps, some people when they become obese become insulin resistant and some do not. And, actually we plotted so that if someone becomes obese, but not insulin resistant, then in the multivariant model their insulin resistance is what's going to dominate not the obesity. We went back to the comparison of the control group and the offspring group, and if you plot the relationship between their relative body weight and their insulin resistance you find that the insulin resistance goes up much more steeply. You get very different slopes in the controls and in the offspring. You get a very general slope in the control population, but in the offspring population there's a very steep increase in insulin resistance as the percent of ideal body weight increases. And, so maybe this obesity is a trigger for whatever the underlying mechanism is, but the underlying mechanism is what seems to be more important in terms of predicting who is going to go on to develop diabetes.

J. HOET: Dr. Camerini, what was the weight of your prediabetics?

R. CAMERINI-DAVALOS: We studied only those within 15% of ideal body weight.

G. GRODSKY: Two investigators showed us today that by 40 or 50 minutes, in a glucose tolerance test, the levels of insulin that were measured were normal or sometimes higher than normal and it's an old observation. It's that delayed hyperinsulin response. We would anticipate that any time you have a defect in final terminal release of insulin, that the provisionary phenomenon, the potentiating phenomenon, goes on and will fight its way against that terminal release and later you'll get insulin release. You may get the same area of insulin in a 45 or 60 minute glucose tolerance test in someone with a terribly abnormal release system, terminal release, compared to a normal. And, so I think that those people who are measuring late insulin release have to be very careful in how they interpret that data since that represents the bulk of the insulin that goes into the blood. Then, you have to worry about measuring the total area. I appreciate the problem, but one should understand the weakness of late measurements of insulin.

R. CAMERINI-DAVALOS: Dr. Grodsky, what do you call late?

G. GRODSKY: I would say anything after 30 minutes is late. And, I'm sort of taking the outside time.

R. CAMERINI-DAVALOS: Dr. Soeldner and I have been going through two IV's in a short time.

G. GRODSKY: I was very sensitive of the fact that you were not doing what I'm talking about, but I'm just making a general remark. I think a short IV tells you whether you're going to have impairment or not. A longer tells you about the second phase. But, anything other than that, I think, is very difficult. Any measurements that are solely into the second phase tell you very little unless they're low. If they're low, then you know you've got an impairment. But, if they're normal, that doesn't mean that you have had a normal response of the beta cell. It means that you could have had a delayed response caused by a defect.

A. REDDI: Dr. Warram, you have identified those offspring who are at increased risk for diabetes. What steps are you taking to prevent the progression of diabetes and its complications?

J. WARRAM: I'm doing nothing, Dr. Reddi.

A. REDDI: I mean, are you suggesting a dietary control?

J. WARRAM: I think that we will reach the point where we would like to do something 13 years before the onset of diabetes, rather than at the time it starts. And, it would be nice if this study would lead to that kind of information on which to base that rationally, but at the moment we don't have enough understanding to intervene at this point.

In looking at some of these individuals over 15 or 20 years, there are individuals who become very insulin resistant, have very high fasting insulins, very high insulin response to the oral glucose tolerance test, very high insulin on the IVGTT and they don't become diabetic, at least they haven't yet. They clearly have beta cells that are able to withstand this continued pressure. There are others where seemingly their beta cells collapse fairly quickly. Some people seem to be able to endure enormous insulin resistance so that there must be some additional defect when the beta cell fails and this, too, may be genetically determined.

F. PUCHULU: Dr. Efendic, any relationship between the low insulin responders and the insulin gene polymorphism? Did you find some relationship between both?

S. EFENDIC: It's just the low insulin response during the early phase, which is interesting. It would imply that the insulin gene can be in some way related to secretion coupling mechanisms.

C. DOMINGUEZ: About 10 years ago, we measured glucose tolerance and insulin production during oral glucose tolerance tests in about 70 patients that were offsprings of at least one diabetic parent. What we did was to feed that patient at least 350 gms of carbohydrate during the 5-7 days prior to the test and we found the following: First, the offspring are slightly hyperglycemic although none of them reached the level of diabetes. Second, the 30 minute insulin was lower in the offsprings of diabetics than in the controls. Third, the level of insulin at 30 minutes was positively correlated with the level of blood sugar, relative body weight and the basal insulin. If you compare insulin at 30 minutes with these three variables, the offspring always have lower insulin secretion at 30 minutes. At 120 minutes, things get complicated. It appears that those that have a low insulin secretion at 30 minutes, have a little higher blood sugar at 120 minutes, and at that time serum insulin is high, too. But, in our population we found more frequent low insulin production than normal insulin production. To complicate things a little more, if we did comparisons for the same level of serum insulin the offspring had slightly higher blood sugars. The offspring also had slightly, but significantly lower, serum insulin. So, it looks like two things are going on together here. Or, perhaps type 2 diabetes is a heterogeneous disease and the offspring are not the same.

J. BARBOSA: I think we already know now that obesity is heterogeneous. We know that there are the apples and the pears, and I think this is very important, because apparently insulin resistance is quite different in the apples, versus the pears, so I think it is time to take that into consideration in any of these studies.

J. WARRAM: The data that I was presenting just now was recorded 8-23 years ago, but it is the only way that you can get a clear picture of the sequence of things.

R. RAMERINI-DAVALOS: Dr. Efendic, I was a little bit confused about your terminology, because you called gestational diabetics prediabetics, and I really was confused about what was normal and what was abnormal. I think

182

Stu Soeldner and I have a large number of normal control subjects. In fact, I have now almost 400. We always compare our prediabetics with controls by age and sex. Now, I like to be sure that when you call your patients prediabetic you are talking about subjects with normal blood sugars, whatever test you use, compared with the controls of similar age and sex.

S. EFENDIC: They have diabetes during pregnancy and at the moment when we investigate them they have completely normal glucose tolerance and they have always impaired insulin response. Most of them have completely normal insulin sensitivity. We take as strong evidence that the insulin release defect precedes insulin resistance.

R. CAMERINI-DAVALOS: You see I have been penalized. I have been using the term, prediabetics, for those subjects before any abnormal tolerance to glucose. Now, you've called gestational diabetics subjects with normal blood sugar.

S. EFENDIC: No, no, no. You see diabetes is a dynamic state. You start with prediabetes, you go to manifest diabetes, but from manifest diabetes you can go to prediabetes if you have a normal glucose tolerance. Prediabetes to us is arbitrary criteria where a patient has completely normal glucose tolerance. If somebody has had gestational diabetes, then has a completely normal glucose tolerance, then we call it prediabetes.

R. CAMERINI-DAVALOS: I think the audience should be clear about that. That they call, at least Dr. Efendic calls, subjects prediabetes who already had an abnormal tolerance to glucose or even abnormal blood sugars that went back to normal. We never use that criteria. For us, when a subject crosses the barrier he can never be, again, a prediabetic. In fact, we published a paper with Drs. Marble and Soeldner about this. Many of them go back and forth, but once they cross, we never call them prediabetics anymore. So, it's all right if you define that, but the audience should be aware that we're talking about different groups of people.

ANTECEDENT EVENTS FOR NON-INSULIN DEPENDENT DIABETES MELLITUS

¶Peter H. Bennett, Clifton Bogardus, William C. Knowler, and Stephen Lillioja

National Institutes of Health, National Institute of Arthritis
Diabetes and Digestive and Kidney Diseases
Phoenix, Arizona Epidemiology and Clinical Research Branch

During the past decade there has been a proliferation of knowledge concerning non-insulin dependent diabetes. International acceptance of a classification of diabetes has contributed to this development in that non-insulin dependent diabetes (NIDDM) was clearly separated from insulin-dependent diabetes (IDDM), and the term impaired glucose tolerance (IGT) was introduced to describe a category of subjects who had glucose tolerance which was above the limits seen in normal healthy young adults, but which fell below the levels considered diagnostic of NIDDM (1). The diagnostic criteria for NIDDM were also reconsidered, first by the National Diabetes Data Group (NDDG) and later by the World Health Organization (WHO). This resulted in internationally accepted criteria for the diagnosis of diabetes.

Both these developments were important insofar as they introduced a degree of uniformity in characterizing these diseases and provided a framework for prospective epidemiological and clinical investigations that has served to advance knowledge of the etiology and pathogenesis of both forms of the disease. NIDDM was subdivided in the NDDG and WHO classifications into a non-obese and an obese form. While the distinction between these two types in etiologic terms is probably not clear-cut, the obese type is certainly the predominant form in most populations.

PHASES IN DEVELOPMENT OF NIDDM

The pathogenesis of NIDDM can be conveniently divided into four phases: genetic susceptibility, insulin resistance, IGT and NIDDM itself. Each of these phases occurs in all subjects who ultimately develop the disease.

GENETIC SUSCEPTIBILITY

While the exact mode of inheritance of NIDDM is uncertain there is overwhelming evidence that the majority of persons with NIDDM inherit a susceptibility which predisposes them to the disease. While NIDDM is certainly a heterogeneous disorder, the nature of the genetic susceptibility for some of the rarer NIDDM syndromes has been elucidated. Such syndromes include diabetes associated with Leprechaunism, Type A insulin resistance and those forms of the disease which result from genetic disorders of either the insulin or insulin-receptor gene, or the manner in which the precursors

of insulin are processed. However, the identity of the genetic susceptibility that leads to NIDDM in the majority of subjects is currently lacking, although there are several lines of evidence which indicate its presence.

Evidence that NIDDM is primarily a genetic disorder first emerged from
studies of twins (2). The rate of disease concordance in identical twins is
considerably greater than that seen in non-identical twins or siblings.
This indicates that there is genetic susceptibility to the disorder but
gives no information about whether or not the disorder is caused by one
or many genes, and whether or not it follows a dominant or recessive mode
of inheritance. Futhermore, evidence from the twin studies does not preclude the possibility that there are several distinct disorders that lead
to the same phenotype. There are, however, populations, such as the Pima
Indians and Nauruans, that are relatively homogeneous and isolated, who have
inordinate prevalences of the disease suggesting that the majority of those
affected in the same population have the same type of NIDDM. While twin
studies have not been possible in these populations because of their limited
size, other evidence of genetic susceptibility among them has been obtained.

In both the Nauruans (3) and the Pima, NIDDM shows familial aggregation and the prevalence of diabetes is a direct function of the degree of
genetic admixture. The age-sex adjusted prevalence of diabetes in full-
blooded Pima Indians is much higher than seen in subjects of Caucasian ancestry. Even though living in the same environment, those of non-Indian
ancestry have an age-sex adjusted prevalence of the disease which is only
one-half that of full-blooded Pima Indians and those of half-Pima, half-
Caucasian ancestry have an intermediate prevalence. Very similar findings
have been reported in Nauru. The occurrence of a disease in high frequencies in one ethnic group and much lower frequencies in another ethnic group
and intermediate frequencies in mixed bloods when living in the same envir-
onmetn is evidence that the disease has a genetic basis.

Other evidence of the genetic nature of the susceptibility to NIDDM
comes from studies of associations between the disease and other genetically determined characteristics. There are many examples of such studies.
In Mexican-Americans, for example, the prevalence of diabetes is a function
of several genetic markers such as the haptoglobin and rhesus blood groups,
and these point to the relative frequency of American Indian and non-Indian
genes as a determinant of the frequency to NIDDM (4). In the Pima Indians,
as well as some other populations such as the Xhosa of South Africa and
Asian Indians from South Africa and Fiji, associations between the frequency
of NIDDM and certain HLA markers have been demonstrated (5). In the Pima
Indians HLA-A2 is associated with higher frequencies of NIDDM than other
HLA types and this is true even among putatively full-blood Pima Indians.
This association, which so far has not been supported by genetic linkage
studies, suggests that there is a gene in linkage disequilibrium with the
HLA locus which either confers susceptibility or modifies the expression
of the diabetes gene or genes.

Other features of NIDDM which provide additional support for genetic
susceptibility as a prerequisite to the development of the disease come
from studies of pedigrees in the populations with high NIDDM frequencies.
In both the Pima and Nauruans the familial pattern of disease according to
segregation analysis is best explained by the inheritance of a major gene
with a dosage effect, i.e. co-dominance (6). Although the interpretation
of pedigree data in populations where the disease is so frequent is difficult, if these conclusions are correct, it should be possible to map the
chromosomal location of the putative gene or genes concerned by using restriction fragment length polymorphism analysis. Such studies have not
yet been performed.

INSULIN RESISTANCE

Insulin resistance was found to be characteristic of subjects with NIDDM in the late 1960s. It was shown that subjects with latent or chemical diabetes, who would now be described as having IGT, showed evidence of insulin resistance (7). Thus, the question as to whether insulin resistance might be the pathophysiological basis for the development of NIDDM was raised. Plasma insulin levels following a glucose load were found to follow an inverted U-shaped distribution when mean levels were plotted against the level of glucose tolerance. On average serum insulin levels among those with IGT or mild diabetes were higher than in persons with unequivocally normal glucose tolerance. Futhermore, it was recognized that obesity was associated with even higher insulin levels than seen among the non-obese (8). However, at this time the mechanism underlying insulin levels represented mutant insulins, an excess of insulin precursors, or whether the high insulin levels were the response to abnormalities of the target tissues, and in particular the insulin receptor. Primarily through a tedious process of exclusion, it became apparent that the most likely explanation for insulin resistance was that target tissues were less responsive to insulin and that insulin-mediated glucose disposal was defective. The development and application of the techniques for glucose and insulin clamping showed that the mechanism of insulin resistance in most subjects with IGT and mild diabetes was a post-binding receptor defect in insulin action 99). In the meantime, however, abnormalities of insulin action that were due to abnormalities of the insulin itself or its processing, e.g. mutant insulin and hyperproinsulinemia, the presence of anti-insulin receptor antibodies and abnormalities of the insulin receptor itself were described. These causes of hyperinsulinemia and insulin resistance, however, were found to be rare syndromes that were often associated with IGT or NIDDM. Nevertheless, the msjority of those with IGT and NIDDM could not be explained by the presence of abnormal insulins or insulin receptor abnormalities, and a post-receptor binding defect of insulin action appeared to be the most likely explanation for the most prevalent forms of insulin resistance.

In the Pima Indians, and subsequently in other populations at high risk of developing NIDDM, insulin levels for a given degree of glucose tolerance were found to be excessive relative to those found in Caucasians. Insulin levels in nondiabetic Pima Indians when matched for a degree of glucose tolerance were approximately 50% higher in the fasting state and 100% higher in the post-load state than observed in Caucasians. This finding ultimately led to the hypothesis that hyperinsulinemia due to peripheral insulin resistance at the post-receptor target tissue level provided a possible basis for the propensity of the Pima to develop NIDDM. More recently it has been shown that fasting and post-load insulin levels among those with normal glucose tolerance strongly predict the development of NIDDM (11). Hyperinsulinemia among subjects with normal glucose tolerance has also been described in other populations with a high likelihood of developing NIDDM, such as Asian Idians, Mexican Americans and the Australian Aborigine.

While the mechanism of insulin resistance is beyond the scope of the present paper, studies from the Pima Indians implicate abnormalities in the non-oxidative pathway of glucose disposal that lead to glycogen synthesis. Insulin resistance as measured by hyperinsulinemia-euglycemic clamps also shows evidence of familial aggregation and the frequency distribution of insulin-stimulated glucose uptake rates has a trimodal distribution, consistent with insulin mediated glucose uptake being determined by a single codominant gene. It is tempting to speculate, therefore, that the genetic basis for NIDDM may lie in an inherited abnormality in the glycogen synthetic pathway.

Subjects who develop NIDDM presumably all pass through a phase in which they have IGT (1). The category represents a group of subjects who fall in the upper part of the first component of the distribution of glucose tolerance levels in populations where bimodal glucose frequency distributions are seen, such as in the Pima Indians, the Mexican-Americans, and various groups of Pacific islanders (see Figure). The designation primarily indicates that such subjects are at an increased risk of developing diabetes rather than

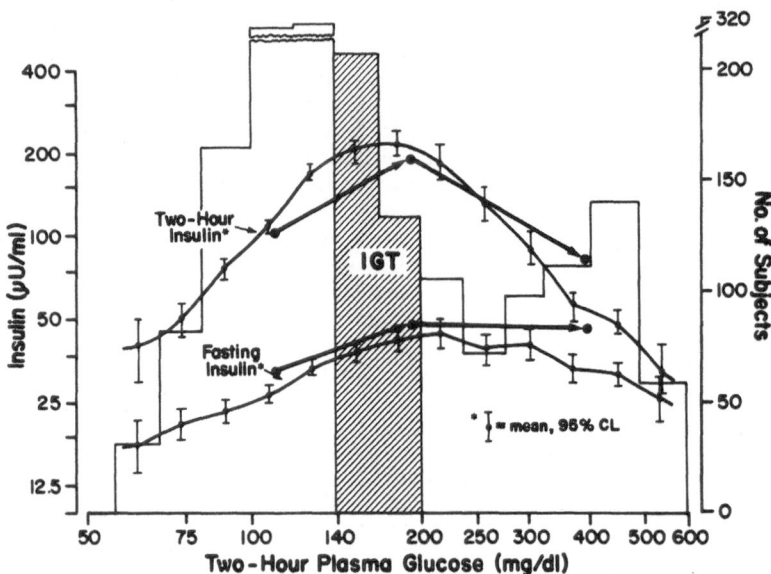

Fig. 1.   The frequency distribution of two-hour post-75 g oral load plasma glucose concentrations (on a logarithmic scale) in 1845 Pima Indians aged 25 years and over, none of whom were receiving oral hypoglycemic agents or insulin, is shown. The bimodal characteristics of the distribution can be seen. The mean two-hour post-load and fasting insulin levels, and their 95% confidence limits on a logarithmic scale are plotted in the same intervals of glucose tolerance for the same subjects. In this cross-sectional analysis both mean fasting and post-load insulin levels increase with increasing degrees of glycemia in those with normal and impaired glucose tolerance, whereas the insulin levels, especially the two-hour levels, fall progressively in those with NIDDM. The highest insulin levels are seen in subjects with impaired glucose tolerance and mild diabetes.

The mean two-hour fasting insulin levels and the corresponding mean two-hour plasma glucose level in nine subjects who progressed from normal glucose tolerance to NIDDM are also shown by the heavy line. Their insulin levels measured longitudinally, in general, follow those seen in the cross-sectional data, with the highest insulin levels occurring at the point of transition from IGT to NIDDM. The mean fasting insulin level remained high after NIDDM developed, whereas the two-hour level fell considerably. These data indicate that hyperinsulinemia is present at the time of transition from IGT to NIDDM and that fasting hyperinsulinemia persists even after NIDDM has appeared.

having a particular disease state. Subjects with impaired glucose tolerance, as documented in many studies, may subsequently develop NIDDM, may
return to normal, or may retain IGT. Although all studies indicate an increased risk of the development of diabetes this risk appears to be a function of the severity of IGT and the duration of its persistence. Furthermore, since many subjects with IGT will subsequently revert to normal it is
postulated that subjects with impaired glucose may represent a high risk
group within whom intervention strategies may offer the possibility of prevention of worsening to diabetes.

There are a number of factors which predict the worsening of normal
glucose tolerance and the developement of IGT. Those with higher fasting
and two-hour post-load glucose levels and with the highest fasting and post
glucose load insulin levels for a given degree of glucose tolerance and who
therefore exhibit relative insulin resistance are more likely to develop IGT.
The development of IGT is accompanied by worsening of peripheral insulin resistance and possibly the development of hepatic insulin resistance. Other
factors which hasten worsening of glucose tolerance include obesity.

The natural history of IGT has been studied in several populations.
Many of these have been represented by quite small numbers of persons, but
there is general agreement that the development of NIDDM is most likely
among those who have the more severe degrees of IGT. Among the Pima Indians
with IGT those who have the higher glucose levels, the higher fasting insulin levels, but lower two-hour post-load insulin levels are most likely to
decompensate to diabetes. Also, those who are more obese and who are of 35
to 54 years of age are more likely to decompensate than either younger or
older subjects.

IGT is characterized by the presence of greater degrees of insulin resistance than seen in subjects with normal glucose tolerance. Among those
with IGT those with the greatest degree of insulin resistance are most prone
to develop diabetes. The degree of hyperinsulinemia seen in subjects with
impaired glucose tolerance, however, appears to be appropriate for their
degree of glucose intolerance. In other words, among the Pima Indians there
is no evidence of a defect in insulin secretion among those with normal glucose tolerance and among those with impaired glucose tolerance.

TRANSITION TO NIDDM

Subjects with IGT have severe insulin resistance and elevated insulin
secretion compared to normals. In those with NIDDM insulin resistance is
even more severe, but insulin secretion is relatively reduced. Hence the
transition from IGT to NIDDM is distinguished from the transition from normal to IGT primarily by the fast that insulin secretory failure develops in
the progression to NIDDM. It appears that either worsening insulin resistance and/or an inability to further increase insulin response is an important determinant of progression to NIDDM. Within the hyperinsulinemic insulin resistant group with IGT those with below average insulin responses
are more likely to develop NIDDM. Such subjects typically have extremely
high fasting insulin levels. In a recent study the geometric mean fasting
insulin level in subjects with IGT who developed NIDDM was 291 pM (41 uU/ml)
which rose to 1368 pM (192 uU/ml) two hours after a glucose load. On the
other hand those who continued with IGT had a lower geometric mean fasting
serum insulin level of 241 pM (34 uU/ml) and two-hour post-load levels of
1639 pM (229 uU/ml). Thus, in those who progressed to NIDDM, even though
the post-load response was very substantial, it appeared that the level of
hyperinsulinemia may have been unable to control the glycemia in the face
of severe and possibly worsening insulin resistance. In these circumstances the degree of glycemia would worsen, and as we have shown previously

the development of NIDDM is accompanied by a marked deterioration in glucose tolerance over a short period of time. On the other hand fasting insulin levels remain extremely high and tend to be even higher at the time of diagnosis of NIDDM than they were at the time IGT was present. Among those with NIDDM fasting insulin levels do fall to some degree with increasing duration of diabetes, but remain higher than in subjects with normal glucose tolerance, whereas insulin responses to glucose fall considerably after NIDDM develops and fasting hyperglycemia supervenes.

The mechanism by which the post-load insulin response fails to suffice to maintain glucose homeostasis is unknown. There are several possible explanations. High glucose levels themselves may lead to impaired pancreatic responsiveness. This may be an effect on the glucose sensing mechanisms of the islets or the higher glucose levels may have a direct toxic effect on the pancreatic beta cell. Alternatively the pancreatic beta cell may already be operating at maximum capacity to maintain the supranormal basal insulin levels and becomes unable to respond in a timely manner because it no longer has reserves of preformed insulin and must resort to increased de novo insulin synthesis to respond to stimuli. It is also possible that some individuals have less reserve of beta cells which prevents them from manufacturing greater amounts of insulin and limits the insulin secretory capacity of the pancreas. IF so they would decompensate at levels of glycemia that could be maintained by others. The population studies suggest this possibility in that those with IGT and a lower than average insulin response may already be undergoing the transition to insulin secretory failure that is induced by insulin resistance.

NON-INSULIN DEPENDENT DIABETES MELLITUS

NIDDM in obese subjects, therefore, appears to represent the end result of a series of changes that occur over many years that culminate in the failure to maintain glucose homeostasis. At this point they become members of the hyperglycemic component in populations with bimodal frequency distributions of glucose tolerance. The internationally agreed criteria for diabetes define a group who are then subject to the development of a number of sequelae such as the classical microvascular complications of diabetes as well as other vascular and metabolic complications. These ultimately result in blindness, renal failure, amputation, increased frequencies of atherosclerotic heart disease, cerebrovascular disease, etc. and increased mortality.

MECHANISMS FOR THE DEVELOPMENT OF NIDDM

The events that lead to NIDDM in the Pima Indians, and probably in obese subjects from other populations who develop NIDDM, include as a primary event the development of insulin resistance. Insulin resistance is probably a genetically determined characteristic, as is suggested by the observations of familial aggregation, but it is also influenced by environmental factors. Obesity for example can result in exacerbation of insulin resistance, but in our view cannot account for it in its entirety. An insulin resistant subject, upon becoming obese will develop worsening insulin resistance, and this in turn will lead to some deterioration of glucose tolerance and the establishment of a new glucose equilibrium that is associated with higher fasting and post challenge insulin levels. However, as long as glucose tolerance remains within the normal range, and even in the IGT range in the majority of subjects, the levels of insulinemia achieved appear appropriate to the degree of glucose intolerance based on projections made from those with entirely normal glucose tolerance. However, among those with IGT, a substantial fraction will eventually develop NIDDM.

Among the IGTs who are hyperinsulinemic but who have lower than average insulin responses glucose homeostasis may fail and a relatively rapid transition to much higher glucose levels will occur and NIDDM will develop. Even with NIDDM, basal insulin levels remain extraordinarily high, but the insulin response to the glucose challenge is blunted and protracted, and insufficient to bring the glucose levels back to the range seen in normal glucose tolerance and IGT.

The antecedent events leading to NIDDM, therefore, appear to be insulin resistance accompanied by the development of hyperinsulinemia. If the degree of insulin resistance is sufficient, glucose levels increase and serve to stimulate further hyperinsulinemia. Eventually, especially in the face of worsening insulin resistance, this is followed by a failure of insulin secretion. At this time the degree of glycemia will worsen rapidly and NIDDM will supervene.

RELATIONSHIP TO NIDDM IN OTHER POPULATIONS

Whether or not the mechanism and pathogenesis or NIDDM described among the Pima Indians is similar in all populations is open to debate. In Caucasian populations a substantial proportion of those developing NIDDM are not obese, and it has been suggested that in such persons NIDDM represents a primary deficiency in insulin secretion. Prospective studies of the development of NIDDM in such populations, however, have not been performed. In some populations, such as in northern Europe, a much higher proportion of the NIDDM may be attributable to the process that typically leads to insulin dependent diabetes. For example, a recent study by Groop and his colleagues in Helsinki has shown that a considerable proportion of NIDDMs have islet cell antibodies and other autoantibodies at the time of diagnosis, as well as often being of the HLA DR3/DR4 type (10). In such populations, it seems likely that many cases of NIDDM have a pathogenesis analogous to that which occurs in IDDM, with autoimmune destruction of the pancreatic beta cell as the primary pathophysiologic basis for the development of diabetes. Obesity related NIDDM, however, constitutes the majority of NIDDM seen in most parts of the world. It is likely, therefore, that the findings among the Pima Indians may be used as a model for the pathogenesis of obesity-related NIDDM in most populations.

The proposed pathogenetic mechanisms for NIDDM include a primary defect relating to the development of insulin resistance and a secondary defect relating to pancreatic insulin secretory failure. If means to prevent insulin secretory failure or maintain beta cell responsiveness in those with IGT, or to reduce insulin resistance, and thus protect the pancreas from the development of secretory failure, can be found and applied, then NIDDM may become a preventable disease.

REFERENCES

1. World Health Organization, Geneva, 1985, Report of a Study Group: Diabetes Mellitus. World Health Organization Technical Report Series 727.

2. Barnett, A.H., Eff, C., Leslie, R.D.G., Pyke, D.A., 1981, Diabetes in identical twins: a study of 200 pairs. Diabetologia 25: 13-17.

3. Serjeantson, S.W., Owerbach, D., Zimmet, P., Nerup, J., Thoma, K., 1983, Genetics of Diabetes in Nauru: effects of foreign admixture, HLA antigens and the insulin-gene-linked polymorphism. Diabetologia 25: 13-17.

4. Stern, M.P., Ferrell, R.E., Rosenthal, M., Haffner, S.M., Hazuda, H.P., 1986, Association between NIDDM, Rh blood group and haptoglobin phenotype: results from the San Antonio heart study. Diabetes 35: 387–391.

5. Williams, R.C., Knowler, W.C., Butler, W.J., Pettitt, D.J., Lisse, J.R., Bennett, P.H., Mann, D.L., Johnson, A.H., Terasaki, P.I., 1981, HLA-A2 and type 2 (insulin independent) diabetes mellitus in Pima Indians: an association of allele frequency with age. Diabetologia 21: 460–463.

6. Yamashita, T.S., Mackay, W., Rushforth, N.B., Bennett, P.H., Houser, H., 1984, Pedigree annlyses of non-insulin dependent diabetes in the Pima Indians suggest dominant mode of inheritance. Am J Hum Genet 36: 183S.

7. Reaven, G., Miller, R, 1968, Study of the relationship between glucose and insulin responses to an oral glucose load in man. Diabetes 17: 560–569.

8. Savage, P.J., Dippe, S.E., Bennett, P.H., Gorden, P., Roth, J., Rushforth N.B., Miller, M., 1975, Hyperinsulinemia and hypoinsulinemia. Insulin responses to oral carbohydrate over a wide spectrum of glucose tolerance. Diabetes 24: 362–368.

9. Bogardus, C., Lillioja, S., Howard, B.V., Reaven, G., Mott, D., 1984. Relationship between insulin secretion, insulin action, and fasting plasma glucose concentration in nondiabetic and noninsulin-dependent diabetic subjects. J Clin Invest 74: 1238–1246.

10. Groop, L., Miettinen, A., Groop, P-H., Meri, S., Koskimies, S., Bottazzo, G.F., 1988, Organ specific autoimmunity and HLA-DR antigens as markers for B cell destruction in patients with type II diabetes. Diabetes 37: 99–103.

HEMOSTASIS AND ENDOTHELIAL DISORDERS IN PRE-DIABETES

¶Pierre Drouin[+] and Pierre-Jean Guillausseau[++]

[+]Hopital Jeanne d'Arc, Nancy, France
[++]Hopital Lariboisiere , Paris, France

Vascular complications represent today the main causes underlying morbidity and mortality in diabetic patients. The role of hemostasis disorders, as well as disturbances in endothelial cell function and hemorheologic abnormalities have been suggested by a great amount of evidence in diabetic microangiopathy and in atherogenesis. The aim of this chapter is to review the abnormalities in hemostasis, endothelial cells function and in hemorheology observed in patient with pre-diabetes.

PLATELET FUNCTION ABNORMALITIES
In vitro studies
Numerous studies have precisely documented the existence of an enhanced platelet adhesiveness in diabetic subjects. In the same way, platelets hyperaggregability has been found in diabetics, after platelet activation by ADP, epinephrine or collagen. The prevalence of these abnormalities is extremely high when severe micro and/or macrovascular damages are present. On the other hand, platelet hyperactivity has been evidenced in patients with latent (or chemical diabetes (1) or in patients without vascular complications. Among patients with occlusive lower-limb arterial disease, platelet abnormalities are more severe in diabetic patients when compared to non diabetic subjects.

In vivo studies
More recently in vivo platelet hyperactivity index have been described. β thromboglobulin is a platelet alpha granule compound which is secreted during the release reaction. β thromboglobulin assay in plasma is reliable as index of in vivo platelet hyperactivity. β thromboglobulin plasma levels are markedly elevated in diabetic patients. The same results have been observed for platelet factor 4 another in vivo platelets hyperactivity - index. Indirect evidence of platelet hyperactivity is also given by the reduction in platelet life-span which has been observed in diabetic patients.

PLATELET AND ENDOTHELIAL PROSTAGLANDINS DISORDERS
Halushka et al (2) have demonstrated an increase in PGE-like material release from diabetic platelets after stimulation by various inducers. The hyperactivity of thromboxane-pathway in diabetic platelets has also been shown. This impairment in arachidonic acid metabolism seems to be related to an increase in platelet membrane phospholipids release. A defect in prostacyclin (PGI_2) release from endothelial cells has been observed in diabetic animals and in diabetic patients. The imbalance between PGI_2 synthesis and thromboxane A_2 formation is thought to be responsible for a lower threshold for platelet aggregation.

PLATELET-DERIVED GROWTH-FACTOR AND DIABETES

Recent studies indicate that diabetic serum contains an increased growth-promoting activity for vascular smooth-muscle cells, for fibroblasts and for human umbilical vein endothelial cells. Conflicting results have been presented concerning platelet-derived mitogenic activity. Hamet et al (3) have shown in a recent symposium that platelet mitogenic activity for vascular smooth muscle cells and for human fibroblasts was high in the supernatant of platelets from diabetic subjects. Using washed platelets (to eliminate a contamination from other growth factors such as insulin or IGF I or II), we have reported a loss in alpha granule content (β thromboglobulin and platelet-derived mitogenic activity for mouse fibroblasts) in diabetic patients with proliferative retinopathy.

ENDOTHELIAL CELL FUNCTION ABNORMALITIES

Many substances relevant for diabetic angiopathy are synthetized and released by endothelial cells: prostacyclin (PGI_2), factor VIII_{VWF} and plasminogen activator. An increase in factor VII_{VWF} levels has been shown in diabetic subjects, mainly in the presence of severe retinal damage but also in the absence of any retinopathy. Plasminogen activator activity release induced by venostasis has been found consistently low in diabetic subjects. This finding indicates another endothelial cell function abnormality.

Hemorheological Abnormalities in Diabetes

Type 1 diabetes has been shown to be accompanied by abnormalities in the rheological behavior of blood. As far as macrorheology of blood is concerned, several groups using rotational viscometers have clearly demonstrated an increased whole blood viscosity. Differencies in viscosity are larger at low shear rates suggesting that red cell aggregation has an important role in the hyperviscosity of diabetes.

Plasma viscosity which contributes to whole blood viscosity is also elevated in juvenile Type I diabetes. The elevated levels of fibrinogen and of acute phase reactant proteins and also the marginal depression of albumin are associated with plasma hyperviscosity. The parameters of blood microrheology are red blood cell deformability, aggregation and adhesion. With regard to red blood cell deformability, the results observed remain controversial. Numerous in vitro studies using the filtration technic have been made but the contaminating factors influencing blood filtration are well known. The use of micro-pipettes led also to conflicting results. The same holds true when other technics are used such as viscometry or flexibility measurements. Red cell aggregation has been found to be increased in Type I diabetes. This abnormal aggregation is likely to be responsible for the raised blood viscosity at low shear rates. The adhesion of erythrocytes to endothelial cells has been found to be increased and related to the extent of vascular complications. But further studies are needed to confirm these results observed in vitro.

Finely abnormalities of molecular rheological parameters (e.g. membrane fluidity) have not yet been clearly demonstrated. Most of the investigations undertaken involving the fluorescence polarization technic with the DPH probe embedded in the deep region of the lipid bilayer have given conflicting results which could quite possibly be due to a lack in standarization of the methods used. We are not aware of any study conducted in pre-diabetic patients.

PLATELET AND ENDOTHELIAL FUNCTION STUDIES IN PRE-DIABETES

In contrast with the great amount of studies concerning diabetes, only a few studies have been performed in pre-diabetes (1,4,5,6) (Table I). These results indicate that platelet aggregation is normal in pre-diabetes with low or high ADP dosage, or with epinephrine. Circulating aggregates are

TABLE I

PLATELET STUDIES IN PREDIABETES

·	Sagel(1)	Colwell(4)	Colwell(5)	Gensini(6)
NUMBER OF SUBJECTS				
Control subjects	15	18-25	25	35
Prediabetics	7	8-10	10	7
METHODS				
Platelet aggregation				
ADP 0.125 umol	N			
ADP 0.250 umol	N			
ADP 0.500 umol	N	N	N	
ADP 1.000 umol	N		N	
Epinephrine		N	N	
Plasma factor activity		N	N	
Circulating aggregates				N
MDA formation				N

N: Not different from control subjects

not elevated nor megathrombocytes. Malondialdehyde release from platelet (which is an index of thromboxane B_2 formation) has been shown to be not different from control platelets. The only abnormality is a slight increase in factor VIIIvWF levels, while factor VIIIRAG and factor VIIIAHF activity are normal (6). This last finding may suggest an early dysfunction of endothelial cells in pre-diabetes. These studies need however to be confirmed and extended to another endothelial cells functions.

REFERENCES

1. Sagel, J., Colwell, J.A., Crook, L. and Laimins, M., 1975, Increased platelet aggregation in early diabetes mellitus. Ann Intern Med 82: 733-738.

2. Halushka, P.V., Lurie, D. and Colwell, J.A., 1977, Increased synthesis of prostaglandin-E-like material by platelets from patients with diabetes mellitus. Engl J Med 297: 1306-1310.

3. Hamet, P., Fugimoto, H., Umeda, F., Lecavalier, L., Franks, D.J., Orth, D.N. and Chiasson, J.L., 1985, Abnormalities of platelet-derived growth factors in insulin-dependent diabetics. Metabolism 34 (suppl. 1): 25-31.

4. Colwell, J.A., Halushka, P.V., Sarji, K., Levine, J., Sagel, J. and Nair, R.M.G., 1976, Altered platelet function in diabetes mellitus. Diabetes 25 (Suppl 2): 826-831.

5. Colwell, J.A., Sagel, J., Crook, L., Chambers, A., and Laimins, M., 1977, Correlation of platelet aggregation, plasma factor activity, and megathrombocytes in diabetic subjects with and without vascular disease. Metabolism, 26: 279-285.

6. Gensini, G.F., Abbate, R., Favilla, S. and Neri Serneri, G.G., 1979, Changes of platelet function and blood clotting in diabetes mellitus. Thrombos Haemostas (Stuttg.), 42: 983-993.

MICROCHANNELS IN PREDIABETES

¶R.A. Camerini-Davalos[+], A.S. Reddi[++],
J.M.B. Bloodworth[*], and C.A. Velasco[+]

[+]Department of Medicine, New York Medical College
Metropolitan Hospital Center, New York, New York
[++]Department of Medicine, UMDNJ-New Jersey Medical School, Newark, N.J.
[*]Department of Pathology, University of Wisconsin Medical School
and Middleton Veterans Hospital, Madison, Wisconin

In humans, diabetic microangiopathy affects arterioles, capillaries and venules throughout the body. This fact signifies the unity of the vascular occurrences. The pathology of the microchannels functional or structural, has a variable dynamic natural history where localized abnormalities are commonly found at different stages of their development.

It is generally agreed that heredity plays an important role in determining susceptibility to diabetes and the accompanying disease of the microchannels. Disagreements arise when the nature of the transmission of this susceptibility and the time of onset in the offspring are discussed. It is necessary then to distinguish between genetic pre-disposition (liability, susceptibility) which is inherited but has not yet become manifest, and microangiopathy present as an expression of the progressing disease.

The nature of the inherited factor may be variable, and perhaps expressed in diverse, genetically determined, immunologic, metabolic, hormonal, and/or enzymatic deviations from normal; which may have a common end - point that we call diabetes with microangiopathy. At what stage can we find abnormalities in the microchannels of diabetic patients? Only at the end stage of overt symptomatic diabetes, with "permanent" hyperglycemia? Or, are they already present in subjects highly predis-posed to diabetes but with normal tolerance to glucose? Is hyperglycemia an absolute necessity for the development of the diabetic microangiopathy?

This work was supported in part by General Research Support Grant RR-05398 from the General Research Support Branch, Division of Research Resources NIH. Health Research Council of the City of New York. Diabetes Research Fund, New York. The Michael J. Bilotto Research Fund of HOPE for Diabetics Foundation, New York.

MATERIALS AND METHODS

As described in chapter 19, only Caucasian, identical non-diabetic twins of diabetic patients, offspring of proven conjugal diabetic parents with normal tolerance to glucose: genetic prediabetics (GP); and, non diabetic controls (C); within 15% of ideal body weight, were included.

For the in vivo observations of the microcirculation of the bulbar conjunctiva a concentrated stroboscopic light for improved speed and resolution with Eastman fine grain positive film and a 40mm macroscopic single lens reflex system was used. Estimates of linear blood velocity are possible because the normal eye movements displace the granular pattern during the interval between duplicate flashes of the light source. Displacement of the aggregate is corrected for vessel movement and divided by the interval between flashes to calculate human blood velocity.

For the studies of retinal circulation, fluorescein photography has been utilized, with a Zeiss fundus camera with recycling of the flash power pack at 1-second intervals.

For the recording of the arterial pulse of the right index finger the Lax and Feinberg electric vasculograph was used. Morphologic surface microvessels studies of the finger's nailbed was demonstrated and quantitated by capillary microscopy. Capillaroscopy of the end-row capillaries of the nailfold permits a percentile determination of the number of capillaries with nodular apical elongations. Originally, 500 capillaries were counted in each case. Since there was excellent numerical correlation from finger to finger, however, each determination now is made on the basis of visualization and counting of fifty consecutive capillaries within a given nailfold. The third and fourth fingers of each hand are examined (ie., a total of four fingers). The percentage of nodular apical elongations (NAE) is based on a minimum count of 200 capillaries in any given individual. An examination and count of a single nailfold takes ten minutes. During the examination of a given nailfold, the appearance of NAE does not change (1).

Examination of the vascular basement membrane was done according to the method of BLoodworth (2) which is similar to the Siperstein one. Muscle biopsies were performed with a modified Vim-Silverman needle in the right lateral aspect of the quadriceps femoris, exactly midway between the hip and knee, 10 minutes after 5 ml of lidocaine (Xylocaine) had been injected in the area (3).

RESULTS

Retina and conjunctiva

No statistical significant difference was found between C and GP when the ratio of the width of the vessels (venule/arteriole and venule/ capillary) in photographs of the retina and conjunctiva was determined. No difference in the estimates of linear blood velocity in the bulbar conjunctiva was found between the two groups, but an apparent venular and capillary dilatation was found in the GP when compared to C (Table 1).

TABLE I

BULBAR CONJUNCTIVAL VESSEL DIAMETERS (u).

	Venules (Maximum ± S.E.)		Capillaries (Maximum ± S.E.)	
	Radius (u)	Velocity (u/sec.)	Radius (u)	Velocity (u/sec.)
Normals (n=25)	77 ± 2.1	390 ± 36	9 ± 0.3	410 ± 36
Prediabetics (n=25)	148 ± 3.6	388 ± 37	15 ± 0.6	390 ± 41
P	< 0.001		< 0.001	

Finger pulse wave

In young persons, the recorded arterial pulse wave of the fingers should be dicrotic (Figure 1). Prediabetic patients below the age of 40 years revealed abnormal monocrotic pulse wave in 21 of the 32 studied: 65%, compared to 37% abnormals in C.

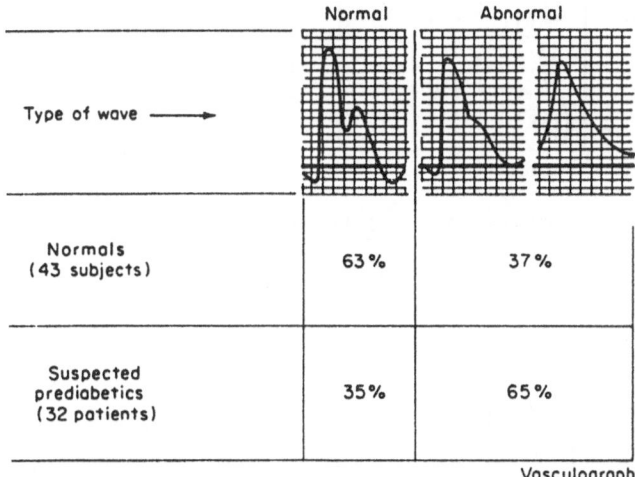

Type of wave ⟶	Normal	Abnormal	
Normals (43 subjects)	63%	37%	
Suspected prediabetics (32 patients)	35%	65%	

Vasculograph

Figure 1. Arterial pulse waves of the finger.

Nailbed capillaries

Morphologic surface microvessel studies of the nailbed of GP have shown significant increased prevalence of abnormalities (Figure 2). (4) In the GP there was also a positive statistical correlation between the nodular apical elongation of the nail capillaries or "knobs" and glucose area (Figure 3).

PREVALENCE OF "KNOBS"

MORPHOLOGICAL CLASSIFICATION		CONTROLS	PRE-DIABETICS
% APICAL KNOBS *		12	26
% SIDE KNOBS		4	9
TOTAL		16	36

p VALUES *

MORPHOLOGICAL CLASSIFICATION	CONTROLS / PRE-DIABETICS
APICAL	0·002
SIDE	0·002
TOTAL	0 002

PREVALENCE OF WIDENING

MORPHOLOGICAL CLASSIFICATION		CONTROLS	PRE-DIABETICS
% OVERALL WIDENING		9	52
% WIDE EFFERENT LIMB		9	30
% WIDE TRANSITIONAL LIMB		10	35

MORPHOLOGICAL CLASSIFICATION	CONTROLS / PRE-DIABETICS
OVERALL WIDENING	0·002
WIDE EFFERENT LIMB	0·002
WIDE TRANS. LIMB	0·002

CAPILLARY PATTERN

MORPHOLOGICAL CLASSIFICATION		CONTROLS	PRE-DIABETICS
% WITHIN NORMAL LIMITS		71	59
% TORTUOUS		25	37
% MEANDERING		2	2
% GENERAL ENLARGEMENT		2	2

MORPHOLOGICAL CLASSIFICATION	CONTROLS / PRE-DIABETICS
WITHIN NORMAL LIMITS	0·002
TORTUOUS	0·002
MEAND.	
GEN. ENL.	

MEANS

$$ p = \frac{\text{PERCENT DIFFERENCE}}{\text{S.E. OF THE DIFFERENCE}} $$

Figure 2. Nailbed capillaries.

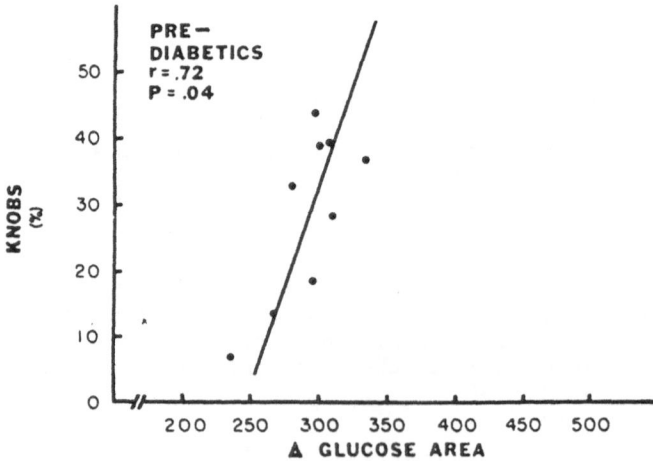

Figure 3. Correlation between the knobs and the glucose area.

Muscle capillaries basement membrane width

A statistically significant difference (p < 0.01) was found when
the mean of the observed values for muscle capillary basement width
(MCBMw) of 30 GP was compared with the one of 40 C: Figure 4. Adjusted
mean values for age and sex for both groups was even more significantly
different: p < 0.001   (1137 v 1418A.)

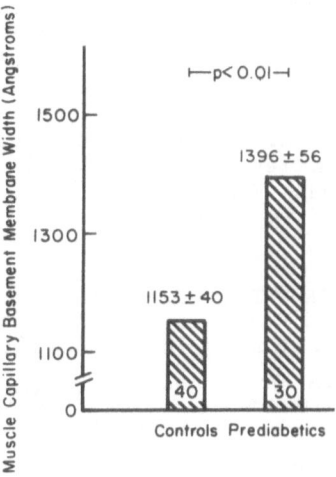

Figure 4. Muscle capillary basement membrane width.

Seven GP patients had thickening of basement membrane (BMT) (above
the upper limit for age and sex of C) and 8 had increases in the standard
deviation (ISD). Two GP with BMT had normal SDS and 3 with ISD had normal
mean MCBMw. A log transformation was applied to both MCBMw and the SDS.
Analysis of these data did not change the results. The MCBMw and SD were
highly correlated. This is confirmed by the fact that almost no difference
was found when the mean coefficients of variation of C and GP were compared. The distribution of the values were similar.

Accepting that both BMT and ISD reflect abnormal MCBMw, one criterion
of abnormality or the other was found in 10 (33%) GP patients and in 3
(7.5%) C. This is in agreement with findings of Aronoff et al, and
Siperstein et al (5). Recently Williamson also found abnormal MCBMw in
patients from the Joslin Center (6):

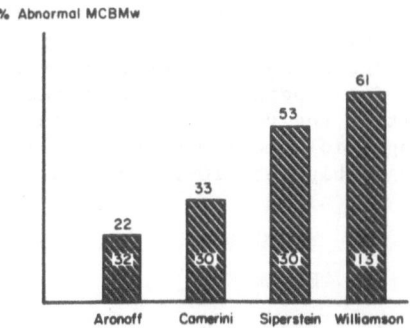

Figure 5. Percentage of abnormal muscle capillary basement membrane
width according to different investigators.

Blood glucose and serum insulin levels during the OGTT for the 10 GP with abnormal MCBMw were compared to the controls and to the GP with normal MCBMw, the only significant difference (P < 0.05) was found between the 180-min immunoreactive insulin of the controls (10.9 ± 2.8) and that of the GP with abnormal MCBMw (16.2 ± 2.8).

Ten of 30 had BMT suggesting a bimodal frequency distribution and this may be interpreted as an indication that there are two different groups of GP: one with normal and the other with abnormal MCBMw. Are those in the latter group the ones that develop clinical vasculopathy at a later date? Are they the ones who will progress to chemical or even to overt diabetes?

Fifty percent of those with abnormal MCBMw originally, progressed to chemical (CD) or overt diabetes (OD) in 10 years compared to 35% of those with normal MCBMw, Table II. None of them developed recognizable clinical vasculopathy so far.

TABLE II

MUSCLE CAPILLARY BASEMENT MEMBRANE WIDTH VERSUS BLOOD GLUCOSE.

1978	1988
10 pt. normal OGTT but abnormal MCBMw	5 (50%) abnormal BG 3 C.D. 2 O.D.
20 pt. normal OGTT with normal MCBMw	7 (35%) abnormal BG 6 C.D. 1 O.D.

DISCUSSION

The findings, in subjects highly predisposed to diabetes, of morphological changes in the microchannels, are another indication of insult to the vasculature <u>before</u> hyperglycemia. It should also be mentioned that biochemical and hormonal abnormalities have been found by us and other investigators in GP (7), and some of the abnormalities may be related, directly or indirectly, to the early changes of the vasculature.

We postulate that the presence of abnormalities of the microchannels in subjects with a high index of predictability for diabetes but normal carbohydrate metabolism suggests that the pathophysiological mechanisms responsible for the microangiopathy are already acting at that time, and if they progress to the stage of chemical or even overt symptomatic diabetes, as many of them do, hyperglycemia, then becomes an aggravating and/or accelerating insult to the vasculature. This concept would be consistent with the pathophysiological mechanism acting in a nondiabetic pregnant mother delivering a big baby 10-30 years before she herself develops overt diabetes.

REFERENCES

1. Terry, E.N., Messina, E.J., Schwartz, S.M., Redish, W., Steel, J.M., 1967, Manifestation of diabetic microangiopathy in nailfold capillaries. Diabetes 16: 595-97.

2. Bloodworth, J.M.B., Jr., 1963, Diabetic microangiopathy. Diabetes 12: 99-114.

3. Camerini-Davalos, R.A., Velasco, C.A., Glasser, M., Bloodworth, J.M.B., Jr., 1983, Drug-induced reversal of early diabetic microangiopathy. N Engl J Med 309: 1551-1556.

4. Redisch, W., Rouen, L.R., Terry, E.N., Oppermann, W., Kuthan, F., Clauss, R.H., 1973, Microvascular Changes in Early Diabetes Mellitus. In: Camerini-Davalos, R.A., Cole, H.S., Eds., Vascular and Neurological Changes in Early Diabetes. New York and London, Academic Press: 383-390.

5. Camerini-Davalos, R.A., Oppermann, W., Rebagliati, H., Glasser, M., Bloodworth, J.M.B., Jr., 1979, Muscle capillary basement membrane width in genetic prediabetes. J Clin Endocrinol Metab 2: 251-259.

6. Ganda, O.P., Williamson, J.R., Soeldner, J.S., Gleason, R.E., Kilo, C., Kaldany, A., Miller, J.P., Garovoy, N.R., Carpenter, C.B., 1983, Muscle capillary basement membrane width and its relationship to diabetes mellitus in monozygotic twins. Diabetes 32: 549-556.

7. Camerini-Davalos, R.A., 1978, Early diabetes. Concept. Terminology. In: Camerini-Davalos, R.A., Hanover, B., Eds., Treatment of Early Diabetes. New York and London, Plenum Press 119: 1-6.

DISCUSSION

C. HOWARD: Dr. Bennett, have any samples of the pancreas of these patients that you've studied become available and been examined? And, is there any evidence of islet pathology of any sort? And, finally, do you have any non-obese Indians that you've been able to study that follow the same course; for example, hyperinsulinemic not associated with obesity? I'm unclear what's occurring first here since most of the population is obese. What kind of controls could you have that would be the non-obese?

P. BENNETT: We have examined a reasonable number of pancreas, postmortem of course, from Pimas, both diabetic and non-diabetic. In terms of the islet pathology in the diabetics, there's a very wide variation. Some of the diabetics even after 10, 12, 14 years of diabetes have an abundance of beta cells, large islets, and obviously a lot of insulin in those cells. At the other extreme, there are individuals with small islets, quite a lot of fibrous tissue and amyloid is present in quite a number of those diabetics. In the non-diabetics, in general, the impression is one of a very adequate islet cell mass. We have not done careful morphometry with Caucasian controls measured blindly and simultaneously, but taking the numbers at face value the Pima islets are at the upper end.

I'd like to mention just one other very intriguing observation. We've had the opportunity to have pancreas of five Pima who died within the first year of life. Those islets were extremely large and typical of the islets of the infants of a diabetic mother. They had a lot of beta cells, but a very low quantity of delta cells.

In terms of the non-obese, yes, not all of the Pima Indians are obese, and we do see diabetes in the non-obese in rates that are very appreciably greater than those in Caucasians of similar non-obese weights. The non-obese that we see also have hyperinsulinemia.

J. HOET: Just to make things clear, when you speak about hyperinsulinism this is not hyperproinsulin?

P. BENNETT: No, we have measured proinsulin levels and typically the proinsulin constitutes about 8% of the immunologically active insulin.

J. HOET: Insulin antibodies?

P. BENNETT: We have encountered occasional insulin antibodies during the old assays, but we have not systematically studied insulin antibodies using the modern techniques.

S. EFENDIC: Dr. Bennett, I have an idea that you are really talking about two different types of diabetes and I would like to know what is the role of the liver in the development of glucose intolerance in your patients?

P. BENNETT: We believe that the liver does become resistant and maybe resistant out of proportion in those with severe impairment of glucose tolerance. Our evidence for that is that the insulin levels are over and above those predicted from the normal population. And, secondly, we have failed to see complete suppression of hepatic glucose production measured crudely in some of those subjects.

B. WAJCHENBERG: Dr. Bennett, you just mentioned that in the muscle biopsy of your patients you have noticed a decrease in glucose synthesis in glycogen synthetase. How come considering your findings of decreasing glucose disposal? Did you see a compensatory gluconeogenesis and glucose oxidation or not?

P. BENNETT: The differences between Pimas and Caucasians are primarily attributable to differences in the non-oxidative glucose disposal. And, that was, of course, the reason why we then started to concentrate on the events in glycogen synthesis and tried to isolate the defect.

H. LAUBE: Dr. Bennett, the Pima Indian story reminds me very much of the spiny desert mice in Israel which are perfectly normal so long as they live in the desert. At the moment they have normal laboratory chow, they develop diabetes. Do you have any experience or are there any studies done with different kinds of nutrition in the Pima Indians? Do they influence the rate of diabetes?

P. BENNETT: I can't tell you whether nutrition influences the rate of diabetes on the basis of experimental evidence. On the other hand, we believe that the Pimas have developed their inordinate rate of diabetes in relatively recent times. There's no question that things have changed a lot and changes in diet are certainly one of the prime suspects at this point. I mean the other thing that's really changed a lot is the amount of physical activity for daily living and working and so forth on the reservation. So, I think those are the two things that we can say have certainly changed, the traditional diet has now been replaced by a western diet.

J. HOET: What about increasing the physical activity? Because physical activity can not really induce the insulin resistance that they have.

P. BENNETT: Well, it's very interesting. We have done physical activity assessments and Pima Indians, in spite of their obesity, have very high VO2 max, and we've been unable to differentiate any important relationship between VO2 max and insulin resistance. Now, what we have not done is started an intensive aerobic exercise program to try to see what increased exercise over a prolonged period of time would do. It's certainly a factor. And, we're trying to gather a lot of baseline information for future prospective work.

One very brief comment that while the Pimas have been sort of notable, there are many other tribes of American Indians in the United States, who have high and seemingly increasing rates of diabetes at this time. So, it's certainly not something that is uniquely restricted to the Pima tribe.

V.   POPULATION STUDIES

ISELT-CELL AND INSULIN AUTOANTIBODIES IN FIRST-DEGREE RELATIVES
OF TYPE I DIABETICS:
A 5-YEAR FOLLOW-UP STUDY IN A SWISS POPULATION

¶G.A. Spinas*, L. Matter**, T. Wilkin+, O. Staffelbach*, W. Berger*

*Department of Internal Medicine, University Hospital of Basle, Switzerland
**Clinical Immunology, Kantonsspital, St. Gallen, Switzerland
+General Hospital, Southhampton, Great Britain

It is widely accepted that autoimmune mechanisms are involved in the pathogenesis of type I (insulin-dependent, IDDM) diabetes mellitus. (1)Islet cell antibodies (ICA) reacting with antigens in the cytoplasma, or on the surface of islet-cells (ICSA), or against a 64 kD human islet-cell protein, as well as insulin autoantibodies (IAA) are present years before the onset of clinical diabetes. They probably serve as serologic markers of ongoing beta-cell destruction in predisposed individuals. In monozygotic twins initially discordant for type I diabetes, loss of beta-cell function has been shown to be temporarily associated with the presence of ICA (2). Several studies in discordant monozygotic twins or first-degree relatives of type I diabetics revealed that ICA-positive relatives are more likely to develop overt diabetes than are the ICA-negative (3). Moreover, the presence of both ICA and IAA in these individuals confers an even higher risk of progression to IDDM (1)

We report here the results of a family study which was set up in 1981 in order to evaluate prevalence and time course of ICA in unaffected first-degree relatives of type I diabetics.

SUBJECTS AND METHODS

Subjects: Sixty six unrelated families with at least one IDDM family member participated in the study (4). One hundred seventy nine nondiabetic healthy first-degree relatives (average age: 39.8 years; 89 siblings, 34 parents and 56 offspring) were recruited over a period of 5 years (April 1981 to April 1986) and followed up regularly, i.e. after 6,12,24,36,48 and 60 months (mean follow-up: 50.6 months). Blood was drawn to determine blood glucose, HbA1c and ICA at each visit. HLA-DR phenotypes were determined in 144 subjects. Five hundred fifteen serum samples (2 - 5 per proband) were tested for the presence of insulin autoantibodies.

Eighty-nine healthy normal volunteers with no family history of diabetes mellitus were HLA-DR typed and used as control subjects.

Islet-cell antibody assay: Cytoplasmic islet-cell antibodies were determined by indirect immunofluorescence on unfixed cryostat sections of blood group O human pancreas specimens. ICA-titers were assessed by serial dilu-

tion to end-point starting with a dilution of 1:2. For this study all positive sera were retested using the same pancreatic specimen, and only consistent results are reported as positive. Positive samples were further
tested for complement-fixing ability using an anti-human-C3-conjugate.

Insulin autoantibodies: Sera were examined for IgG autoantibodies to human
insulin by means of a direct, immunospecific enzymelinked immunosorbent assay
(ELISA) as previously described (5).

HLA typing: 144 first-degree relatives, all diabetic family members as well
as the control subjects were HLA-DR typed. HLA-DR antigen determination was
performed as previously described (15).

Statistical analysis: The chi-square-test was used for statistical evaluation, and 5% was chosen as the level of significance.

RESULTS

HLA-DR antigens: Table 1 shows the HLA-DR haplotypes of the diabetic family
members. Two families with more than one diabetic are not considered. The
control population consisted of unrelated blood donors with no family history
of diabetes. The haplotype HLA-DR3, - DR4 and DR3/4 were significantly more
frequent in diabetics as compared to the control population ($p < 0.001$). In
fact, 90% of the diabetics were HLA-DR3 and/or 4.

On the other hand the frequency of the haplotypes HLA-DR2 and HLA-DR5
was found to be significantly decreased in the IDDM patients (8% vs 22% and
2% vs 21% of controls, respectively).

Islet-cell antibodies (ICA): A total of 1024 sera (5.7 per proband) were
tested for ICA. Fifty four (5.2%) were ICA-positive and 2 showed complement-
fixing ability. Fourty-four percent of the sera were positive only at a
dilution of 1:2 (borderline, but confirmed by at least 2 observers and on
two different pancreatic specimens), 41% of the titers were 1:4, and in 15%
ICA-titers were higher than 1:4 (7 patients). Thus, during the observation
period of 50.6 months ICA were found in 13% of the first-degree relatives
However, the prevalence rate on initial screening was 5% and constantly remained between 3.4% and 5.6% in following screenings, i.e. after 6, 12, 24,
36, 48, 60 months.

ICA have been found regularly in 5 subjects (1 sibling, 2 parents, 2
offspring) since their entry to the study. Four of them have remained ICA-
positive for at least 49 months without showing any signs of glucose intolerance. One of these 4 probands had low titers between 1:2 and 1:4, whereas
the other three had titers in the range of 1:8 to 1:64 with one of the subjects showing complement-fixing ICA. One individual (father of a diabetic)
after having been ICA-positive for 18 months (titer 1:4 - 1:8) developed
IDDM 3 years after tne disease had become manifest in his child. The
father is HLA-DR1/4, tne son 3/4.

Five subjects (4 siblings, 1 parent) who have been ICA-positive for 12
to 36 months since their entry to the study have lost the ICA and remained
negative since (2 to 6 occasions). All but one (1:16) had ICA in the low
titer range of 1:2 to 1:4.

Two siblings who were negative at the time of entry to the study have
acquired ICA after 4 to 6 months and remained positive since.

TABLE I

HLA	Diabetics (n=64)	Controls (n=89)	p
DR2	8 %	22 %	< 0.05
DR3 (incl. DR4)	49 %	16 %	< 0.001
DR4 (incl. DR3)	67 %	27 %	< 0.001
DR5	2 %	21 %	< 0.001
DR3/4	26 %	1 %	< 0.001

In a further analysis, 10 relatives (6 siblings, 3 parents, 1 offspring) ICA developed during follow-up but have now disappeared. Eight had ICA titers of 1:2 - 1:4 on 1 - 3 occasions, 2 were positive 1:8 and 1:16, respectively.

"Fluctuating" ICA were found in 2 subjects with low ICA-titers (1:2 to 1:4). Fluctuation was defined as disappearance and reappearance of ICA on at least 2 occasions. The fluctuation was confirmed by retesting both positive and negative samples on the same pancreatic specimen.

All but 2 of the ICA positive subject were HLA-DR typed. As shown in table 2, all ICA-positive subjects have at least one HLA-DR haplotype in common with the diabetic proband. As yet, none of the ICA-negative subjects has developed diabetes mellitus.

TABLE II

I C A	Relatives			HLA-DR compared to diabetic		
	siblings	parents	offspring	identical	haplo-identical	non-identical
Persistent for more than 48 months* (or until IDDM developed)	1	2	2		5	
Positive for 12 - 36 months but negative now	4	1		1	3	
Acquired after 6 - 48 months and persistent since	2			1	1	
Acquired during study but lost now	6	3	1	2	6	
Fluctuating	2				2	

* 1 out of these 5 subjects developed IDDM after having been ICA-positive for 18 months

Insulin autoantibodies (IAA): IAA defined as an insulin-binding value of 10 binding units and above were found in 23 subjects (13%). Three were persistently positive, and 5 became positive during the study. Eleven subjects being IAA positive at entry lost their IAA, and in another 5 individuals IAA were found intermittently. In most of the IAA positive cases insulin-binding values of 10-20 units were found. Only 3 individuals had insulin binding values greater than 20 units. There was no correlation between IAA- and ICA-positivity.

Association between HLA-specificities and ICA or IAA: As shown in table 3, no correlation between any HLA-DR specificity and ICA or IAA was found. Additionally, there was no association between ICA or IAA and DR3/4, DR3 and/or 4, non-DR3 or 4, DR2 and/or 5 (exclusive 3,4) and DR2 and/or5 (inclusive 3/4), respectively.

TABLE III

DR type	Islet cell antibodies (ICA)		Insulin autoantibodies (IAA)	
	positive (n)	negative (n)	positive (n)	negative (n)
DR1	5	20	3	7
DR2	3	22	0	8
DR3	10	36	1	18
DR4	14	48	5	25
DR5	1	22	2	6
DR6	4	19	2	12
DR7	3	14	2	3
DR8	0	8	0	0
DR3/4	4	12	0	6
DR3 and/or 4	17	91	6	39
DR non 3 or 4	4	30	4	11

DISCUSSION

In our family study 13% of healthy first-degree relatives of IDDM patients were ICA-positive at some point in time, but in as few as 2.7% ICA were present throughout the entire observation period. One out of 5 persistently ICA-positive probands developed IDDM, whereas, as yet, none of the ICA negative did. IAA were found in 13% of unaffected relatives regardless of ICA-status or HLA-DR phenotypes.

The overall ICA-frequency in our series is comparable with the ones reported in the literature. ICA-prevalence rates of 26 and 27% have been described in first-degree relatives and non-diabetic identical twins (5), but in most of the studies considerably lower ICA-prevalence rates ranging from 0.9 to 12% are reported (6). Since in our study population ICA were transient or fluctuated, the real ICA-prevalence, calculated on initial or subsequent screening or as a percentage of the total amount of screened serum samples, was not higher than 3.4 - 5.6%.

Fluctuation of ICA-positivity has been reported in healthy first-degree relatives (3). However, this finding was not confirmed by others, suggesting that fluctuation may well be related to variation in the sensitivity of different human pancreatic substrates (7). Our findings showing ICA-fluctuation in the low titer range only also indicate that this may reflect inherent differences in the quality of the human pancreatic substrate. On the other hand, the observed fluctuation could be confirmed using the same pancreatic specimen for all the samples indicating that this could indeed represent weak and transient signs of islet cell autoimmunity, e.g. as a consequence of viral islet infection.

The one relative who developed IDDM shares one DR haplotype with the diabetic family member and had been persistently ICA-positive for 18 months. This corresponds to the results of the Barts Windsor study (3), where 7 out of 685 unaffected first degree relatives became diabetic. All had at least one haplotype in common with the diabetic proband and all had ICA prior to diagnosis.

Several reports demonstrate that IDDM develops in about 30% of ICA-positive first-degree relatives (2). However, IDDM may develop in ICA-negative unaffected monozygotic twins as well (2). The fact that only 30% of ICA-positive family members progress to overt diabetes and that ICA may be transient (3) indicates that some susceptible individuals may indeed overcome autoimmune processes directed against the beta cell.

Studies on association between ICA and the major histocompatibility complex (MHC) have revealed conflicting results. The presence of ICA has been shown to be correlated with HLA-B8 (8) in IDDM, with DR3 and B14 in diabetics with secondary oral hypoglycemic agent failure, and with D14, B18 in first-degree relatives. Recently Kobayashi et al. found HLA-DR4 antigens to be more frequent in ICA-positive diabetics with progressive beta cell dysfunction than in patients who lost ICA and whose beta cell function recovered. However, in most of the studies, no association between HLA-antigens and the presence of ICA was demonstrable (4, 7). Also in the present study, no evidence was found to establish a correlation between the occurrence of ICA and certain HLA-DR specificities.

Insulin antoantibodies occur in up to 47% of first-degree relatives (5, 1) and have been found to precede IDDM development by several years. They may represent an additional marker of impending IDDM, since it has been demonstrated that individuals positive for both IAA and ICA are more likely to develop IDDM than subjects positive for either of the markers alone (1). Furthermore, IAA may be related to the presence of ICA(1), but conflicting evidence has been published (5, 10). In our series IAA were not associated with ICA, nor were they related to any HLA-DR types.

In summary, our study has shown that ICA and IAA develop in a large proportion of unaffected first degree relatives of type I diabetics. However, in most of the cases ICA were transient, and only 1 out of 5 probands with persistent ICA progressed to IDDM. Thus, ICA may reflect episodic islet cell autoimmunity, but their value for predicting the development of IDDM is rather poor. The presence of IAA is not related to ICA, indicating that antibodies to islet-cells and their products arise independently.

ACKNOWLEDGEMENT

We thank Professor G. Thiel, Division of Nephrology, University Hospital, Basel, and Professor T.M. Neri, Institute of Immunology, Basel, for performing the HLA typing.

REFERENCES

1. Srikanta, S., Ricker, T., McCulloch, D.K., Soeldner, J.S., Eisenbarth, G.S., and Palmer, J.P., 1986, Diabetes 35: 139-142.

2. Srikanta, S., Ganda, O.P., Jackson, R.A., Gleason, R.E., Kaldany, A., Garovoy, M.R., Milford, E.L., Carpenter, C.B., Soeldner, J.S., and Eisenbarth, G.S., 1983, Type 1 diabetes mellitus in monozygotic twins: chronic progressive beta cell dysfunction. Ann Intern Med 99: 320-326.

3. Spencer, J.M., Tarn, A., Dean, B.M., Lister, J., and Bottazzo, G.F., 1984, Fluctuating islet-cell autoimmunity in unaffected relatives of patients with insulin-dependent idabetes. Lancet, i: 764-766.

4. Spinas, G.A., Keller, U., Neri, T.M., Matter, L., Staffelbach, O., and Berger, W., 1985, HLA-Antigene and Inselzellantikorper bei Typ-1-Diabetikern verschiedener Altersgruppen und ihren Verwandten 1. Grades Schweiz Med Wschr 115: 48-54.

5. Wilkin, T.J., Hoskins, P.J., Armitage, M., Rodier, M., Casey, C., Diaz, J., Pyke, D.A., and Leslie, R.D.G., 1985, Value of insulin autoantibodies as serum markers for insulin-dependent diabetes mellitus. Lancet i: 480-482.

6. Srikanta, S., Ganda, O.P., Rabizadeh, A., Soeldner, J.S., and Eisenbarth, G.S., 1985, First-degree relatives of patients with type 1 diabetes mellitus. Islet-cell antibodies and abnormal insulin secretion. N Engl J Med 313: 461-464.

7. Marner, B., Agner, T., Binder, C., Lernmark, A., Nerup, J., Mandrup-Poulsen, T., and Waldorff, S., 1985, Increased reduction in fasting C-peptide is associated with islet-cell antibodies in type I (insulin-dependent) diabetic patients. Diabetologia 28: 875-800.

8. Irvine, W.J., McCallum, C.J.M., Gray, R.S., Campbell, C.J., Ducan, L.J.P., Farquhar, J.W., Vaughan, H., and Morris, P.J., 1977, Pancreatic islet-cell antibodies in diabetes mellitus correlated with the duration and type of diabetes, coexistent autoimmune disease, and HLA type. Diabetes 26: 138-147.

9. Gleichmann, H., Zoercher, B., Greulich, B., Gries, F.A., Henrichs, H.R., Bertrams, J., and Kolb, H., 1984, Correlation of islet-cell antibodies and HLA-DR phenotypes with diabetes mellitus in adults. Diabetologia 27: 90-92.

10. Sochett, C., McKey, M., Yoon, J.W., and Daneman, D., 1986, Insulin antibodies in IDDM children before insulin therapy: relationship to islet-cell antibodies, C-peptide and antibody response to human insulin. Diabetes 35: 93 A.

CHILDHOOD INSULIN-DEPENDENT DIABETES

¶Yoshio Goto and Jo Satoh

Third Department of Internal Medicine
Tohoku University School of Medicine, Sendai, Japan

Before 1960, childhood diabetes was very rare. In 1961 we sent questionnaires to all the departments of medicine and pediatrics of the medical schools. This survey detected only 39 cases of childhood diabetes at the 46 university hospitals during the years 1956-1960. This figure is an unbelievable one if compared with those in European countries and even with those at the present time in Japan. Annual urine examinations of elementary and junior high school children has been legally obligatory for the early detection of renal disease since 1973 and urine glucose has been screened in addition to urine albumin. This nationwide detection survey has provided information not only on the incidence or prevalence but also about the natural history and clinical features of diabetes among children. Mimura (1) reviewed the reports on glucose tolerance tests during 1973 to 1978, and collected 47 cases of IDDM and 37 cases of NIDDM among 967,919 examinees (age 6-15 years old). The prevalence was 4.9 per 100,000 for IDDM and 3.8 per 100,000 for NIDDM. Kitagawa et al. (2) have been continuing the review for the diabetes detection in Tokyo and estimated the incidence of asymptomatic IDDM as 0-0.9 (average 0.4) per 100,000 population and that of asymptomatic plus symptomatic IDDM as 1.2-1.6 per 100,000 children per year.

Since 1976, medical expenses for the treatment of diabetes in children under 18 years old have been covered by the government. The numbers may be slightly overestimated if they were all IDDM. However, the prevalence rate per 100,000 children may be lower if compared with those of European countries. Most of the reports show that the frequency of diabetes is greater in females than males. Similar female preponderance was also found in our series of 113 childhood diabetics (Toyota et al,, (3)). The Childhood Diabetes Research Committee of the Ministry of Health and Welfare sent questionnaires to hospitals and collected clinical records of 1,572 diabetics from hospitals (Hibi, et al. 1982). There were 633 boys and 936 girls and the female to male ratio was 1:48 and the seasonal distribution of diabetes-onset showed the highest in February and the lowest in July. Family history of diabetes was positive in 480 of the 1560 cases (30.8%).

The incidence of IDDM is high in Scandinavian countries in comparison with France and Israel and clear correlation between the incidence and distance from Equator was pointed out by La Porte et al. (1985). The prevalence of childhood diabetes in Japan, however, shows no clear north-to-south gradient (Goto et al. (4).

As stated above, childhood diabetes was rare in the past but it has been increasing during the last 20 years in Japan as well as in other Asian countries. What are the reasons? It is unlikely that the diabetic gene(s) or diabetes-associated genes have been accumulating among the people. It is possible to assume that B-cell affinitive toxic substances have increased in our environment, although we do not know what the substances are. The most probable explanation for the increase in IDDM especially among the younger generation may be made from immunological studies. This hypothesis seems to be supported partly by our experiments on NOD mice. The development of insulitis and hyperglycemia of the NOD mice is completely prevented by injection of the substances obtained from streptococci or E. coli via normalization of the deviated immune response network (Toyota et al. 1986, Sato et al. 1988). Decrease of bacterial infections due to the improved living environment may cause less chance of immune system response and may result in the increase of immune-associated IDDM.

HISTOCOMPATIBILITY ANTIGENS

The discovery of major histocompatibility complex system reevealed the definitive difference in genetics of diabetes that IDDM but not NIDDM was associated with certain types of HLA. The genes coding for HLA are located on the short arm of chromosome 6. Because the HLA system was shown to be linked to the putative immune-response gene, an autoimmune-pathogenesis was also indicated in IDDM as was in the other autoimmune diseases. It was known that HLA-B8 and B15 were positively and HLA-B7 was negatively associated with IDD in the Caucasian race. Later, serological typing of class II HLA showed the stronger association of HLA-DR with IDDM than the class I antigen.

Since Wakisaka et al. first reported association between HLA and juvenile diabetes in Japanese in 1976, the extended studies were performed in the different regions of Japan. There were some variations depending on the reporters in HLA-types that associated with Japanese IDDM. However, it has generally been accepted that HLA-Bw35 and Bw54 were positively associated with Japanese IDDM. There were also positive associations between HLA-DR and DRw9 and IDDM. Negative associations of Bw52 and DR2 with IDDM were observed in Japanese. As summarized in Table 1, there were linkage disequilibriums between Bw35 and DR4, between Bw54 and DRw9, and between Bw52 and DR2 in Japanese.

Table II shows frequencies of selected HLA-DR antigens as reported by Mimura et al. The relative risk for IDDM in HLA-DR4/DR9 heterozygotes (10. 44) in Japanese was significantly higher than that in DR4 (2.44) or DR9 (3.75) alone haplotypes, as HLA-DR3/DR4 hetorozygotes had higher relative risk for IDDM than the homozygotes in Caucasians. Approximately 92% of Japanese IDDM had HLA-DR4 and /or DR9, and 67% in healthy controls. On the other hand, 98% of Caucasian IDDM and HLA-DR3 and/or DR 4, and 59% in controls.

Mimura et al. tested the relationship between HLA-DR and the persistent ICSA in sera from the patients with duration of IDDM for more than 5 years. Prevalence of ICSA was significantly higher in IDDM with HLA-DRw9 homozygote or DRw9/x than with DR4 homozygote as with DR3 reported in Caucasian IDDM. A similar association was observed between HLA-DR9 homozygote and similar association was observed between HLA-DR9 homozygote and IDDM complicated with other autoimmune diseases such as Hashimoto's thyroiditis and Graves disease. This indicates that HLA-DRw9 in Japanese may substitute for DR3 in Caucasians.

TABLE I

ASSOCIATION BETWEEN IDDM AND HLA IN JAPANESE

Linkage disequilibrium of HLA	Frequency in IDDM
Bw35 —— DR4	increase
Bw54 —— DRw9	increase
Bw52 —— DR2	decrease

TABLE II

FREQUENCIES (%) OF SELECTED HLA-DR ANTIGENS AND RELATIVE RISK FOR THESE ANTIGENS (Mimura 1984).

HLA-DR	Patients N=52	Controls N=45	RR
2	0(0)	5(11.1)	
2,X	1(1.9)	3(6.7)	0.27
4	10(19.2)	4(8.9)	2.44
4,X	13(25.0)	11(24.4)	1.03
9	4(7.7)	1(2.2)	3.75
9,X	2(3.8)	2(4.4)	0.86
4,9	17(32.7)	2(4.4)	10.44
4 and/or 9	48(92.3)	30(66.7)	6.00

X=presence of DR3, w6, 7, w8

TABLE III

ASSOCIATION BETWEEN IDDM AND HLA IN VARIOUS ETHNIC GROUPS

	positively associated HLA		negatively associated HLA	
Caucasian	B8 DR3	B15 DR4	B7	DR2
American black	DR3 DR4			DR2
Japanese	Bw35 DR9	Bw54 DR4	Bw52	DR2

TABLE IV

PREVALENCE OF ICA IN JAPANESE IDDM

Duration of IDDM	ICA No.	%	Reporters
< 1y		13	Tanae (1981)
		16	Nagaoka (1975)
		34	Shinjo (1982)
	14/41	40	Kobayashi (1981)
	15/28	53	Kobayashi (1982)
		63	Notsu (1985)
	16/19	84	Ueda (1984)
overall	6/44	14	Kobayashi (1984)
	16/57	28	Kasahara (1984)
	52/162	32	Notsu (1985)
	24/50	48	Ueda (1985)
healthy subjects		0~0.5	

TABLE V

PREVALENCE OF ICA IN FAMILY MEMBERS OF IDDM PATIENTS IN JAPAN

Family	ICA No.	%
parents	5/23	22
siblings	0/15	0
children	1/6	17
	6/44	14
Non-diabetic control	0/177	0

(Kobayashi 1984)

217

Table III shows the association betweeen IDDM and HLA antigens in various ethnic groups. HLA-DR4 is positively and DR2 is negatively associated with IDDM in all ethnic groups. HLA-DR3 is associated with IDDM in Caucasian and American Blacks, and DR9 in Japanese. These ethnic differences in the HLA antigens that are associated with IDDM may account for some of the ethnic variation (e.g., incidence) in the disease. The recently developing techniques of molecular biology may be able to reveal a molecular basis for association between IDDM and IDDM-susceptible genes that link to HLA and for ethnic differences in IDDM-HLA associations.

ICA AND ICSA

Presence of autoantibodies directed against pancreatic islets is another characteristic of IDDM. These anti-islet autoantibodies consist of cytoplasmic and cell-surface antibodies namely ICA and ICSA. ICA is understood as a marker of ongoing B cell destruction rather than a pathogenetic role in IDDM. On the other hand, ICSA reacts with living islet cell-surface of human or rodent origin and ICSA-antigen was indicated to be a species-non-specific, but B cell-specific glycoprotein. ICSA has a cytotoxic effect on B cell in complement-mediated or cell-mediated manner in vitro.

It has been reported from Europe and North America that 70 to 90% of Caucasian patients were positive for ICA and ICSA at the time of onset of IDDM. The prevalence of ICA seems to parallel that of ICSA. However, as shown in Table IV, the reported prevalences of ICA in Japanese IDDM were generally low as compared with those in Caucasian IDDM. In the patients with duration of IDDM for less than one year, the prevalence of ICA varied very much depending on the reporters and the range was from 13 to 84%. The overall prevalence of ICA was 14 to 48%. A similar tendency was observed in ICSA (Table IV).

The differences in prevalence of ICA and ICSA may be due to technical problems rather than to pathogenetic characteristics in Japanese IDDM, because recently Kobayashi et al. reported that the prevalence of ICA in Japanese IDDM was as high as that in Caucasians reported from Europe and North America. He stained the sections of fresh pancreas resected in surgical operations and found ICA in 83% of patients within one month after the onset of IDDM by conventional immunofluorescent staining and in 100% of patients by the three layer immunofluorescent staining method applying a biotin-avidin system. The prevalence of ICA decreased with increasing duration of IDDM. Thus, the prevalence of ICA or ICSA in Japanese IDDM is thought to be essentially the same as in Caucasian.

There are limited numbers of reports on autoantibodies other than ICA and ICSA in Japanese IDDM patients. Approximately 10 to 20% of patients with IDDM had anti-nuclear, anti-pituitary or anti-thyroid antibodies, whereas less than one percent of healthy controls were positive for these autoantibodies. These data indicate that the prevalence of polyendocrine types of IDDM, namely type la classified by Irvine, in Japanese is similar to that in Caucasian.

AUTOANTIBODIES IN FAMILY MEMBERS OF IDDM PATIENTS IN JAPAN

We have no conclusive data on the prevalence of autoantibodies in family members of Japanese IDDM patients, because there have been very few reports on this study. In Table V, approximately 20% of non-diabetic parents or children of IDDM patients had ICA, whereas none of non-diabetic controls were positive for ICA. As for the other autoantibodies, one of 18 parents of IDDM patients was positive for anti-thyroid or anti-nuclear antibody.

These studies on epidemiology, genetics and immunology in Japanese IDDM suggest that although the incidence of IDDM is obviously lower in the Japanese population in comparison to the Caucasian, the significance of autoimmune component in the pathogenesis of IDDM in Japanese is as high as in the Caucasian race.

REFERENCES

1. Mimura, G., 1985, Epidemiology of childhood diabetes in Japan. Tonyobyogaku no Shinpo 19: 162–168.

2. Kitagawa, T., Mano, T., Fujita, H., 1983, The Epidemiology of childhood diabetes mellitus in Tokyo Metropolitan area. Tohoku J Exp Med, 141 Suppl: 171–179.

3. Toyota, T., Kikuchi, T., Abe, Y., et al., 1979, Childhood diabetes in Tohoku area. Eds., G. Mimura, T. Kitagawa, I. Hibi, Tokyo: Childhood diabetes in Asia. Medical Journal Sha: 126–130.

4. Goto, Y., 1986, Epidemiology of diabetes mellitus. Nihon Rynsho, 44, suppl: 116–124.

5. Wakisaka, A., Aizawa, M., Matsuura, W., et al., 1976, HLA and juvenile diabetes mellitus in the Japanese. Lancet 2: 970.

6. Kobayashi, T., Sugimoto, T., Itoh, T., et al., 1986, The prevalence fo islet cell antibodies in Japanese insulin-dependent and non-insulin-dependent diabetic patients studied by indirect immunofluorescence and new method. Diabetes 35: 335–340.

CHILDREN AT HIGH RISK OF DIABETES MELLITUS:
NEW YORK STUDIES OF FAMILIES WITH DIABETES
AND OF CHILDREN WITH CONGENITAL RUBELLA SYNDROME

¶Robert C. McEvoy[1,2], Barbara Fedun[3], Louis Z. Cooper[3],
Nancy M. Thomas[2], Santiago Rodriguez De Cordoba[4],
Pablo Rubinstein[4], and Fredda Ginsberg-Fellner[1]

Departments of Pediatrics[1] and Anatomy[2], Mount Sinai School of Medicine
of the City University of New York; Developmental Disabilities Unit[3]
Department of Pediatrics, St. Luke's Roosevelt Medical Center
and Laboratory of Immunogenetics[4], Lindsley F. Kimbell Research Institute
New York Blood Center, New York, New York, USA.

The frequency of Type I, or insulin-dependent mellitus (IDDM) in the general population is approximately 1 in 600 individuals. By contrast, in families where one child has IDDM, the likelihood that another child will develop IDDM is about 100 times higher. This population, at high risk for the development of IDDM, seemed an ideal group in which to identify some of the factors which might precede the development of clinically apparent IDDM. IDDM is clearly a multifactorial disease. The existence of a gene or genes predisposing to diabetes and mapping within or very near the HLA locus on chromosome six has been suggested by several different investigators. In addition, environmental agents also appear to be needed to "trigger" the predisposition towards overt disease since concordance for monozygotic twins is estimated at only approximately 30%. Convincing evidence has accumulated over the last several years that the mechanism of the expression of the genetic susceptibility is an autoimmune destruction of the pancreatic beta cells.

Numerous reports, beginning in the mid-1800's, have implicated viruses as an environmental agent which might play a role in the triggering of such an autoimmune process. In man, RNA viruses such as mumps, rubella, and Coxsackie, have been strongly implicated in the subsequent development of diabetes. Mumps and other viral infections have also been associated with the rapid development of transient islet cell and insulin autoantibodies, although short-term studies to date have not demonstrated a significant increase in IDDM. There have been reports of an association between intrauterine infection with rubella virus (Congenital Rubella Syndrome, CRS) and diabetes since 1949 when Menser et al. published the first of a series of reports which have subsequently pointed out that 40% of individuals with

The studies have been supported by grants from the National Institutes of Health (DK-19631, DK 39286), the Juvenile Diabetes Foundation International, the American Diabetes Association, the National Foundation/March of Dimes, the New York Diabetes Association, and the Diabetes Research and Education Foundation.

CRS, if followed longitudinally for significant periods of time, demonstrate either overt IDDM or significant carbohydrate intolerance by the second to third decade of life. Consequently. we have also followed a group of subjects with CRS from the last rubella epidemic in New York, during 1964-66. We will summarize here our work to date on these two interesting human populations and report in some detail our most recent genetic data further localizing the diabetes susceptibility gene, and epidemiological data documenting an association between the presence of insulin autoantibodies, presence of islet cell surface antibodies, and glucose intolerance in the subjects with CRS.

METHODS

STUDY GROUPS

Since 1977, we have studied a group of families in which at least one child has IDDM. Through 1987, a total of 328 such families have been studied in detail including 566 siblings who initially did not have diabetes. In this report, these individuals will be designated as the Family Study. During and immediately after the 1964-66 rubella epidemic in New York City, over 600 infants were born with stigmata of CRS. Subsequently, many of these children have been followed at the Developmental Disabilities Center of St. Luke's-Roosevelt Medical Center. Since 1982, we have studied this well-characterized cohort of individuals with CRS, examining the same markers for predisposition to diabetes that we had identified in the Family Study. These include: HLA type including identification of polymorphisms at the HLA DR, DQ, and DP loci; estimation of glucose tolerance by hemoglobin A_1c determination, by oral and, in some cases, intravenous glucose tolerance testing measuring both glucose and serum insulin responses, and by C peptide responsiveness; evidence for islet cell autoimmunity measuring either islet cell cytoplasmic antibodies (ICA) or islet cell surface antibodies (ICSA) and insulin autoantibodies (IAA), as well as autoantibodies against other organs including the thyroid and adrenal glands. The techniques employed in these studies have been reported in previous publications (1-10) except for the current methodology for the IAA which is given in greater detail below.

INSULIN AUTO-ANTIBODY DISPLACEMENT ASSAY

Any endogenous insulin in sera to be tested for IAA was extracted with acid charcoal as previously described (9) and the sera were incubated with ^{125}I-porcine insulin (1.0 uU/ml) at a final dilution of 1:10 in the presence or absence of biosynthetic human insulin (Novolin, Squibb-Novo, 4ug/-ml). The sera were incubated for 72 hours at 4° C when the antibody-bound radioactivity was precipitated by polyethylene glycol (PEG, final concentration 10.6% w/w). After centrifugation, the PEG-precipitated radioactivity was quantitated in a gamma counter and the antibody-bound insulin displacable by this excess of unlabeled human insulin was expressed as uU/ml of whole serum. The results in these two diabetes-prone populations were compared to results obtained from two normal populations: 160 normal blood donors (Mean ± 1 SD, 0.07 ± 0.06 uU/ml), and 101 normal children without a family history of diabetes mellitus (0.07 ± 0.06 uU/ml). No sample from either group exceeded 0.19 uU/ml (Mean +2 SD), so any samples with insulin binding of 0.20 uU/ml or greater were considered positive for IAA.

RESULTS AND DISCUSSION

STUDY OF FAMILIES WITH IDDM

Genetics   Since the discovery of significant association between particular HLA antigens and IDDM, but not non-insulin dependent diabetes mellitus, progress in the understanding of the baffling genetics of this disease has been considerable. Thus, genetic linkage between disease susceptibility and the HLA system has been proven. Although disagreement on some aspects remains, a conclusion that is probably acceptable to everyone is that a gene or genes in linkage disequilibrium with Class II HLA alleles (DR, DQ, and/or DP) contributes solely or predominantly to the genetic component of the susceptibility to IDDM. The association between these Class II histocompatibility markers (in higher association - HLA DR4, and to a lesser extent, DR7) and diabetes is highly relevant to a study of a large group of individuals. However, we and others have previously shown that it is also highly predictive in an individual family as well. In our Family Study, no significant deviation from Mendelian ratios has been observed in the inheritance of the HLA genes where 23.5% of siblings share two haplotypes with the diabetic proband, 55.5% shared one and 21.0% shared no haplotypes (Chi square = 1.57, NS). This information has been particularly helpful in predicting the onset of diabetes in additional members of these families in which one member was already diabetic. Through 1987, of the 566 initially non-diabetic siblings enrolled in our Family Study, 16 had developed Type I diabetes. Of these 16, 12 shared HLA identity with their previously-diabetic sibling. Fifteen of the 16 were either HLA DR3, DR4, or both. The single exception was a child with Down's Syndrome.

MHC CLASS II GENE PRODUCTS

These genetically well-characterized families have been an ideal population to further define the location of the putative diabetes susceptibility gene on Chromosome 6, apparently very near the MHC Class II genes. Use of high resolution isoelectric focusing methods has greatly facilitated the systematic analyses of biochemical variability in the HLA-Class II products to unequivocally identify DR, DQ, DP products in 157 individuals from 27 multiplex IDDM families. Using these techniques, we have recently described a significant association between DP beta C and DP beta F with DR3 and DR4 haplotypes, where DP beta C occurs more frequently than DP beta F among DR3, and the reverse among DR4 haplotypes.

In order to determine whether these DR/DQ-DP associations could be secondary to the selection of HLA haplotypes caused by the association with IDDM, the 106 haplotypes were separated into 67 "IDDM-affected" and 19 "control" haplotypes based on the criteria that "control" haplotypes were those exclusively present in healthy siblings of IDDM patients. The most striking association was observed among the DR3 haplotypes (N=18). All 18 of the DR3 haplotypes encoded identical DR3-specific DR3 beta I, DQ alpha, and DQ beta chain variants, but differed in their DR beta II chains. Thus, two different groups, each including 9 DR3 haplotypes could be established based on the isoelectric focusing variations of DR3 beta II. All DR3 haplotypes including DR3 beta II B were also found to be HLA B8. No differences in the IDDM association of these two subsets of haplotypes were found and, in fact, identical numbers of "affected" and "control" haplotypes were observed among the DR3-DR3 beta II A and the DR3-DR3 beta II B haplotypes.

MHC CLASS II DP PRODUCTS

DR3 haplotypes can also be distinguished by isoelectric patterns of DP products independent of the variation at the DR beta II locus and, interestingly, all DR3 haplotypes carrying the DP beta C allele (N=9) were found among DR3-IDDM affected haplotypes (P < 0.05 by Fisher's exact test). Similarly among DRw6 haplotypes, DP beta C again associated exclusively with "affected" status. The same was true for DP beta B and "affected" DR7 hap-

lotypes. Because the relevant DP variants are different in DR3 and DR7 haplotypes, we have concluded that DP may not itself be the "disease gene" but,
rather, the centromeric bound of the region that contained this susceptibility gene. These data suggest that the polymorphic variations at the DP
locus represent genetic markers useful in the discrimination between high-
and low-risk for diabetes, but otherwise indistinguishable, DR3, DRw6, and
DR7 Class II haplotypes. These observations, together with those of other
investigators demonstrating a similar role for DQ variations in DR4 haplotypes, strongly suggest that HLA-linked, IDDM susceptibility genes are located centromeric to DR, and, most likely, between the DQ and DP loci.
They also reinforce that the susceptibility factor is not one of the currently recognized HLA Class II gene products.

ISLET CELL ANTIBODIES

The presence of antibodies in the sera from newly diagnosed patients
with IDDM which bind to islet cells has been widely recognized as an important autoimmune marker in IDDM. Reports from our Family Study (1,3,7,8,
10) and by others have confirmed that these islet cell antibodies also mark
the non-diabetic individuals at risk for development of diabetes. Fifteen
of the 16 siblings who developed diabetes over the 10 year follow-up period
ending in 1987 had evidence of islet cell antibody prior to the diagnosis
of IDDM. It is of note that while the presence of the islet cell antibody
is predictive of the eventual development of IDDM, the majority of the
non-diabetic siblings who share one or more HLA haplotypes with their
affected sibling and who are islet cell antibody-positive have not yet
developed diabetes. Thus, the presence of islet cell antibody is not,
itself, directly related to a pathologic process in the islets.

IMPAIRED INSULIN SECRETION

The third predictive marker for the eventual development of diabetes
has been an impairment of insulin secretion in response to either an oral
or intravenous glucose load. On the basis of the data from our Family
Study on insulin secretion, we conclude that, at least in these families,
impairment of beta-cell function can become detectable many months or even
years before the onset of clinically apparent diabetes, even in very young
children. Of the 16 siblings who decompensated to diabetes during our 10
year follow-up from 1977 to 1987, 14 had been found to have impaired insulin secretion prior to the onset of clinical diabetes. Thus, our data
suggest that a triad of 1) HLA identity, 2) islet cell antibody positivity,
and 3) an impaired insulin secretion are useful markers for identifying
children at high risk for development of IDDM. In fact, of 6 non-diabetic
children who had this triad in 1984, two became diabetic by 1987. At present, of the remaining non-diabetic siblings in our family study, 18 are
HLA-identical to their diabetic probands and have islet cell antibodies
and impaired insulin secretion. It will be of continuing interest to determine what percentage of these children develop diabetes in the future.

INSULIN AUTOANTIBODIES

We and others are continuing to examine other markers which may be
helpful in further defining the family members at risk for the development
of diabetes. Others have suggested that autoantibodies against insulin,
which have been shown to be present at the onset of clinical diabetes by
several groups including our own (9), are predictive of the eventual development of IDDM. We have been unable, at least in our Family Study, to
support this finding. Sera were available for 6 of the siblings who decompensated the diabetes, at some point prior to the clinical development
of diabetes and at the time of diagnosis of the diabetes. Of these 6 siblings, 4 (67%) were IAA-positive at the time of diagnosis of diabetes,

whereas none of these individuals were positive on the previous samples which were taken from 3 to 111 months prior to the beginning of insulin treatment. At the time that these data were published, we had been unable to demonstrate the presence of IAA in any individuals who did not have clearly impaired glucose tolerance. Subsequently we have refined the insulin autoantibody assay and can now demonstrate the presence of IAA in individuals who are metabolically normal. These data will be discussed below under the CRS study.

STUDY OF CHILDREN WITH CONGENITAL RUBELLA SYNDROME

Genetics. It seems clear that environmental factors are needed to "trigger" the state of genetic susceptibility into one in which IDDM is expressed clinically, at least as shown by the 70% lack of concordance in studies of identical twins. Thus, it is reasonable to assume that the frequency, extent, and severity of exposure to such environmental "trigger(s)" may determine the penetrance of the genotype confirming susceptibility to IDDM. We have studied the children with CRS in this regard, since previous studies have indicated that up to 40% of such individuals develop IDDM. We reported a study (4) in which the HLA antigens of 173 patients with CRS were examined. Twenty-one of these individuals (12.1%) were clinically diabetic at the time of the study when the average age of the patients was approximately 17 years. This study confirmed the extremely high incidence of diabetes in the CRS population. The frequency of HLA antigens DR2 and DR3 were significantly lower and higher, respectively in the diabetic CRS patients as opposed to the CRS patients without diabetes or in control individuals. These data suggest that the genes that control susceptibility to IDDM in the general population appear also to be necessary for the development of glucose intolerance in CRS patients.

ISLET CELL ANTIBODIES

Antibodies against the islet cells were also determined in the CRS population. In our initial report of 173 such patients (5), 20.2% of the CRS individuals were positive for islet antibodies versus 3.4% of a population of control children without diabetes. Recently we have examined an additional 187 sera from the non-diabetic CRS population for the presence of islet cell surface antibodies, and 47 sera (25.1%) were positive for such antibodies. Thus, islet cell antibody-positivity in the CRS population will be much less discriminatory in identifying individuals who will develop IDDM, unless the incidence of diabetes in this population will be extraordinarily high.

INSULIN AUTOANTIBODIES, HYPERINSULINEMIA

With the modification in the insulin autoantibody assay as described above, we examined the same 187 sera for presence of IAA. Surprisingly, 57 (30.5%) of the sera were positive for the presence of IAA by this more sensitive assay. Twenty-seven of the CRS patients were positive for both islet-cell and insulin autoantibodies and glucose tolerance tests have been performed on twenty of these individuals. Twelve of these individuals met criteria of the National Diabetes Data Group as having either diabetes or impaired glucose intolerance. However, and of continuing interest, only one of these individuals had a diminished insulin secretory response to the oral glucose challenge. The remaining individuals, and several of those that were not glucose intolerant, had an increased total insulin response to the oral glucose challenge. This cannot be explained as an artifact of the insulin assay caused by the endogenous insulin antibodies as free insulins were measured. Whether these individuals are presently in an hyperinsulinemic state preceding a decompensation toward hypoinsulinemia is a question which awaits further follow-up. The presence of elevated glucose

in the face of hyperinsulinemia, however, suggests a state of insulin resistance which is uncommon in IDDM.

We have no satisfactory explanation for the increased autoimmune responsiveness in these CRS patients, but autoimmune phenomenon are not limited to those relevant to diabetes mellitus. Many of the CRS patients (41%)
have diminished total T lymphocytes and 56% have an abnormally low OKT4/OKT8
cell ratio. In addition, anti-thyroid microsomal or anti-thyroglobulin antibodies were found in 26% of the CRS patients versus less than 15% in a
control population. The influence of this profound intrauterine infection
with rubella virus and the subsequent development of these autoimmune phenomena in later life is a focus of continuing intensive study in our laboratories. As both the immune and several endocrinological systems seem to be
involved, a multidisciplinary approach will be needed to elucidate the complex interactions between this viral infection and the profound immuno-dys-
regulation in these unfortunate patients.

In summary, the analyses of the development of diabetes in non-diabetic
family members of an individual with diabetes mellitus have defined a triad
of markers which seem to identify individuals at high risk for the development of diabetes. These include HLA identity or haplo-identity with the
diabetic proband, the presence of antibodies to the pancreatic islets, and
diminished insulin secretory response to an oral or intravenous glucose
challenge. The CRS patients have a very high incidence of diabetes which
seems to be genetically similar to that of the general population in that
the same HLA markers for diabetes are found in the CRS patients with diabetes
as in the general diabetic population. However, the presence of islet cell
antibodies, of insulin autoantibodies, and of glucose intolerance in these
individuals is much higher than the general population and continued study
will be necessary to determine whether these markers indeed identify risk
for the development of insulin-dependent diabetes in these very special individuals. Similarly, it remains unknown as to whether these markers, which
seem so predictive in these diabetic families, will be applicable to the population at large. This is particularly relevant since the majority of individuals who present with IDDM have no first degree family history of diabetes
mellitus.

REFERENCES

1. Dobersen, M.J., Scharff, J.E., Ginsberg-Fellner, F. and Notkins, A.L.:
Cytotoxic autoantibodies to beta cells in the serum of patients with insulin dependent diabetes mellitus. New Engl. J. Med. 1980; 303:1493-1498.

2. Rubinstein, P., Ginsberg-Fellner, F. and Falk, C.T.: Genetics of Type
I diabetes mellitus: a single, recessive, predisposition gene mapping between HLA-B and GLO. Amer. J. Hum. Genet. 1981; 33:865-882.

3. Ginsberg-Fellner, F., Dobersen, M.J., Witt, M.E., Rayfield, E.J., Notkins, A.L. and Rubinstein, P.: HLA antigens, cytoplasmic islet cell antibodies and carbohydrate tolerance in families of children with insulin-
dependent diabetes mellitus. Diabetes 1982; 31:292-298.

4. Rubinstein, P., Witt, M.E., Fedun, B., Walker, M.E., Cooper, L.Z. and
Ginsberg-Fellner, F.: The HLA system in congenital rubella patients with
and without diabetes. Diabetes 1982; 31:1088-1091.

5. Ginsberg-Fellner, F., Witt, M.E., Yagihashi, S., Dobersen, M.J., Taub,
F., Fedun, B., McEvoy, R.C., Roman, S.H., Davies, T.F., Cooper, L.Z., Rubinstein, P. and Notkins, A.L.: The congenital rubella syndrome as a model
for Type I diabetes mellitus (IDDM): Increased prevalence of islet cell
surface antibodies. Diabetologia 1984; 27:87-89.

6. Ginsberg-Fellner, F., Witt, M.E., Fedun, B., Taub, F., Dobersen, M.J., McEvoy, R.C., Cooper, L.Z., Notkins, A.L. and Rubinstein, P.: Diabetes mellitus and autoimmunity in patients with the congenital rubella syndrome. Rev. Infect. Dis. 1985; 70 (Suppl. 1)-:S170-S176.

7. Toguchi, Y., Ginsberg-Fellner, F., and Rubinstein, P.: Cytotoxic islet-cell surface antibodies (ICSA) in patients with Type I diabetes and their first degree relatives. Diabetes 1985; 34:855-860.

8. Ginsberg-Fellner, F. Witt, M.E., Franklin, B.H., Yagihashi, S., Toguchi, Y., Dobersen, M.J., Rubinstein, P. and Notkins, A.L.: Triad of markers for identifying children at high risk for the development of insulin-dependent diabetes mellitus. J. Amer. Med. Assoc. 1985; 254:1469-1472.

9. McEvoy, R.C., Witt, M.E., Ginsberg-Fellner, F., and Rubinstein, P.: Anti-insulin antibodies in children with Type I diabetes mellitus: Genetic regulation of production and presence at diagnosis prior to insulin replacement. Diabetes 1986; 35:634-641.

10. Ginsberg-Fellner, F., McEvoy, R.C., Rubinstein, P. and Notkins, A.L.: Ten-year longitudinal study of children at high risk of insulin-dependent diabetes mellitus. New Eng. J. Med 1987; 317:1352-1353.

FAMILY STUDIES OF INSULIN-DEPENDENT DIABETES: THE UK EXPERIENCE

¶E.A.M. Gale, P.J. Bingley, and A.C. Tarn

Department of Diabetes and Immunogenetics
St. Bartholomew's Hospital, London

The presentation of insulin-dependent diabetes (IDDM) in children and young adults usually appears to be sudden (1), suggesting an acute pathology, but we now know that this is only the final step in a process of cumulative beta-cell damage extending over months or even many years. By the time of diagnosis some 80-90% of beta cells have been destroyed. Clinical trials have shown that immunosuppression of newly diagnosed patients may prolong the survival of the remaining beta cells, but it would be log al to intervene at an earlier stage, when the majority of these cells are still viable. This approach could only be considered if it were possible to predict accurately the onset of diabetes in a given individual.

POPULATION STUDY

The Family Study Approach

Prospective analysis of individuals at increased risk offers the best chance of developing and testing a predictive index. The highest risk of all is present in twins discordant for diabetes. Some 30-50% of unaffected twins will develop IDDM, usually within the first ten years from diagnosis of their cotwin (2). Children of two parents with IDDM have an almost equally high risk - around 33% - but they and discordant twins are of course extremely rare. First degree relatives of a child with diabetes offer a more convenient cohort for prospective study. This approach, now widely employed, allows continuing analysis of genetic, immunological and metabolic markers of risk, as well as permitting investigation of possible environmental factors. A large population base is needed before susceptible individuals can be identified in sufficient numbers; intensive study of this group may, in time, allow simpler and more precise markers to be developed.

The Bart's Windsor Family Study

This was started by the late Professor Andrew Cudworth in 1978. The rationale for prospective follow-up was provided by the recognition of HLA associations (3), the observation that siblings HLA identical with the proband were at increased risk (4), the discovery of islet cell antibodies in newly diagnosed diabetic patients (5) and the possibility of prospective screening for viral infections suspected of being implicated in the pathogenesis of Type I diabetes (6).

The original study was based on a clinic register developed by Dr. John Lister, with a number of other families being recruited from other local clinics, making a total of 204 families. All the families were caucasian, contained a diabetic proband diagnosed before the age of 20 and at least one unaffected sibling under that age. The families have been visited regularly at home by field workers over the past 10 years and, following initial tissue typing, blood has been taken at 4-6 monthly intervals for organ-specific antibodies, viral studies and a variety of other investigations. Of the original total, some 185 families remain in contact with the study, though many are now only under postal follow-up.

In 1984 the Bart's Windsor cohort was frozen at 204 families but maintained under long-term surveillance. Since then a new family study known as the Bart's Oxford Study has been established. This is based on a defined population of 2.4 million people in the Oxford Region. Newly diagnosed diabetic patients under the age of 21 (approximately 120 cases per year to date) will be ascertained over a 5 year period, and their families recruited for the study. Surveillance is maintained by 4 locally based nurses who have taken over the role of field workers, and regular blood samples are taken from all the family members. For reasons of cost screening is based upon measurement of ICA and HLA typing is restricted to families with an ICA positive non-diabetic member and an equal number of control families. The central aim of the new extended study is recruitment of high risk individuals in sufficient numbers for prospective study.

METHODOLOGY

Genetic Markers

Diabetes develops on a basis of genetic susceptibility, but is not simply a disease of genetic predestination. The classic demonstration of this comes from the study of identical twins. If one twin develops IDDM diabetes, the other has a 50-70% change of avoiding the disease completely. In contrast only 10% of twins are discordant for non-insulin-dependent diabetes (NIDDM) indicating a much stronger genetic component in this variety of diabetes. Further evidence that the genetic contribution to NIDDM is of greater importance than that to IDDM comes from analysis of the frequency of diabetes within first degree relatives. The life-time risk of developing IDDM has been calculated as 2.9% for parents, 6.6% for siblings and 4.9% for children of an individual with IDDM (7).

Despite many efforts, the mode of inheritance of IDDM remains unclear. The HLA associations of Type I diabetes have been studied extensively, and powerful links with HLA-DR3 and DR4 have been established. A study of 123 subjects diagnosed before the age of 20 (8) found that 98% possessed either DR3 (relative risk = 5.0), DR4 (relative risk = 6.8) or both (relative risk = 14.3) The relative risk conferred by DR3 is more than merely additive with that conferred by DR4, suggesting that each makes a separate contribution in predisposing to diabetes, but that they also have an unexplained complementary effect in combination.

HLA analysis has a more specific role in predicting risk within first degree relatives. Siblings who are HLA identical with the proband are most at risk. This risk has been put as high as 30% (9,10), but our current estimate is rather lower, giving a cumulative risk by Life Table analysis of 15.7% of developing diabetes by the age of 25 for HLA identical siblings and 8.6% for haploidentical siblings, while none of the non-identical siblings were in our sample projected to be diabetic by that age. The Pittsburgh group (11) suggest rather lower figures of 10.3% in HLA identical and 2.2% in haploidentical siblings.

Autoimmunity and Type I Diabetes

The first evidence that autoimmunity might be involved came from the description of mononuclear cell infiltrates in the islets of patients dying soon after developing juvenile diabetes. A detailed study of a large number of post-mortem pancreatic specimens has emphasized the diversity of the changes within a single pancreatic specimen, often varying markedly from lobule to lobule, so that some islets contain virtually no beta cells, others show marked cellular infiltration, and others appear relatively normal. This histological picture is entirely consistent with immunological and metabolic evidence of a protracted disease process preceding onset of diabetes.

A large number of autoimmune abnormalities, both humoral and cellular, have been described in association with IDDM. These include a variety of circulating antibodies directed against surface and cytoplasmic components of islet cells. Methodological differences introduced considerable confusion but this now promises to be resolved by introduction of an international standard expressed in JDF units. Complement fixation has been described, and was originally felt to be more specific for beta cell damage. It is now thought to represent high titers of ICA rather than a different class of antibody but remains a valuable marker of risk. In our study 13 of 24 (54%) of relatives positive for complement fixing ICA (CF-ICA) on 3 or more occasions developed IDDM, as against 1 of 30 (3%) with non-complement fixing ICA alone and 2 of 665 (0.3%) of those who were ICA negative. Life Table analysis suggests that the risk of developing IDDM within 8 years are 76% for CF-ICA, 3% for non-complement fixing ICA and 0.6% for those ICA negative. The relative risk of CF-ICA (compared with ICA negative family members) is 188.5.

The cellular component of the immune attack on beta cells may be of greater importance in the pathogenesis of the disease, but methods of study are relatively undeveloped at present. The major research effort is directed towards isolation and characterization of lymphocyte subsets directed against islet tissue. A recent advance has come from the demonstration of HLA-DR expression on islet cells; their appearance on target tissue might explain the importance of HLA associations in the onset of diabetes, and it has been suggested that their aberrant expression may invite immune attack, representing a form of cellular "suicide."

Is diabetes inevitable once high titer or CF-ICA have appeared? Opinions differ on this vital issue, but our own experience suggests that both the strength and the persistence of the reaction should be taken into account. We classify a complement-fixing reaction as positive when demonstrated on 3 separate occasions, and using this criterion alone a slow but almost inexorable progression to diabetes would seem likely. Metabolic testing in the "survivors" has however allowed us to identify a group with normal glucose tolerance and first-phase insulin secretion 8-10 years after CF-ICA were first detected. Only long-term follow up in this group will answer the question we have posed.

Abnormalities of Insulin Secretion

An important recent development has been the identification of abnormalities of insulin secretion in the pre-diabetic period. The most prominent of these changes has been impairment of the first phase insulin response to intravenous glucose. A linear fall in first phase insulin secretion over time can be demonstrated and it was hoped that this might provide a marker of beta cell loss just as, for example, falling glomerular filtration rate indicates a loss of functioning nephrons. In practice the intra-subject variability of this technique is so great as to limit its usefulness, at least in the early stages of the development of diabetes. A clearly sub-normal response is strongly predictive of diabetes but probably represents a late stage in the attack.

Abnormalities of insulin secretion are likely to form an essential part of any predictive index, expecially since they potentially introduce a dynamic component and might allow the rate of change to be estimated. A major limitation is that childhood diabetes develops in children, and physiological tests applicable to this age group need to be developed. One particular problem is that fasting and stimulated insulin levels rise about the time of puberty, probably because of increasing insulin resistance at this time, and further exploration of this phenomenon is needed.

Carbohydrate Intolerance and "Pre-diabetes"

Several studies have shown that glucose tolerance testing in siblings of a child with IDDM will reveal a number with impaired glucose tolerance, although the rate of progression to IDDM within this group is low. Earlier studies are difficult to interpret because modern criteria for IDDM were not used, and probably included individuals with "maturity onset diabetes of the young" (MODY). Rosenbloom et al (12) examined the 10 year prognosis of impaired glucose tolerance in siblings of children with diabetes and found that 5 of 19 required insulin within 7 years, as against 1 of 86 with normal tolerance.

Another indication of a prolonged metabolic abnormality came from the study of identical twins discordant for diabetes. When height at diagnosis was considered, and one twin had developed diabetes under the age of 19 (i.e. during growth), the diabetic twin was shorter by a mean of 3.5 cm in 8 of 16, corresponding to a growth delay of 35 weeks. The mean duration of symptoms in the same individuals was only 6 weeks. No differences in height were found at diagnosis when diabetes developed over the age of 19.

We have accumulated a large number of sequential blood samples within our family study population, and examined these to find if random blood glucose levels were increased in those who progressed to diabetes. Analysis of around 800 samples from non-diabetic family members (parents and children) showed that the 97.5th percentile was 6.3 mmol/l (115 mg/dl). Nine of 13 who subsequently developed diabetes had a raised random blood glucose 6-34 months prior to diagnosis. Six of the 13 had also had an oral glucose tolerance test, and 5 of these showed a diabetic curve 4 - 21 months before insulin was needed. These findings strongly suggest that the development of carbohydrate intolerance is gradual rather than abrupt, although terminal decompensation with symptoms of thirst and polyuria understandably gives the impression of a disease of sudden onset.

The indications are that the progression to diabetes, via appearance of auto-immune changes, development of abnormalities of insulin secretion and evidence of carbohydrate intolerance, is variable but surprisingly slow. As blood glucose levels rise above the renal threshold physiological changes occur which lead to clinical diagnosis in some, whereas others present more abruptly when challenged by an acute illness such as a viral infection. Most patients have residual insulin secretion when studied soon after diagnosis, but this usually declines to almost unmeasurable levels within a few years. If this view of the natural history of "pre-diabetes" is correct, current emphasis on the importance of the "remission" or honeymoon period would seem to be misplaced.

232

REFERENCES

1.   Hamilton, D.V., Mundia, S.S., Lister, J., 1976, Mode of presentation of juvenile diabetes.   British Medical Journal ii, 211-212.

2.   Barnett, A.H., Eff, C., Leslie, R.D.G., Pyke, D.A., 1981.   Diabetes
in identical twins.   A study of 200 pairs.   Diabetologia 20: 97-93.

3.   Nerup, J., Platz, P., Andersen, O.O. et al, 1974, HLA antigens and
diabetes mellitus.   Lancet i: 864-866.

4.   Walker, A., Cudworth, A.G., 1980, Type 1 (insulin-dependent) diabetic multiplex families: mode of genetic transmission.   Diabetes 29: 1036-
1039.
5.   Lendrum, R., Walker, G.J., Gamble, D.R., 1975, Islet cell antibodies
in juvenile diabetes mellitus.   Lancet i: 880-882.

6.   Gamble, D.R., 1980, The epidemiology of insulin dependent diabetes
mellitus with particular reference to the relationship of virus infections
to its etiology.   Epidemiologic Reviews 2: 49-70.

7.   Tillil H., Kobberling, J., 1987, AGe-corrected empirical genetic
risk estimates for first degree relatives of IDDM patients.   Diabetes 36:
93-99.

8.   Wolf, E., Spencer, K.M., Cudworth, A.G., 1983, The genetic susceptibility to Type I (insulin-dependent) diabetes - analysis of the HLA-DR
Association.   Diabetologia, 1983, 24: 224-230.

9.   Gorsuch, A.N., Spencer, K.M., Lister, J., Wolf, E., Bottazzo,
G.F., Cudworth, A.G., 1982, Can future Type I diabetes be predicted?
A study in families of affected children.   Diabetes 31: 862-866.

10.   Ginsberg-Fellner, F., Witt, M.E., Bonita, H.F., et al., 1985, Triad of markers for identifying children at high risk of developing insulin-
dependent diabetes mellitus.   Journal fo the American Medical Association
254: 1469-1472.

11.   Cavender, D., Wagener, D.K., Rabin, B.S. et al., 1984, The Pittsburgh insulin-dependent diabetes mellitus study.   HLA antigens and haplotypes as risk factors for the development of IDDM in patients and sibling.
Journal of Chronic Disease 37: 555-568.

CAN THE HIGH RISK OF TYPE I DIABETES IN FINLAND BE EXPLAINED
BY FAMILIAL AGGREGATION AND BY HLA HAPLOTYPE DISTRIBUTION?

Eva Wolf, Jaakko Tuomilehto, Raisa Luonamaa and
The Study Group on Childhood Diabetes in Finland*

*Principal Investigators: H.K. Akerblom and J. Tuomilehto

Finland is the country which has the highest incidence of Type I (insulin dependent) diabetes in the world. The age-adjusted annual incidence
in 1977 to 1984 was 30 per 100,000 in the age group 0-15 years (1). Finland is also one of the countries in the world where the incidence of Type
I diabetes is rapidly increasing. The latest data from 1986 to 1987 indicate that the incidence is now about 40 per 100,000 which means about 350
new cases per year.

In September 1986 a nationwide epidemiologically based study into Type
I diabetes called "DiMe" study was started in Finland which has a population
of 4.5 million. The aim of the "DiMe" study is to find out more about the
genetic and environmental factors involved in Type I diabetes and their
interaction in order to plan the appropriate preventive measures for the
future. All families with a newly diagnosed Type I diabetic child aged
0-14 years were invited to take part in the nationwide study which began
in September 1986. As of April 1988, 430 new cases have been reported from
the 33 collaborating hospitals. More than 90% of the families have agreed
to participate.

GENETIC STUDY

The major genetic susceptibility to Type I diabetes is conferred by
genes in the HLA region which is located on the short arm of chromosome 6
in the distal portion of the 6p21.3 band (for review see 2). Linkage between the HLA system and the genes coding for susceptibility to Type I diabetes has clearly been demonstrated (3).

Therefore, HLA antigens and HLA genes can be taken as markers for Type
I diabetes. Whether one uses conventional serological methods for determining HLA antigens or one uses the recently developed techniques of RFLP
(restriction fragment length polymorphism) analysis or oligonucleotide
typing or whether one determines the aminoacid sequence of the HLA genes
themselves it remains the HLA haplotype which carries the disease susceptibility allele that is important.

This study has been done with the support of the NIH grant DK-37957 and
also with grants from the Sigrid Juselius Foundation, the Association of
the Finnish Life Insurance Companies and the Nordisk Insulinfond.

235

The aim of the genetic part of the DiMe study was to collect HLA genotype and haplotype data from all participating newly diagnosed Type I diabetic children and their first degree relatives i.e. parents and siblings.

FAMILIAL AGGREGATION

The majority (87.7%) of the first 400 Finnish families with a newly diagnosed Type I diabetic child reported to the DiMe study by March 1988 were simplex families or so called sporadic cases where only one child had diabetes, and 49 (12.3%) were multiplex families or so called familial cases where at least one other first degree relative had also Type I diabetes (Table 1). Of these 400 families 19 had more than one Type I diabetic child; 18 had 2 and one family had 3 Type I diabetic children. Of the newly diagnosed DiMe probands 14 had a Type I diabetic sibling diagnosed before the DiMe study started in September 1986 and were therefore secondary cases, one DiMe proband was a tertiary case and up till now 5 of the "healthy" siblings of the newly diagnosed DiMe probands also developed Type I diabetes during the study.

At the time of the present analysis in 292 of the participating families the information on family history of Type I diabetes in first and also in second degree relatives was complete and computerized. Twelve fathers and 9 mothers had Type I diabetes which means that 7.2% of the diabetic children had an affected parent, 9.6 % had an affected grandparent and 37.7% had at least one second or third degree relative with Type I diabetes.

HLA HAPLOTYPE DISTRIBUTION

Out of the 43 HLA genotyped multiplex families participating in the DiMe study 60% were families with one diabetic child and one diabetic parent and 30% were families with 2 affected children. Those HLA haplotypes which had been transmitted from the affected parent to the affected child were studied in more detail.

Due to the dominant "en bloc" inheritance of the HLA antigens parent and child are by definition haplo-identical. The haplotype which the affected child has inherited from the affected parent has to carry the disease susceptibility gene for Type I diabetes except in the rare event of recombination.

There were 19 such haplotypes of which 11 (58%) were DR4 positive and 5 (26%) DR3 positive. These percentages were very similar to the gene frequencies found in the newly diagnosed Type I diabetic probands of the DiMe study, i.e. 50% for DR4 and 20% for DR3.

Table 2 shows which B locus antigens were found together with DR4, DR3 and DR1 on these 19 haplotypes. Whereas, as expected, 3 out of 5 of the DR3 positive haplotypes carried B8 as expected only 3 out of 11 DR4 positive haplotypes carried Bw62. Four of the DR4 positive haplotypes carried the B locus antigen Bw56 which was a completely unexpected finding. All these DR4, Bw56 positive haplotypes carried the A locus antigen A2 and the C locus antigen Cw1. This A2, Cw1, Bw56, DR4 haplotype has not been reported to be increased in Type I diabetes in any other study or in any other ethnic group.

Bw56 is a subgroup of the broad antigen Bw22 which also consists of Bw55 which is the major subgroup of Bw22 in Caucasoid populations and of Bw54 which is only found in Mongoloid populations. Bw54 has been described to be increased in Japanese Type I diabetic patients (4).

TABLE 1

MULTIPLEX FAMILIES FOUND AMONG FIRST 400 REPORTED DIME FAMILIES
GROUPED ACCORDING TO FAMILY HISTORY OF TYPE I DIABETES
IN FIRST DEGREE RELATIVES

Groups of multiplex families	n	%
1. PROBAND AND ONE PARENT	30	7.5
2. PROBAND AND BOTH PARENTS	0	0.0
3. PROBAND AND ONE SIBLING	14	3.5
4. PROBAND AND TWO SIBLINGS	1	0.3
5. PROBAND AND ONE PARENT AND ONE SIBLING	4	1.0
6. PROBAND AND ONE PARENT AND TWO SIBLINGS	0	0.0

TABLE II

HAPLOTYPES OF TYPE I DIABETIC PROBANDS INHERITED FROM
A TYPE I DIABETIC PARENT (12 FATHERS, 7 MOTHERS).

DR ANTIGEN	B LOCUS ANTIGEN								Total
	Bw56	Bw62	B18	Bw60	B8	B7	B44	Bx	
DR4	4	3	3	1	–	–	–	–	11
DR3	–	–	–	–	3	–	1	1	5
DR1	–	1	–	–	–	2	–	–	3
Total	4	4	3	1	3	2	1	1	19

237

TABLE III

ETIOLOGIC FRACTION OF HLA-A,B,C AND DR ANTIGENS WHICH
WERE FOUND SIGNIFICANTLY MORE FREQUENT ON DIABETIC
THAN NON-DIABETIC HAPLOTYPES

HLA ANTIGEN	ETIOLOGIC FRACTION
DR4	0.34
Cw3	0.18
A2	0.15
B8	0.12
Bw62	0.11
DR3	0.10
Bw60	0.05
Bw56	0.05

The HLA-A,B,C and DR gene frequencies found in the Type I diabetic probands of the DiMe study were calculated and those HLA antigens which were found more frequently on diabetic than on non-diabetic haplotypes were determined. In each family the four parental haplotypes were divided into diabetic haplotypes which were found in the Type I diabetic children or Type I diabetic parents and into non-diabetic haplotypes defined as those parental haplotypes which never occurrred in a Type I diabetic child or Type I diabetic parent or affected sibling(5).

Table III lists all HLA antigens whose frequencies were significantly increased on 237 diabetic haplotypes expressed in terms of their etiologic fraction which is a measure for the strength of the association between an HLA antigen and the disease susceptibility gene (6). As expected DR4 and DR3 and Bw62, B8 and Bw60 were significantly increased. In addition A2 was increased and so was Bw56 with an etiologic fraction of the thirty-nine diabetic haplotypes were found in the DiME probands which carried Bw56 and 43 of them (87%) of them also carried A2, Cw1 and DR4 (5). These antigens were in strong linkage disequilibrium on diabetic haplotypes. In contrast, only 8 non diabetic haplotypes were found with Bw56 and none was DR4 positive.

This A2, Bw56, Cw1, DR4 haplotype was not found in the Bart's Windsor family study done in England between 1978 and 1983 (7). The antigens Bw56 was defined with the same HLA antisera in both studies and the data analyses were done exactly in the same way. Not a single A2, Bw56, Cw1, DR4 haplotype was found in 282 diabetic haplotypes and in 158 non diabetic haplotypes derived from the Bart's Windsor family study. Only 2 haplotypes carried Bw56 and one was DR7 and the other DRw6 associated.

Compared to the Bart's Windsor family study the frequency of DR3, DR4 heterozygosity was much lower in the DiMe study (48.6% versus 24.6%). The high frequency of DR3, DR4 heterozygosity found in the English study fitted best with the hypotheses that two disease susceptibility genes exist one in linkage disequilibrium with DR3 and one with DR4 which potentiate each other and which have a more than additive effect on relative risk. In contrast, haplotype might just be enough to determine susceptibility to Type I diabetes in Finnish children.

CONCLUSION

The existence of a new and specific HLA haplotype – the A2,Bw56, Cw1, DR4 haplotype – which is increased in Type I diabetes in Finland and which has not been described in any other study before was demonstrated. The finding that 4 out of 19 diabetic haplotypes which were transmitted from a diabetic parent to a diabetic child were such A2, Bw56, Cw1, DR4 haplotypes together with the significantly increased gene frequency of Bw56 on diabetic versus non diabetic haplotypes show that this newly found haplotype provides a genetic explanation for about 10% of the Type I diabetic cases and is partly the reason why Finland has a higher frequency of Type I diabetes than for instance England where this A2, Bw56, Cw1, DR4 haplotype has not been found.

Investigators at the local collaborating hospitals:

A. Hakulinen, L. Herva, P. Hiltunen, T. Huhtamaki, N-P. Huttenen, A. Nuuja, T. Huuponen, T. Joki, R. Jokisalo, S. Kallio, E. Kaprio, M-L Kaar, L. Laine, J. Lappalainen, j. Maenpaa, A-L. Makela, K. Niemi, P. Ojajarvi, M-R Stålber, M. Sillanpaa, S. Pontynen, J. Sankala, T. Uotila, P. Varimo.

REFERENCES

1. Åkerblom, H.K., Reunanen, A., 1985, The epidemiology of insulin-dependent diabetes mellitus (IDDM) in Finland and in Northern Europe. Diabetes Care 8:Suppl. 1: 10–16.

2. Crumpton, M.J, 1987, HLA in medicine. Br Med Bull, 43: 1–240.

3. Walker, A., Cudworth, A.G., 1980, Type 1 (insulin dependent) diabetic multiplex families: Mode of genetic transmission. Diabetes 29: 1036–1039.

4. Wakisaka, A., Aizawa, M., Matsura, N. et al., 1976, HLA and juvenile diabetes mellitus in the Japanese. Lancet 2: 970.

5. Wolf, E., Tuomilehto, J., Cepaitis, Z., et al, (in preparation), A2, Cw1, Bw56, DR4 – a new haplotype increased in Type 1 diabetes in Finland.

6. Bentsson, B.O., Thompson, G., 1981, Measuring the strength of associations between HLA antigens and diseases. Tissue Antigen 18: 356–363.

7. Wolf, E., Spencer, K.M., Cudworth, A.G., 1983, The genetic susceptibility to Type 1 (insulin dependent) diabetes: Analysis of the DR association. Diabetologia 24: 224–230.

GENETIC AND HUMORAL MARKERS IN IDDM PATIENTS AND THEIR FAMILIES

¶Maximino Ruiz, Felix E. Puchulu, Alejo Florin Christensen

Fundacion Argentina de Diabetes y Enfermedades Metabolicas (FADEM)
Seccion Diabetologia of Hospital de Clinicas "Jose de San Martin "
Centro de Educacion Medica e Investigaciones Clinicas (CEMIC)

The association between some HLA and insulin-dependent diabetes was demonstrated by Nerup et al[1] when they observed a high prevalence of HLA B8 B15 in this type of diabetes. Afterwards, several authors[2] demonstrated that there are a linkage disequilibrium of the HLA B8 and B15 and the HLA DR3 and DR4, and that these are the principal genetic markers.

Islet cell antibodies (ICA) were described in 1974 by Botazzo et al.[3] Islet cell antibodies are IgG immunoglobulins that fix complement and react against the different cells of the Langerhans islet (alpha, beta, and delta). The specific antigens are probably microsomal particles composed of lipoproteins of subcellular fractions membrane of the endoplasmic reticulum.

Different kinds of ICA antibodies, against the microsome, cell membrane antigens (ICSA), and against the different cells of the pancreatic islets have been demonstrated.[4] There is a relationship between IDDM and ICA, especially during the first two years after diabetes. During this period the presence of ICA was demonstrated in 60 to 80% of the patients decreasing to 20% after this time.

These antibodies are markers of an autoimmunity mechanism described as one of the main pathogenic factors in insulin-dependent diabetes.[5]

Hypothesis:
    1. The Argentinian insulin-dependent patients with diabetes have the same HLA pattern observed in the Caucasian population, taking into account the ethnic composition of the country.
    2. The HLA composition are useful as markers for persons with high risk of developing insulin-dependent diabetes.
    3. The prevalence of ICA in IDDM in Argentina is similar to that observed in the same type of patients with diabetes in other countries.
    4. The combination of HLA and ICA are clinical markers useful in defining different subtypes of IDDM and to detect persons at high risk for diabetes.

Aims:
    The aim of this study was to find 1) the prevalence of genetic (HLA) and humoral (ICA) markers in Argentinians with insulin-dependent diabetes 2) the relationship with different characteristics pertaining to age of

onset and duration of diabetes, and 3) the possibility of demonstrating the importance of these markers in a) the determination and characterization of subtypes of IDDM, b) the probable pathogenic mechanism, and c) as predictors of high risk for diabetes.

MATERIAL AND METHODS

The material was divided into two groups

I. HLA studies
This group includes three subgroups:
   a. Persons with insulin dependent diabetes
      n = 60 Age (mean ± S.D.) 25.4 ± 13.1 years
      Age of onset: 20.8 ± 11.5 years
      Sex: M = 40, F = 20
      Duration of diabetes: 3.5 ± 6.04 years

   b. Relatives of persons with insulin-dependent diabetes
      n = 14 Age (mean ± S.D.) 30.7 ± 20.5 years
      Sex: M = 5, F = 9

   c. Controls
      n = 257 Age and sex matched

II. ICA studies
      n = 85 Age (mean ± S.D.) 22.9 ± 10.7 years
      Sex: M = 36, F = 49
      Age of onset: 19.8 ± 10.3 years
      Duration of diabetes: 1.79 ± 2.54 years
      Type of diabetes: IDDM 70
                        NIDDM 15

A. HLA-A,B and C antigens were detected by complement-dependent standard microlymphocytotoxicity testing of T-lymphocytes against antisera following Terasaki et al. method.[11]
HLA-DR, and DQ antigens were detected by prolonged incubation micro-lymphocytotoxicity testing of B lymphocytes against International Histocompatibility Workshop B-cell antisera.

B. The determination of the ICA was done by the indirect immunofluorescence technic, using recent post-mortem human pancreas (blood group O) as antigen. The patient's serum antibody was marked with an anti IgG conjugated with isothiocyanate of fluorescein. A reaction was considered positive when the islets took a uniform green fluorescence.[3]

C. The statistical methods used were the x^2 and the Student's test.

RESULTS

I. HLA studies.
The prevalence of HLA alleles Class I in 60 persons with insulin dependent diabetes was for locus A: A2 35%, A3 16.6%, and locus B: B8 16.6%, B12 13.3% and B18 13.3%. The B15 was observed in only 4 patients (6.6%). In the locus C the more frequent types were Cw 3, Cw 4 and Cw 5 (8.3% in each one).

The comparison of these results with the control group (6,7) demonstrated a high prevalence of the HLA B8 and B18 and Cs 3, Cw 4 and Cw 5.

In the HLA-Class II we studied the subtypes DR and DQ. In the first

TABLE I

COMPARATIVE FREQUENCIES OF HLA A, B AND C ALLELES IN IDDM AND IN CONTROLS IN ARGENTINA

	A			B			C	n (%)
	Diabetics n: 60	Controls [1] n: 275		Diabetics n: 60	Controls [1] n: 275		Diabetics n: 15	Controls [2]
A_2	21 (35.0)	113 (43.9)	B_8	10 (16.6)	28 (10.9)	Cw3	5 (33.3)*	(23.0)
A_3	15 (25.0)	44 (17.1̄)	B_{12}	8 (13.3)	55 (21.4)	Cw4	5 (33.3)*	(19.6)
A_1	10 (16.6)	48 (18.6)	B_{18}	8 (13.3)*	27 (10.5)	Cw5	5 (33.3)*	(12.0)
A_9	6 (10.0)	75 (29.1)	Bw6	7 (11.6)	N.D.	Cw2	2 (13.3)	(8.6)
A_{28}	6 (10.0)	12 (4.6)	B_{14}	6 (10.0)	15 (5.8)	Cw6	2 (13.3)	(14.4)
A_{24}	5 (8.3)	N.D.	B_{21}	6 (10.0)	17 (6.6)	Cw7	2 (13.3)	(6.1)
A_{10}	4 (6.6)	32 (12.4)	Bw4	5 (8.3)	N.D.			
A_{29}	3 (5.0)	20 (7.7)	Bw35	5 (8.3)	52 (20.2)			
A_{30}	3 (5.0)	N.D.	B7	(6.6)*	26 (10.1)			
Aw32	2 (3.3)	25 (9.7)	B_{15}		21 (8.1)			
A_{11}	1 (1.6)	25 (19.7)	B_{17}		19 (7.3)			

N.D.: Non determined   * $p < 0.05$

1 Morales V.H., García Morteo O., Salvioli J.E., Cédola N., et al. Histocompatibility Laboratory - La Plata Buenos Aires, 1981
2 Verruno L., Haas E., Raimondi E., Argentine Society of Clinical Research - Mar del Plata - Argentina, 1983

TABLE II

PREVALENCE OF HLA ALLELES CLASS I IN IDDM RELATIVES AND CONTROLS IN ARGENTINA

	A			B			C	n (%)
	IDDM relatives n: 14	Controls [1] n: 257		IDDM relatives n: 14	Controls [1] n: 257		IDDM relatives n: 14	Controls [2]
A_2	6 (42.8)	113 (43.9)	B_8	3 (21.4)**	28 (10.9)	Cw3	5 (35.7)*	(23.0)
A_3	3 (21.4)	44 (17.1)	B_{12}	1 (7.1)	55 (21.4)	Cw4	1 (7.1)	(19.6)
A_1	3 (21.4)	48 (18.6)	B_{18}	5 (35.7)**	27 (10.5)	Cw5	4 (28.5)*	(12.0)
A_9	1 (7.1)	75 (29.1)	Bw6	13 (92.8)	N.D.	Cw2	3 (21.4)	(8.6)
A_{28}	2 (14.2)	12 (4.6)	Bw4	5 (35.7)	N.D.	Cw6	3 (21.4)	(14.4)
A_{10}	3 (21.4)	32 (12.4)	B_7	2 (14.2)	26 (10.1)	Cw7	1 (7.1)	(6.1)
A_{29}	2 (14.2)	20 (7.7)	B_{15}	2 (14.2)	21 (8.1)			

N.D.: Non determined.   * $p < 0.05$ ** $p < 0.01$

1 Morales V.H., García Morteo O., Salvioli J.E., Cédola N. et al. Histocompatibility Laboratory- La Plata - Buenos Aires, 1981
2 Verruno L., Haas E., Raimondi E.. Argentine Society of Clinical Research - Mar del Plata - Argentina, 1983

TABLE III

PREVALENCE OF HLA ALLELES CLASS II (DR AND DQ) in IDDM,
THEIR RELATIVES AND CONTROLS IN ARGENTINA

| | DR | | | | DQ | n (%) |
	IDDM n: 17	Relatives n: 7	Controls n: 57		IDDM n: 10	Relatives n: 7
DR3	13 (76.4)	5 (71.4)	13 (22.8)	DQw2	8 (80)	4 (57.1)
DR4	9 (52.9)	3 (42.8)	13 (22.8)	DQw3	5 (50)	2 (28.5)
DRw52	11 (64.7)	3 (42.8)	N.D.	DQw1	1 (10	0
DRw53	10 (58.8)	2 (28.5)	N.D.			
DR7	3 (17.6)	2 (28.5)	14 (24.5)			
DR1	1 (5.8)	0	7 (12.2)			
DR2	1 (5.8)	0	11 (19.2)			
DR5	1 (5.8)	1 (14.2)	15 (26.3)			
DR6	1 (5.8)	0	13 (22.8)			

group, the phenotypes DR3 and DR4 were more frequent and DR2 was less frequent in persons with IDDM than in the controls.

In relation to the subtype HLA DQ we studied 10 insulin dependent diabetics in which the DQw2 appeared in 8, and DQw3 in five. We do not have a control group for this subtype as yet.

Their relatives had similar frequencies of the alleles in the loci DR and DQ as in the patients with IDDM.

In relation to the relative risk, we found that subjects B8, B18, DR3 and DR4 have a higher risk than controls. On the contrary, people with B7 or DR2 have lesser risk in comparison with the controls.

II. ICA studies.
The presence of ICA was detected in the serum of 48 of the 85 patients (56.5%). Twenty five were females and 40 had IDDM. ICA was more frequent (65%) in those with diabetes less than two years ($p = 0.01$), and onset of diabetes before age 20 (73%).

Among the 15 patients with non-insulin dependent diabetes at the time of the study, 10 developed IDDM during the follow-up period of ten years, 8 of them had ICA positive at the first examination.

TABLE IV

HLA AND INSULIN DEPENDENT DIABETES n (%)

	IDDM n: 60	Controls [1] n: 275	Relative Risk
LOCUS B			
B8	10 (16.6)	28 (10.9)	1.76
B18	8 (13.3)	27 (10.5)	1.41
B7	4 (6.6)	26 (10.1)	0.63
LOCUS DR	n: 17	n: 57	
DR3	13 (76.4)	13 (22.8)	6.01
DR4	9 (52.9)	13 (22.8)	3.80
DR2	1 (5.8)	11 (19.2)	0.26

1 Morales V.H., García Morteo O.,Salvioli J.,Cédola N.
et al. La Plata. Buenos Aires, Argentina, 1981

TABLE V

Relation between the ICA positive and the duration of diabetes in persons with diabetes with an onset before 20 years.

Duration	ICA positive	ICA negative	Total
Less than 2 years	22 (84,6%)	4 (15,4%)	26
2 years or more	2 (28,6%)	5 (71,4%)	7
p 0.01			

Relation between the ICA positive and the duration of diabetes in persons with diabetes with an onset after 20 years.

Duration	ICA positive	ICA negative	Total
Less than 2 years	20 (51,3%)	19 (48,7%)	39
2 years or more	4 (30,8%)	9 (69,2%)	13
P 0.40			

The difference between the two types of diabetes and the two sexes are not statistically significant.

The analysis of the combined data was done to verify the hypothesis that there are two types of insulin-dependent diabetics (Table V).

In the patients with diabetes with an onset before 20 years, the ICA positive was more frequent in those with a duration less than two years; in the persons with diabetes with an onset after 20 years, there was not any statistical difference between groups.

Considering the results in relation to the duration of diabetes, we observed that the prevalence of ICA positivity in those with less than 2 years was higher in the juvenile type (age of onset before 20 years), than in the adults. On the other hand, in the group with two or more years duration, there was no difference between both groups, and the percentage of ICA positivity was smaller than in the patients with less than two years duration.

DISCUSSION

In our HLA studies, the prevalence of DR3 and DR4, and the relative risk is higher than the controls, and the differences are more important than the alleles of the loci B and C.

These results are coincidental with other research done in Argentina by Morales et al (5), and with other authors in Caucasian population. Other ethnic groups have a different distribution (9).

HLA DR3 and DR4 appear to be genetic markers of predisposition for IDDM, and the HLA B8 and B18 would be in linkage disequilibrium with them (1,2).

When we studied the different phenotypes of the subtypes DR and DQ, we observed two haplotypes or the association of both. The first is DR3 DRw52 DQw2, and the second is DR4 DRw53 DQw3 and the association is DR3 DR4 DRw52 DRw53 Dqw2 DQw3. Because of our small sample of DQ, and the lack of a control group, we do not have the possibility of knowing the importance of this subtype as a marker of genetic predisposition to IDDM.

We agree with Barbosa et al al (7) and others that first degree relatives of our patients with IDDM are pre-type I diabetics, and it would be useful to study the ICA to know the evolution of the disease during the pre-hyperglycemic period.

According to several authors there was no difference in the prevalence of ICA in the two sexes, in contrast with the high frequency of autoimmune endocrine pathology in women. An explanation may be that the demonstration of ICA in the serum of persons with diabetes was the expression of two pathogenic mechanisms.

In patients with non insulin dependent diabetes that became IDDM, half of them were ICA positive during the time when they didn't need insulin therapy. This means that the ICA would be a predictor of IDDM, and that the insulinodependence is not an exclusive parameter in defining this type of diabetes.

The high prevalence of ICA positivity in persons with juvenile diabetes of less than two years duration, in contrast with the adult onset group in which there was no difference between recent and long duration of diabetes, allows us to suggest the probably existance of two pathogenetic types of diabetes. One of them observed in two thirds of the persons with juvenile diabetes in which the autoimmune mechanism is secondary to some aggressors, like virus or other substances. In the other third, there is probably a primary autoimmune disease, as in the IDDM of adult onset in which there is no difference between those with less than two years and those with more years. According to Cudworth et al. the first corresponds to type I, and the second to type II.

The ICA negative persons with diabetes from the onset of the disease was 15.6% in the juvenile group and 48.7% in the adult one.

These data supposed the idea of a group with different etiopathogenic mechanism like pancreatopathies, etc.

We consider that IDDM is an heterogeneous disease in relation to the pathogenic mechanism, and to the non insulin dependent period after the onset of the diabetes.

We can speculate in the differentiation into three etiopathogenic subtypes:

Type I A: primary virus or toxic and secondary autoimmune.

Type II B: primary autoimmune.

Type I C (or non A, non B): No autoimmune.

Therefore the association of genetic (HLA DR and DQ) and humoral (ICA positive) markers as in relatives of patients with IDDM will be useful in detecting those who have a higher risk of developing this type of diabetes.

REFERENCES

L. Nerup, J., Platz, P., Andersen, O.O., Christy, M., Lyngsol, J., Poulsen, J.E., Ryder, L.P., Nielsen, L.S., Thomsen, M., Svejgaard, A., 1974, HLA antigens and diabetes mellitus. Lancet 2: 864-866.

2. Cudworth, A.G., Woodrow, J.C., 1975, Evidence for HLA-linked clues in juvenile diabetes mellitus. Br Med J 3: 133-135.

3. Bottazzo, G.F., Florin-Christensen, A., Doniach, D., 1974, Islet cell antibodies in daibetes mellitus with autoimmune polyendocrine deficiency. Lancet 2: 1279-1283.

4. Bottazzo, G.F., Pujol-Borrell, R. and Gale, E., 1985, Etiology of diabetes: the role of autoimmune mechanisms <u>In</u> The Diabetes Annual 1 by Alberti, K.G.M.M. and Krall, L.P. Elsevier, Amsterdam: 16.

5. Morales, V.H., Garcia Morteo, O., Salvioli, J.E., Cedola, N., De Marco R., 1983, HLA and insulin dependent diabetes. Analysis in Argentina in Diabetes Mellitus by Salvioli, J. and De Marco, R., Eds., Panamericana Bs. As.: 329.

6. Verruno, L., Haas, E., Raimondi, E., 1983, Frequency of antigens, genes and association between loci A and B in Argentina- XV Meeting of the Argentine Society of Clincial Research-Mar del Plata-Argentina.

7. Barbosa, J., Chavers, B., Dunsworth, T., Michael, A., 1982, Islet cell antibodies and histocompatibility antigens in insulin-dependent diabetics and their first degree relatives. Diabetes 31: 585-588.

8. MacDonald, M., Famuyiwa, O., Nwabuebo, I., Bella, A., Junaid, T.A., Marrari, M., Duquesnoy, R.J., 1986, HLA - Or association in black Type I diabetics in NIgeria. Diabetes 35: 583-589.

9. Pirosky, I., Cantora, M., Vellard, J., Braunstein, J., Alessandria, J., 1983, Genetic analysis in a Toba Indian population. Frequency of HLA-DR Medicina (Buenos Aires) 43: 281-284.

10. Serrano Rios M., Regueiro, J.R., Severino, R. et al. 1983, HLA antigens in insulin-dependent and non insulin-dependent Spanish diabetic patients. Diabetes Metabol 9: 116-120.

11. Terasaki, P.I., McClelland, J.D., 1964, Microdroplet assay of human serum cytotoxins. Nature 204: 998.

DISCUSSION

J. BARBOSA: Dr. McEvoy, I'd like to very strongly support Dr. Gale's
plea that we all get together and do the same thing, because otherwise
it's going to be a terrible mess, and I will meet anybody, anywhere, to
try to perhaps even come up with a registry of prediabetics or diabetics
being followed.

That finding on the DP is certainly very exciting, because I am not yet
used to thinking of the DP as being involved in the susceptibility to
diabetes. That DP beta C that you are talking about, is it seen with
both B18 and B8 haptotypes or just one?

R. MC EVOY: Yes, it's only seen in the B8.

J. BARBOSA: That makes it even more interesting. And, about your congenital rubella patients. You have all those that have a type 2 like
diabetes in addition to ones that have a type 1 like diabetes, right?

R. MC EVOY: Yes. Actually, I showed the glucose tolerance test. None
of those children was being treated for diabetes and none of those children
are being called diabetics at the present time. It you give those children
who have abnormal glucose tolerance tests a normal diet they don't spill
sugar in the urine. Now, one can argue that they should be treated, but
the congenital rubella children are profoundly retarded as a group with
marked impairment of several organ systems and to add something that might
predispose them to hypoglycemia, we felt it was not clinically indicated
until they had significant symptoms of diabetes - polyuria, polydipsia,
etc.

Initially, the first individuals who were identified as having diabetes
had a very, very clear association with DR3. The difficulty is that what
do we call these kids who are hyperinsulinemic and glucose intolerant?
Most of those glucose tolerance tests were done in 1987. If anything,
they're getting more hyperinsulinemic as they get more glucose intolerant.
I don't know what to call them. I think they're an extremely interesting
group. The younger kids on the other hand, the kids that developed diabetes
before they were 15, very clearly are very similar to type 1 diabetics and
7% is not an insignificant percentage of a small population.

E. WOLF: Dr. Gale, with your HLA and risk tables, did you use all the HLA
diabetic siblings and all the HLA haplo-identical siblings to derive these
figures, because if that is the case I think you should re-do it by risk
families, because you duplicate your information. And, if you have two HLA
identical siblings in a family, the chances are completely different for
them to develop diabetes. One might develop diabetes, but the second HLA
identical would develop it, but will be different. I think if you re-do
that you might come up with the right risk figures for the HLA.

When I left the Bob Windsor family study in 1983, I got very excited about
the discordance time, because I thought they had 6 or 7 HLA identical

siblings who had become diabetic, and only one of them had a discordance interval of 22 years and all the others were under one year. That fitted perfectly with the results from the twins, because the concordant ones were DL3, DL4 heterozygotes and, therefore, probably had two susceptibility genes. And, I can't see why that has changed. The Pittsburgh data on concordance are very strange. But, I think we should combine them with the Finnish data and the English data.

E. GALE: Thank you. I didn't give our figures from the study with regard to discordance simply because our numbers are rather small and I quoted two studies which had much larger numbers.

D. PYKE: Dr. McEvoy, 7% of your rubella children have undoubted insulin dependent diabetes. Is the approximate age incidence of these offspring the same as insulin dependent diabetes generally, or is it like the original Australian data relatively late in life?

R. MC EVOY: All of those in the initial study that was reported in 1982 had diabetes below the age of 15. So, that they're different from what was reported by Menzer from Australia where most of the children got diabetes in their 20s.

J. HOET: Dr. McEvoy, in the congenital rubella syndrome, do you have any indication about lesions in the pancreas or in the thyroid?

R. MC EVOY: No. We have had only one death in our group. And, I'm unaware of any other studies.

J. HOET: In your children, did you have hyperproinsulinemia?

R. MC EVOY: No. So these were insulin levels after an oral glucose tolerance test.

R. CAMERINI-DAVALOS: Dr. McEvoy, do you have another group similar to those with rubella that have the same changes? In relation to the metabolic changes of these children, if I understood you correctly, they have hyperglycemia during the OGTT and they have hyperinsulinemia. They fit into what, we like to believe, is chemical diabetes or what you may like to call impaired glucose tolerance tests. There are published studies by us and others showing very clearly that following them for years with an oral compound their degree of morbidity and mortality is significantly less. So, why do you prefer not to treat them?

R. MC EVOY: In answer to the first question, I'm not aware of any large group of toxoplasmosis or herpes or Coxsackie that has been followed like this group. And, I'm not aware, myself, of any specific reports of an increased incidence of diabetes in those other parts of the TORCH syndrome. I might just point out that there have been reports of increased ICA positiviity in children who have, for instance, mumps. And, in fact, we have some preliminary data in the few people in the United States that get measles, that they develop ICA assays or IAA or both after having measles. So, I don't know if there is a comparable group. Metabolically, I think we'd have to really stretch it to find a group of 24 year olds who are metabolically anything like these kids.

I guess one always has to look, clinically, at the cost/benefit ratio of a treatment and I, philosophically at least, if the impaired glucose tolerance test is only detectable on a large oral glucose challenge and is not demonstrable by significantly elevated blood sugars, either fasting or postprandial and is not manifested by glucosuria, I just can't see taking any risk of hypoglycemia during their usual life. It's philosophical, though.

B. WAJCHENBERG: Dr. McEvoy, did you check the IVGTT to see if the early fast phase insulin release was decreased?

R. MC EVOY: The answer is no.

B. WAJCHENBERG: I would suggest not to say that they are insulin resistant until you prove there is some defective insulin release. Would you agree with me?

R. MC EVOY: No. The majority of the children who have profoundly elevated insulins have fasting hyperinsulinemia.

B. WAJCHENBERG: Dr. Spinas, you have mentioned the elevated fasting proinsulin. You have mentioned that 10% of your subjects in that risk have elevated proinsulin. Did you concentrate and which type of antisera did you use to measure proinsulin?

G. SPINAS: Proinsulin levels were measured by the group at the Steno Memorial Hospital with the methodology that has been published and I think it's quite specific for proinsulin, but there is a very, very small cross reactivity with C-peptide. I should say that these data are in fact in keeping with what the group in Denmark finds in subjects at risk for type 1 diabetes, that they have elevated proinsulin levels. So, I think the assay is one of the best available at this time.

P. BENNETT: Dr. Gale, you said that once the insulin response to an intravenous glucose load was abnormal and impaired glucose tolerance was present, there was no return. Is that fact, or fantasy? What is the new medical evidence for it? And, for Dr. McEvoy in terms of the congenital rubella individuals with impaired glucose tolerance and hyperinsulinemia, is there evidence of DR4 ICA or IAA associations or the DQ beta 2 in that group as opposed to the hypoinsulinemic group?

E. GALE: It is pure hypothesis, Dr. Bennett. The facts are that there are very few individuals who have been studied through this phase. None have as yet not progressed to diabetes. So, that's a working hypothesis until proven otherwise.

R. CAMERINI-DAVALOS: Subjects with impaired glucose tolerance (chemical diabetes) and hyperinsulinemia that return to normal tolerance have been described by us and other groups.

R. MC EVOY: Relative to the congenital rubella kids and their genetics, it is very difficult to know whether any variation in this group might be just due to ethnic or some kind of selective influence. For instance, 60% of these kids are Hispanic, about 35% of them Black and 5% are White. The ethnic mix in New York is changing, but it's nowhere near that in the general population. So, we have focused the specific studies of genetics on the family studies so far as we've been able to identify specific markers. We hope now to apply those to selected individuals in the congenital rubella study.

P. BENNETT: What about ICA's and IAA's in the IGT hyperinsulinemic individuals?

R. MC EVOY: Yes, many of them were, in fact, IAA positive and/or ICSA positive.

P. BENNETT: So what you perhaps have here is a non-insulin dependent type *hyperinsulinemic disease possibly associated with IAA and with a viral causation. Obviously, a great dilemma for classification purposes.*

R. MC EVOY: Yes, I should mention that these children have auto-antibodies against almost anything we test for, much higher than the background population. They have a decreased ability to respond against several antigens for both cell mediated and humoral mediated immunity. They're very much like BB rats in some ways.

H. GLEICHMANN: Dr. McEvoy, what kind of tests are you applying to determine ICA in your group? And, in particular, I'm interested if you fix your pancreatic section, or if you use an unfixed one?

R. MC EVOY: These are IC assays using insulinoma cells as the target and complement fixation as the end point.

J. HOET: Dr. McEvoy, we should not forget also cytomegalic virus disease for two reasons. First, because cytomegalic virus disease in the human, as in the experiment animal, provides major changes specifically in the beta cell. So that there we may find another group of children of that kind. Now, it is of interest that in Saudi Arabia, very good observations have been made indicating that about 75% of the newborns have antibodies against cytomegalic virus diseases vs, in the Caucasian population in the same setting, it's about 0.1%. We may have clusters in the world where populations like the congenital rubella syndrome may be occurring.

E. GALE: Dr. Wolf, while you were coming up with a genetic explanation for the difference between Finland and England, you pointed out a very powerful environmental factor with respect to the rising incidence throughout northern Europe. We've recently found in the Barth Windsor area that the frequency has doubled. Do you have any suggestions as to what this unknown genetic factor might be? And, is it presumable that we can anticipate that there is an underlying drift upwards in the frequency of diabetes on genetic grounds so that we could make a genetic correction in terms of the fact that diabetic patients survive to reproduce themsevles?

E. WOLF: To your first question, our study has just started. To the second question, I'm trying not to say that it is genetic disease or anything like that.

P. BENNETT: Dr. Wolf, I thought that the current thing, in relation to DRQ, was a specific DRQ and if you had that, you were protected against developing insulin dependent diabetes. If you didn't have that particular type, then you were susceptible. How does that observation relate to your statement that the whole haplotype is the most predictive thing; and, the specific question is do you have any data on the DRQ situation in Finland at this time and/or association with those haplotypes of high risk?

E. WOLF: I'll answer the second question first. We don't have any DQ data yet. To the first one, it's a difficult problem, but as long as they can't show a difference between a diabetic and non-diabetic haplotype, which carries the same HLA antigens, as long as there's no difference, as long as that is true, you will not find HLA identical sibs. They can't differentiate between them, and that's the main thing. Now, I think the Pittsburgh group is the only one who's got families where they have different markers on HLA identical siblings. Therefore, it's not a better marker; it's there in a different proportion, a different linkage to the equilibrium, but it's there on both sets of haplotypes. If I take the whole HLA haplotype and add up the risk from the A to the DR, I end up with the same amount. I mean each marker is nice to have. We wish we had more in between.

J. BARBOSA: We believe that the susceptible antigen is most likely in the D region, and there are X number of DR haplotypes and some provide risks, but others don't, because the DR point is really different. The serology is a very nonspecific way of looking at the D region. We can find lots of heterogeneity within the DR4 or DR3. So, we think that's why haplotypes are important, not because there are other genes close to D or to A that have anything to do with diabetes.

E. WOLF: I would suggest that the best way of subdividing DR3 and DR4 haplotypes is using the B locus. It has about 86 official antigens and about 110 others. So, it's the best way, the B locus is the most poly-morph locus and it's the best way to D3 or 4 haplotype.

J. BARBOSA: Do you believe there are diabetes susceptible antigens in the B region?

E. WOLF: There's very likely some nearby, which have an addictive effect. You can't rule that out. What sort of population have you got in Gaines-ville? We have a homogeneous population in Finland and Bob Windsor's is homogeneous, right? You have people from all over Europe coming there, so they are different haplotypes. And, that's probably why you derive that your adults have less genetic susceptibility than the young people.

J. BARBOSA: Dr. Wolf, I was also very interested in the DR1. We do find DR1 associated with diabetes and the few DR2 with diabetes have the same RSLP pattern as DR1, so we believe that the diabetic susceptibility factor in DR1 is the same as in the DR2 diabetes.

M. GLEICHMANN: I think just to divide diabetic patients into type 1 and type 2 strictly is an oversimplification of the true natural history of diabetes. And, I think what we depict with the ICA positive within the type 2 patients really might represent a retarded form of the so-called type 1. Just the destructive process of the beta cell is slowed down a little bit and the data I presented are very comparable to the data presented by Dr. Riley previously, where he showed that the slope of the destruction of the beta cells is just not as sharp as in the younger population.

C. HOWARD: I would interject, again, in reponse to your statement that, as I presented, there is evidence for a lesion that is occurring in older people. I would agree that ICA is not really the cause, but it does serve as a marker that can indicate that there is some kind of actual pathological damage that's occurring within the islet. It may not always be the insular lesion. I think a key point here is that we do not get ourselves stuck into this type 1 and type 2, NIDDM and IDDM, until we really know what the etiologies are. And, that we have to look at it as though we have functional lesions in which there are also pathological contributors.

H. GLEICHMANN: Maybe ICA is just marking the spread of the destructive process. This might be a marker for the speed only.

J. BARBOSA: I have three questions for Dr. Gale. I wonder if you have looked at whether fasting blood sugars are any better than postprandials? And, also, are these blood sugars done by patients, finger sticks, or are these laboratory blood sugars? And, the final question is has your group reported that IgG insulin antibodies are predictive but IgM are not? What is the status of that distinction?

E. GALE: You asked about fasting vs random, and the nature of our study is that we can't get access to fasting blood glucoses, except preceding an IVGTT. The Joslin group has, however, looked at the fast blood glucose. They have seen a small, but significant and progressive rise, but only over the last six months or so prior to diagnosis, whereas our observations would indicate things might be going on a long time prior to that. The second question concerns the methodology of the glucose measurement and that is, these are intravenous blood samples taken by a doctor visiting with patients at home and analyzed that same day in a laboratory. The third question was the differentiation between the IgG and IgM insulin auto-antibodies and we would stand by the original observation on that.

D. PYKE: Can I ask Dr. Gale how he would interpret the results he described in his 29 cases with conventional ICA's where only one had gone on to diabetes? Do you think that some of the others will later develop it, or have they lost their ICA's? And, do you think that their presence is non-specific, or do you think it represents some form of perhaps lesser islet attack?

E. GALE: My main point is that I wish we had a less sensitive method, because it would save us the difficulty of trying to understand what is happening to this particular group. And, emperically, they are at relatively very low risk of progression to diabetes. And, there are far more of these individuals in a family study population than they would find in the cross section of the general population, and it is tempting to think that this might represent an aborted attack on the beta cells. We have no evidence of that, and probably never will until we have some direct or indirect way of seeing what is happening in the islets themselves.

I think that most people believe there is a point of no return which is represented around the time where the first phase insulin response is lost. As far as I know, it has not been seen to recover in anyone who's been islet cell antibody positive. That person has not escaped developing diabetes later on. We're dealing with a group who are at the very end stage of a process. They've got diabetes. It's just they haven't got the hyperglycemia.

DEVELOPMENT OF DIABETES IN IDENTICAL TWINS

D.A. Pyke

King's College Hospital, London

The value of studies in identical (monozygotic) twins lies as much in what they refute as in what they confirm. Thus if a pair of twins resembles each other in respect of a condition that does not prove that the condition is inherited, but if they differ from each other then the condition cannot be inherited.

This view assumes that "identical twins" are truly indentical. We know that to a certain extent this is not true. There are apparently spontaneous genetic rearrangements, particularly in the regions controlling immune responses. Their frequency and significance is unknown but it is a consideration in drawing conclusions from studies of "identical twins."

The clinical diagnosis of monozygosity is easy. In most of our cases it has been confirmed by 12-group blood typing but this has never in our experience falsified a clinical diagnosis of monozygosity.

We have collected a series of nearly 300 pairs of identical twins over a period of more than 20 years in the United Kingdom. They were ascertained through our own clinic and through colleagues and the British Diabetic Association. They were ascertained because they were diabetic, not because they were twins and this is likely to have introduced a bias towards the inclusion of concordant pairs, in which both the twins are diabetic and therefore have a double chance of recognition rather than the discordant pairs, in which only one is diabetic. Our total figures are therefore likely to exaggerate the relative frequency of concordant against discordant pairs.

There is another bias. Our series contain more twins with insulin dependent diabetes than non-insulin dependent, which is the reverse of their true relative frequency. There must therefore be a bias in the ascertainment of our twins in favour of insulin dependent diabetes as against non-insulin dependent diabetes, or both.

The results in our series of 282 pairs is shown in Table 1. The pairs have been classified as insulin dependent and non-insulin dependent on clinical grounds. In the great majority there did not seem to be any difficulty in doing so.

It is striking that in all but a few of the concordant pairs, the

TABLE I

IDENTICAL TWIN PAIRS

	CONCORDANT	DISCORDANT	TOTAL
IDD	86	92	178
NIDD	75	20	95
	(IDD/NIDD or doubtful)		282

diabetes is of the same type in each affected twin, i.e. the disease seems, in this series, to breed true.

Non-Insulin Dependent Diabetes (NIDD)

The great majority of these pairs - 70 out of 95 - are concordant. In some cases we were notified of the twins as discordant but on glucose tolerance testing the apparently unaffected twin was found to be diabetic, by conventional criteria.

This high concordance rate was found although in most cases the twins were middle-aged or elderly, were living apart, had different life circumstances and were sometimes of different weight. In one third of pairs in which we have reliable data concerning the weight of each pair at the time of diagnosis of diabetes the twins differed by kilos or more; furthermore, the lighter twin developed diabetes first as often as the heavier.

In most of the discordant NIDD pairs the affected twin has been diagnosed only recently. Of those 37 pairs in which the first twin was diagnosed by 1970, all are now concordant.

It seems from these data NIDD - at least as far as it is reflected by the twins in our study - is predominantly, perhaps entirely, genetically determined. This observation does not explain the role of obesity, which is commonly although by no means invariably a feature of NIDD. Obesity is a common association of NIDD but may not be a causative factor.

Nor do these results throw light on the question of whether NIDD is one syndrome or several. Insofar as the results in such a relatively small number as 95 can be regarded as valid they suggest that if NIDD comprises more than one syndrome they are all inherited.

Insulin Dependent Diabetes (IDD)

The results in the twin pairs with IDD are quite different. Discordance is as common as concordance (despite the presumed bias in ascertainment). It might be argued taht discordance is apparent rather than real, that in time the unaffected twin in the discordant pairs will develop diabetes.

This is unlikely in more than a few cases. In 20% of the concordant pairs the second twin developed diabetes within 5 years of the first, whereas in 60% of the discordant pairs the second twin remains unaffected after this period, in many cases after 20 years. It seems highly probable, therefore, that discordance is real and that the apparent figure of 50% seen in figure 1 is an underestimate.

In an attempt to discover the true concordance rate we have followed the 49 pairs notified to us within a year of the diagnosis in the index

twin. In one year 14 of the originally unaffected twins had become diabetic, but then the rate slowed; by 5 years the number was 25, by 6 years 34.
It seems probable therefore that the true concordance rate for IDD is about
36%.

We have examined the material in the hope of finding an explanation
for concordance in some pairs, as against discordance in others. There is
no clinical or personal difference that we have discovered. Heterozygosity
for HLA DR3 and 4 seems to be more common in the concordant than the discordant pairs. (2). Another is a suggestion of a difference between the
two groups in T-cell receptor (beta chain) polymorphisms (3).

'Activated' T lymphocytes are increased in newly diagnosed cases of
IDD. They presumably reflect the immune process which underlines the destruction of pancreatic beta cells. In the recently diagnosed diabetic twins
the level of activated T-cells is raised, but so it is in 10 out of 12 of
their unaffected co-twins. Assuming that about one third of these co-twins
will develop diabetes this increase must either be genetically determined
or indicate an acquired immune disturbance in the twin. The first explanation is unlikely as in co-twins of diabetics who have had the disease for
11 years or more the level of activated T-cells is close to the normal range.
The likely explanation therefore is that most of the co-twins of recently
diagnosed diabetics also show an immune disturbance but recover from it
without developing diabetes.

This concept of recovery from an immune attack (whatever its cause)
is consistent with reports of islet cell antibodies disappearing in some
cases and in others persisting without the appearance of diabetes. Whether
there is a point at which the immune process is so far advanced that progression to diabetes is inevitable we do not know.

Nor do twin studies throw any light on the nature of the stimulus which
leads to the immune destruction of the beta cells - virus, auto-immune or
other.

Some of our co-twins of IDDs have themselves developed diabetes. We
have been able to follow the process as it develops in these particular
respects: 1) Immunological changes in 6 twins. All showed elevation of
activated T cells before the diagnosis of diabetes on repeated testing over
a period of up to 3½ years. In only one of 20 samples was the level in the
normal range. 2) Repeated oral glucose tolerance testing showed that fasting glucose levels were raised only within one year of diagnosis of diabetes
but 2-hour levels were raised 2 -3 years previously. 3) In 7 child pairs
the co-twin has shown striking arrest of growth, growth velocity dropping
to less than the 3rd centile. The mean period between the nadir of growth
velocity and the diagnosis of diabetes was 1.1 years, much longer than the
duration of symptoms - about 6 weeks. Thus it seems that arrest or delay
of growth is a common feature of the pre-diabetic phase in young children.

I close with some highly speculative conclusions from these studies.
1) The frequency of immune changes in non-diabetic co-twins suggests
that the immune 'attack' is common in genetically susceptible persons.
2) Recovery from this 'attack' is common, occurring in about 2/3
cases.
3) The incubation period of insulin dependent diabetes is long, usually a matter of years.
4) The 'attack' operates over a limited period.
5) Recovery from the 'attack' leads to permanent immunity from IDD.

We do not know what determines whether an individual will recover from
the attack or develop diabetes, nor do we know how to influence the outcome.

REFERENCES

1. Barnett, A.H., Eff, C., Leslie, R.D.G., Pyke, D.A., 1981, Diabetes in Identical Twins: A study of 200 pairs. Diabetologia 20, 87.

2. Johnston, C., Pyke, D.A., Cudworth, A.G., Wolf, E., 1983, HLA-DR typing in identical twins with insulin-dependent diabetes. British Medical Journal 286, 253.

3. Millward, B.A., Welsh, K.I., Leslie, R.D.G., Pyke, D.A. Demaine, A.G., 1987, T-cell receptor beta chain polymorphisms are associated with insulin-dependent diabetes. Clin. exp. Immunol. 70, 152-157.

TYPE-SPECIFIC CONCORDANCE IN YOUNG DIABETIC MONOZYGOTIC TWINS

¶Dinesh Kumar, Nabil S. Gemayel, Sukhpal K. Gill, George A. Bray
Pradip Roy-Burman[1], Dennis Deapen[2], and Thomas M. Mack[2]

Department of Medicine, Division of Diabetes and Clinical Nutrition
Department of Pathology[1], and Department of Preventive Medicine[2]
University of Southern California School of Medicine
Los Angeles County Medical Center, Los Angeles, California

In 1972, Tattersall and Pyke (1) indicated that the level of concordance for diabetes among monozygotic twins depended upon the age of onset of
diabetes in the index twin. If diabetes developed before 40 years of age,
the subsequent concordance was estimated at 53%; it increased to 92% when
the index twin was older than 40 years at diagnosis. It has been realized
subsequently that classification of diabetic patients into Type I (insulin
dependent) and 2 (non-insulin dependent) on the basis of age alone is insufficient (2). Epidemiologic observations in Olmsted County, Minnesota
have revealed that while all cases with the onset of diabetes in the first
decade of life were insulin dependent, those who became diabetic in the
second and third decade included 37% and 50% respectively, who actually were
non-insulin dependent cases (3). In a population study from East Finland,
Laakso and Pyorala (4) also found heterogeneity of the type of diabetes
among young patients. Approximately 7% and 20% of those cases with the
onset of diabetes in the third and fourth decade were non-insulin dependent. It is conceivable that the monozygotic twins with onset of diabetes
before 40 years of age described by Tattersall and Pyke (1) were also a
mixed group.

Barnett and coworkers (5) have enlarged the original British twin
series (1) from 96 to 200 monozygotic pairs, and have more carefully
divided them into insulin and non-insulin dependent groups. Eighty of
the 147 insulin dependent pairs were found to be disease-concordant. However, these authors recognized that their method of ascertainment favored
the collection of concordant pairs. Dr. David Pyke (6) has presented an
update at this symposium. He now estimates the level of concordance for
Type I diabetes to be 35% as calculated by an actuarial analysis.

We present our observations of young diabetic monozygotic twins from
the U.S.A. We have analyzed their clinical characteristics and can estimate diabetes type-specific concordance in that context.

These studies were supported in part, by grants from American Diabetes
Association of Southern California Affiliate, and from National Cancer
Institute (#CA 42581).

TABLE I

UNIVERSITY OF SOUTHERN CALIFORNIA DIABETES TWIN REGISTRY
DISTRIBUTION OF 264 MONOZYGOTIC TWIN PAIRS

	Age at onset of diabetes		
	≤30 years	>30-<40	>40 years
Concordant for diabetes	26	16	76
Discordant	59	26	61

MATERIALS AND METHODS

Ascertainment of Diabetic Twins: The University of Southern California
International Twin Study was initiated by Dr. Thomas Mack in 1980 to con-
duct cotwin studies of various neoplasms, multiple sclerosis and other diseases. In 1983, ascertainment of twins with diabetes was begun and 635
pair had been identified by the end of 1987. Twins are ascertained by news-
paper advertisements placed nationwide. Participants are therefore volunteer
pairs; the young, the female, the well educated and presumably the disease
concordant are therefore over represented. The twins or family members re-
sponding to an advertisement are asked a few identifying questions. Diabetes twin registry coordinator then contacts each twin and/or the family by
phone, explains the goals and solicits full participation in the registry.
During the telephone interview, identifying items (name, address, telephone
number, date of birth, ethnicity etc.) are confirmed and medical characteristics (perceived zygosity, age at and means of diabetes diagnosis, initial
and present therapy, episodes of ketoacidosis, evidence of sequelae, indicators of growth and development) are recorded. A brief family history is
also obtained. This information is then confirmed using a postal questionnaire, and written permission is obtained to request records from doctor
and hospital for the purpose of validating the diagnosis using the medical
records.

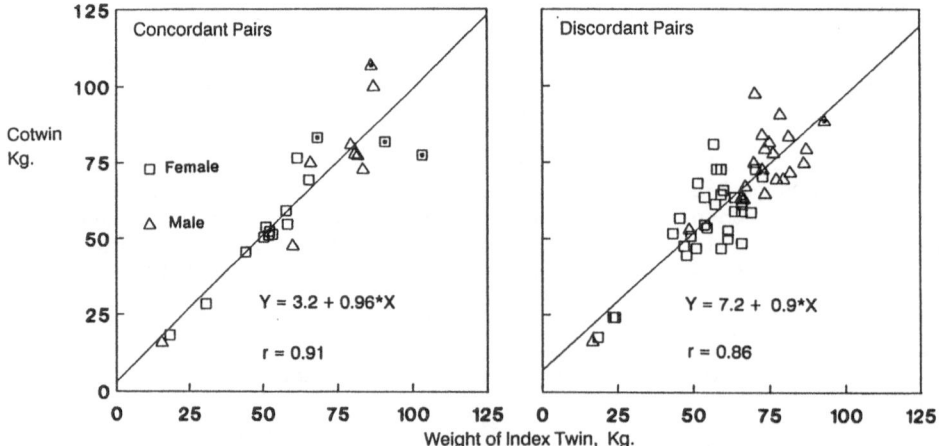

Figure 1. Weights of index and cotwins in diabetes-concordant pairs.
The target points represent overweight (body weight > 120%
of normal) cases. There is close intra-pair correlation,
and concordance for over-weightness.

TABLE II

CLINICAL CHARACTERISTICS OF INDEX AND COTWINS IN DIABETES–CONCORDANT PAIRS

Parameters	Index	Number of cotwins with identical features	Remarks
Weight ≤120% of normal, and insulin treatment within 1 year	19	17	One cotwin overweight, and another with gestational diabetes.
Weight ≤120% of normal, and no insulin treatment	1		Index twin treated with a biguanide for 5 years. Cotwin overweight.
Gestational diabetes	1	1	
Weight >120% of normal	5	5	Only one cotwin treated with insulin within first year of diagnosis

TABLE III

AGE AT ONSET OF DIABETES AND DISCORDANT PERIOD

	Number of pairs	Age of index twin at diagnosis Years	Discordant period Years	Age of cotwin at diagnosis Years
Concordant Pairs				
Index twins*, weight ≤120%	19	9.8 ± 1.6	4.1 ± 0.9	14.0 ± 1.8
Index twins, weight >120%	5	22.4 ± 2.2@$	14.3 ± 4.8@	36.8 ± 6@
Discordant Pairs				
Index twins*, weight ≤120%	57	14.4 ± 1	17.2 ± 1.5	

*   Index twin with characteristics of type 1 diabetes

@   P <0.01 compared to twins with weight ≤120%

$ P <0.03 compared to discordant pairs

TABLE IV

FAMILY HISTORY OF DIABETES MELLITUS

	Number of pairs analyzed	Number of positive family histories	One Parent	Grand Parent
<u>Concordant pairs</u>				
Weights ≤120%	17	6	2	5
Overweight >120%	4	4*	3	2
<u>Discordant pairs</u>	57	23	6	15

*   P <0.05 (Fisher's test)

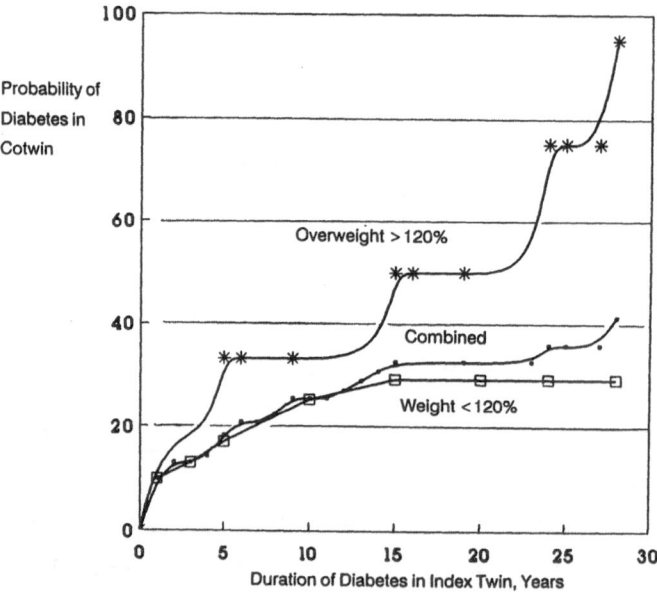

Figure 2.   Calculated cumulative probability of diabetes in a cotwin as a function of duration of disease in index twin. Combined curve represents data of all 85 monozygotic pairs with onset of diabetes in the index twin at age ≤30 years. In overweight (body weight > 120% of normal) twins (n = 6), the probability is much higher and reaches almost 100%. In other pairs (weight ≤ 120%), the probability is 29% at 15 years.

The postal questionnaire includes several modules: twinship characteristics, diabetes diagnosis and treatment, height and weight development, and
family history. It consists of questions asked, to the extent possible, in
both absolute and comparative modes. (That is, the respondent is asked to
estimate his or her weight at graduation from junior high school, as well as
to estimate which twin weighed more, and how much more, at the same age).

DNA Fingerprinting for validation of zygosity: With the cooperation of
twins and their physicians, a blood sample is collected and transported at
ambient temperature to our laboratory by an overnight courier service. Total nuclear DNA is extracted from leukocytes, purified, digested with endo-
nucleases and gel electrophoresed. Each patterns of hybridization to synthetic oligonucleotides specific for mini-satellite DNAs is compared (7) to
that of the cotwin in order to confirm zygosity.

Classification of twin pairs: Of the 635 twin pairs ascertained to date,
264 report monozygosity and 286 dizygosity. For the remaining 85 pairs,
the information is incomplete and zygosity remains undetermined. The distribution of the 264 monozygotic twin pairs according to the age of index
twin at onset of diabetes is given in Table I. We have analyzed 85 monozygotic twin pairs in which the index twin developed diabetes prior to 30
years of age.

According to the classification of diabetes developed by the Early
Treatment of Diabetic Retinopathy Study (ETDRS) group (8), patients fulfilling the following criteria were considered to have Type I diabetes: (a)
age at onset of diabetes $\leqslant$ 30 years, (b) body weight $\leqslant$ 120% of "normal"
(male and female body mass index $\leqslant$ 27.2 kg/m^2 and $\leqslant$ 26.9 kg/m^2 respectively), and (c) insulin therapy initiated within one year of diagnosis and
continued. Of the 261 Type I diabetes patients identified by the EDTRS
group using these criteria, 250 (95.8%) could be confirmed by low post-meal
plasma C-peptide levels ($\leqslant$ 80 fmol/ml), thus validating the diagnostic criteria (8).

Statistical methods: Data were analyzed using Dynastat software on IBM-AT
computer. Student "t" test was used for comparison of group means, and
linear correlations between paired data. Fisher's test (9) was utilized
for evaluation of family history data. The probability of developing diabetes in a cotwin was calculated by Kaplan-Meier (actuarial) survival curve
(9). Data are expressed as mean + SEM.

RESULTS

We report 85 monozygotic twin pairs in which the index twin developed
diabetes before 30 years of age. DNA fingerprinting analyses were performed
in 11 pairs, 9 monozygotic and 2 dizygotic as evidenced by the questionnaire
response. The stated zygosity of all 11 pairs tested was confirmed. Eighty-
four pairs were of European origin; one was Mexican-American. Twenty-six
pairs were concordant and 59 discordant for diabetes at the time of analysis. Fifty-four pairs (17 concordant and 37 discordant) were female, and
the female to male ratio was 1.6.

Onset and duration of diabetes: Mean age of the index twin at onset of
diabetes and duration of diabetes were 13.5 ± 1.7 and 21.7 ± 2.7 years in
concordant pairs, and 14.7 ± 1 and 17.6 ± 1.5 years respectively in discordant pairs. The disease-condordant cotwins developed diabetes 6.3 ± 1.4
years later.

Physical characteristics: We compared the present weights, heights and body
mass indices of twins. In the concordant pairs, heights were 158.3 ± 4.7

and 159.5 ± 4.5 cm, weights were 62.5 ± 4.7 and 62.7 ± 4.3 kg, and body mass indices (BMI) were 25.03 ± 2.77 and 23.62 ± 0.97 kg/m^2 in the index and cotwin respectively. In the discordant pairs, heights of the affected and healthy twins were 164.9 ± 2.1 and 165.4 ± 2.0 cm, weights were 61.4 ± 2.1 and 62.3 ± 2.2 kg, and BMI were 22.32 ± 0.41 and 22.58 ± 0.49 kg/m^2 respectively. There was a significant correlation within pairs for each physical characteristic. The correlation of present weights in our twin pairs is shown in Figure 1. BMI estimates for both twins at the onset of diabetes in the index twin were available for 22 pairs, and showed close resemblance (21.09 ± 0.95 kg/m^2 in index and 22.03 ± 0.56 kg/m^2 in cotwin).

Overweight twins: Five index twins in the concordant group and one in the discordant group were overweight (> 120% of normal) at diagnosis, and thus failed to meet the ETDRS clinical criteria for Type I diabetes (Table II). In addition, only one of them had been treated with insulin within the first year of diabetes. We compared the characteristics of these 5 overweight, disease-concordant twin pairs with those of the remaining concordant pairs, and with those discordant pairs, in which cases met the ETDRS criteria of Type I diabetes. As shown in Table III, the mean age of the overweight index twin was significantly higher at onset of diabetes; four were over 20 years old at onset. In these pairs the period of disease-discordance ranged from one month to 28 years, the group average period was significantly prolonged (P < 0.01), and the onset of diabetes in the cotwin was significantly delayed (P < 0.01).

The incidence of diabetes (Type I or II) in the families of the twins is given in Table IV. A positive family history signifies diabetes in either a parent, a grandparent or a sibling (excluding cotwin). The family history was positive more often in the over-weight disease-concordant pairs (P < 0.05, Fisher's test); the father was diabetic in 3 cases.

Clinical characteristics of index and cotwins in concordant pairs: Nineteen of the 26 index twins in disease-concordant pairs met the ETDRS criteria for Type I diabetes (Table II), as did 17 (89%) of their cotwins. One cotwin was overweight; but after the index twin developed diabetes at age 19 years, the cotwin was diagnosed at 20 years, and both were treated with insulin. BMI values were 26.7 kg/m^2 in the index case, and 28.3 kg/m^2 in cotwin at the time of diagnosis. In another pair, the cotwin developed gestational diabetes at age 25 years following a discordant period of 12 years.

One index twin developed diabetes at age 28 years; while not overweight (BMI 26.4), he used a biguanide drug for 5 years before beginning insulin. His overweight cotwin (BMI 28.56 kg/m^2) developed diabetes at age 40 years. Both members of another pair developed gestational diabetes.

There were 5 pairs who were concordant for both excess weight and diabetes. Four of these cotwins were managed without insulin for > 1 year. The fifth cotwin like her twin (BMI 64.6 kg/m^2), was very obese (BMI 65.8 kg/m^2), and was treated with insulin.

Clinical characteristics of discordant pairs: Fifty-seven of the 59 index twins in discordant pairs met the criteria for Type I diabetes. One had developed gestational diabetes. Another index twin was 24 years old, overweight BMI 32.62 kg/m^2), asymptomatic at the time of diagnosis, and was treated with chlorpropamide for 3 years. His cotwin was overweight (BMI 27.3 kg/m^2), but has not developed diabetes in the 16 years that have elapsed thus far.

Probability of developing diabetes in a cotwin: We analyzed the periods of diabetes-discordancy using the method of Kaplan-Meier, and calculated the cumulative probability that a cotwin would remain nondiabetic. The estimates were 0.82 ± 0.01, 0.75 ± 0.01, 0.68 ± 0.01, 0.68 ± 0.01, 0.65 ± 0.02, and 0.59 ± 0.3 after 5, 10, 15, 20, 25, and 28 years of diabetes in the index twin. The complements of these probabilities represent the cumulative probability of developing diabetes in a cotwin, and are displayed in Figure 2 (see curve labeled "combined"). Note that this curve remains flat at a level of 32% for the eight year period between 15 and 23 years, and then moved to 41% between the 23rd and 28th years. The later inflection in the curve resulted from 2 overweight pairs in which the cotwins became diabetic after discordant periods of 23.7 and 28 years.

We then removed the overweight index twins, and recalculated the estimates. When all index twins weighed ≤ 120% of normal, the cumulative probability of developing diabetes in a cotwin was 16 ± 0.5, 24 ± 0.9, 29 ± 1.2, 29 ± 1.5, 29 ± 2.7% after 5, 10, 15, 20, and 25 years respectively (Figure 2). The group of overweight twin pairs was limited to 6. The calculated probability of developing diabetes in an overweight cotwin was 50% after 15 years, and approached almost 100% after 28 years.

It was observed that 63% of cotwins in the diabetes-concordant pairs had developed diabetes within first 5 years following the onset of Type I diabetes in index twin. Additional 26% became diabetic during 6–10 year period. Thus far no cotwin has developed Type I diabetes at a point beyond 15 years of discordance.

COMMENTS

Diabetes Twin Registry: The twins were ascertained using advertisements, and are therefore unrepresentative of all diabetic twin pairs. The female to male ratio of 1.6 illustrates this bias, and one should therefore be cautious of the observed absolute levels of concordance. There is, however, no reason to believe that young monozygotic cases fulfilling the criteria for Type I diabetes are differentially ascertained in comparison with other young monozygotic cases.

Type of diabetes in young monozygotic twins: We selected twins with onset of diabetes before age 30 years. Nineteen of 26 index twins in the disease-concordant pairs, and 57 of 59 in discordant pairs met the ETDRS criteria of Type I diabetes; remaining 9 (10%) failed to meet these criteria. Gestational diabetes developed in 2 pairs, 6 were overweight and 1 case of normal weight required no insulin. These observations in twins are in agreement with the results of non-twin studies (3,4), where a substantial number of non-insulin dependent cases have been found among diabetics with age at onset prior to 30 years.

In twin pairs concordant for diabetes, the clinical features in both index and cotwin usually suggested concordance for the type of diabetes. For example, 5 index twins were overweight and all of their cotwins were also overweight. Both twins of one pair developed gestational diabetes. The characteristics of Type I diabetes were seen in 17 cotwins of the 19 index twins with Type I diabetes. Nonetheless, some discordance of diabetes type was seen; one cotwin had gestational diabetes and another was overweight (overall 8%). Moreover, we cannot be certain that new cases of Type II diabetes will not yet develop in the unaffected cotwins of the other 57 index cases. Nonetheless, our observations indicate that if any cotwin has been discordant for at least 15 years and develops diabetes, it will most likely be Type II disease.

Overweight and diabetes-concordant pairs: Five of 6 overweight twin pairs were concordant for diabetes. in addition to being overweight, 4 had strong family history and required no insulin within the first year of diabetes; these features suggest non-insulin dependent diabetes (2).

Concordance for diabetes: It is apparent from our observations that a classification of diabetes based solely on age, as applied in the original British twin study (1), may be misleading because young people with onset of diabetes as early as the second or third decade may have features of non-insulin dependent diabetes. We therefore, analyzed the concordance of diabetes in relation to the clinical characteristics of the disease as well as age. Among twin pairs in which the twin had features indicating Type I diabetes, the cumulative probability of developing diabetes in a cotwin reached 29 ± 1.2% by the 15th year of follow up (Figure 2). This estimate is in agreement with that of Pyke reported at this symposium (6). Further, we confirm the previously published observations of Barnett et al (5) that cotwins mostly become diabetic in the first five years after the index diagnosis, and no cotwin appears to develop Type I diabetes after 15 years have elapsed.

These observations, taken together with the observed (all possibly overestimated) pairwise concordance for diabetes in monozygotic twins (29 ± 2.7%) suggest that in addition to the genetic component, environmental factors must play a major role in etiology of Type I diabetes (10).

We found high concordance for over-weightness and five of 6 such twin pairs were also concordant for diabetes. In these pairs, the disease-discordance periods were prolonged, and the probability of developing diabetes in a cotwin was much increased (50% by 15 years and almost 100% by 28 years). We hypothesize that these latter pairs most probably represent obese Type II diabetes. Insulin secretory and immunologic studies would help to confirm this hypothesis.

In summary, our observations show that (1) among the monozygotic twins who developed diabetes before the age of 30 years, there is heterogeneity of the type of diabetes; one group has the clinical features of Type I diabetes while the other group has features consistent with Type II. (2) In twin pairs concordant for diabetes, both the index and cotwin often have type-specific concordance. (3) The probability of developing diabetes in a normal weight (⩽ 120% of normal) cotwin is 29 ± 2.7%, but increases to almost 100% in an overweight cotwin.

ACKNOWLEDGEMENTS

We thank the staff of the International Twin Study, Miss Malak Zacca for their help with telephone interviews, and Mr. Peter Yamashita for data analysis.

REFERENCES

1. Tattersall, R.B., Pyke, D.A., 1972, Diabetes in identical twins. Lancet 2: 1120-1125.

2. National Diabetes Data Group, 1979, Classification and diagnosis of diabetes mellitus and other categories of glucose intolerance. Diabetes 28: 1039-1057.

3. Melton III, L.J., Palumbo, P.J., Chu, C., 1983, Incidence of diabetes mellitus by clinical type. Diabetes Care 6: 75-86.

4. Laakso, M., Pyorala, K., 1985, Age of onset and type of diabetes. Diabetes Care 8: 114-117.

5. Barnett, A.H., Eff, C., Leslie, R.D.G., Pyke, D.A., 1981, Diabetes in identical twins, a study of 200 pairs. Diabetologia 20: 87-93.

6. Pyke, D.A., 1988, Development of diabetes in identical twins. In Early Diabetes: Prediabetes. R.A. Camerini-Davalos, H. Cole, Eds., Plenum Publishing Company, New York: 255-258

7. Yam, P., Petz, L.D., ALi, S., Stock, D., and Wallace, R.B., 1987, Development of a simple probe for documentation of chimerism following bone marrow transplantation. Am J Hum Genet 41: 867-881.

8. Early treatment diabetic retinopathy study classification of Diabetes Working Group: C-peptide and the classification of diabetes patients in the early treatment diabetic retinopathy study (unpublished data).

9. Matthews, D.E., Farewell, V.T., 1985, Using and understanding medical statistics. New York, Karger.

10. Eisenbarth, G.S., 1986, Type 1 diabetes mellitus, a chronic autoimmune disease. N Engl J Med 314: 1360-1368.

PREDIABETES AND THE PATHOLOGICAL LESIONS OF THE PANCREAS

¶J.J. Hoet

Faculty of Medicine, University of Louvain, Brussels, Belgium

In the insulin dependent diabetes (Type I) a specific histological lesion has been described by W. Gepts (1). The lymphocytic infiltration in the islet of Langerhans, known as insulitis, is associated with a progressive disappearance of the Beta cells. Electron microscopy studies in men and animals indicate that an early phase consists of the invasion of the islets by macrophages and a concommitant disruption of the plasma membrane specifically of the Beta cells. At a later stage, lymphocytic infiltration is observed possibly accompanied by polymorphonuclear leucocytes and histiocytes. The progressive destruction of Beta cells is associated in some pancreas with occasional signs of Beta cell regeneration. The impending infiltration disappears when the Beta cells have vanished. The regeneration of the Beta cells seems not to be able to cope with their destruction (2).

Cytokines such as interleukine 1 through their local contacts are toxic for the Beta cells and would be responsible for their disappearance. Antibodies such as ICSA (islet cell surface antibodies) and anti-insulin antibodies may be present as well. They are part of the multiple organ antibodies which are produced by insulin dependent diabetics, characterized by HLA, DR_3, DR_4 and DQ. These antibodies may influence the structure as well as the function of the insulin secreting Beta cell. Therefore, cellular and humoral immune reactions which may be triggered off by viruses are responsible for the destruction of these cells.

However another endocrine gland such as the thyroid gland may be infiltrated by lymphocytes which induce hypothyroidism without accompanying anti-thyroid (microsomal or thyroglobulin) antibodies. It remains to be demonstrated that the sole cellular immune reaction around the Beta cell without a humoral one would be sufficient to induce their destruction (3).

In any event, a time span appears to be necessary in order to achieve a complete Beta cell destruction with absolute insulin dependency. The known aspects of the insulitis lesion evokes a chronic stage which from the clinical point of view would be associated with a period whereby insulin insufficiency would be present without inducing absolute insulin dependency.

A special grant in aid has been provided by N.V. Petrofina S.A. Belgium. The support of the F.N.R.S., Credits aux Chercheurs is also acknowledged.

During this early period, therapeutic interventions could prevent the further destruction of the Beta cells. Hence, the importance of understanding the immunogenics of the diabetes prone subjects which evolution leads to insulin dependency.

The immunohistological observations of Rahier, confirming the disappearance of Beta cells in autopsy material in longstanding non insulin dependent diabetics, indicated as well that they may show a reduced Beta cell mass when compared with non diabetic subjects. However, these islets contained amyloid deposits. The latter are not found in the islets of insulin dependent or haemochromatotic patients. Recent histochemical and electron microscopal observatins have demonstrated amyloid fibrils invaginating the Beta cell membranes and adjacent capillaries (4). In the human, the amyloid connected with the Beta cells consists e.g. of the B-chain of insulin molecule as well as of tubulin. Furthermore, a previously unknown 37 amino-acid peptide has been identified which is similar to calcitonin gene related protein. The latter is known to be present as well in pancreatic epithelial bodies and is being identified also in the Beta cell amyloid of cats. Amyloid deposits in islets of Langerhans has been found in association with diabetes in non human primates where it was a major contributory factor. Interestingly, this lesion was also associated with the appearance of islet cell antibodies usually at an early stage before insulin was required. A similar observation was made in aging human subjects (5).

Another interesting experimental observation may shed further light in the etiology and the slow onset of diabetes. The persistence of experimental viruses in the Beta cell and in thyroid cells as well may lead to endocrine disease without inducing major histological lesions at the islet cell level.

The vertical transmission of viral diseases to the fetus is also a clinical recognized fact. Congenital rubella is associated with several diseases, diabetes included. It may be the same for cytomegalic disease in communities where the latter is endemic. Experimentally, diabetes in the NOD mice is associated with the passage of viral particles from mother to fetus which will be located in the fetal pancreas. The latter event will lead to lymphocytic infiltration 6 weeks later.

The transplacental effects of disturbed maternal metabolism on fetal health and on the development of the fetal beta cell may also intervene as etiological factors in diabetes.

In animal investigation, the maternal metabolism has been disturbed by moderate or severe streptozotocin induced diabetes during pregnancy. The multiplication rate of the fetal Beta cell indicated a major increased rate in the former and a reduced one in the latter. When protein malnutrition was provoked in otherwise normal mothers, the multiplication rate of the neonatal Beta cell was also reduced confirming the induced histological changes in the neonatal insulin secreting cells. In humans, the islets of Langerhans of 60% of the neonates of diabetic mothers who were overweight and died featured eosinophilic infiltration even if the mother had not been treated with insulin. This could be related to the transplacental passage of immunogenic elements such as antibodies or viruses which would provoke during the fetal stage a specific immune reaction at the Beta cell level.

In conclusion, the analysis of the pathologic alterations of the diabetic pancreas suggests a period of latency between the initiating events and the established lesions. The Beta cells do go through progressive changes which in the course of time result in their destruction or disappearance of the appropriate B cell mass. Persistence of virus without manifest histological alterations may still be another event affecting the function of the Beta cell and lead to diabetes.

Congenital viral infections or disturbed maternal metabolism may through their transplacental effects alter as well the development and the integrity of the fetal or neonatal insulin secreting cells.

In each of these instances, there is a time sequence which is associated with a delay in the clinical consequences of these alterations. The further insight in the time sequence of the histopathological changes of the islets of Langerhans will give a better understanding of the prediabetic period and may lead to the elaboration of interventions which may prevent the prediabetic from becoming a diabetic (6).

REFERENCES

1. Gepts, W., 1965, Pathological anatomy of the pancreas in juvenile diabetes mellitus. Diabetes 14: 619-633.

2. Hoet, J.J., Reusens-Billen, B., and Remacle, C., 1987, Lessons from the pathology of the diabetic pancreas. Horm Metab Res 19: 523-525.

3. Betterle, C., Presotto, F., Pedini, B., Moro, L., Slack, R.S., Zanette, F., Zanchetta, R., 1987, Islet cell and insulin autoantibodies in organspecific autoimmune patients. Their behaviour and predictive value for the development of Type I (insulin dependent) diabetes mellitus. A 10-year follow-up study. Diabetologia 30: 292-297.

4. Westermark, P., Wilander, E., Westermark, G.T., Johnson, K.H., 1987, Islet amyloid polypeptide-like immunoreactivity in the islet B cells of Type II (non-insulin-dependent) diabetic and non-diabetic individuals. Diabetologia 30: 887-892.

5. Clark, A., Copper, G.J.S., Lewis, C.E., Morris, J.F., Willis, A.C., Reid, K.B.M., Turner, R.C., 1987, Islet amyloid formed from diabetes-associated peptide may be pathogenic in Type II diabetes. The Lancet, August 1st Issue: 231-234.

6. Hoet, J.J., and Remacle, C., 1987, Pancreatic Islets, Organization of the pancreatic Islets with Special References to Diabetes, Endocrinology 1987, Eds. L.J. DeGroot et al., Grune & Stratton, New York, San Francisco and London.

DISCUSSION

R. RODRIGUEZ: Dr. Hoet, how do you get the diabetes in the rat? I understand your determinations were done the day the pups were born. Do you have determinations afterwards?

J. HOET: Diabetes resulted from Streptozotocin and we looked at pups 21½ days old. The follow-up study shows that there is an insulin secretion, which remains very defective. We have some results for the protein deprived animals and they are not able to cope well at least three months after delivery.

J. BARBOSA: About the twin studies, I'd like to congratulate Dr.Kumar for including dizygotic twins, because I think that will be a very important feature of any registry of twins. Dr. Pyke, I think you mentioned that the 3, 4 twins are more often concordant than the non 3, 4 twins. Did you mention that?

D. PYKE: Yes.

J. BARBOSA: Can you give us some statistics on that?

D. PYKE: Yes, I only didn't go into detail, because it was published some time ago. The proportion of concordant pairs which were HLA, DR3 and 4 heterozygotes was twice that of the discordant pairs. That statistic is significant to the 5% level, but the number we'ge got since then is very small and I suppose that could be interpreted simply as meaning that the concordant pairs have a greater genetic component to their diabetes than the discordant pairs. I take your point about genetic rearrangement. It seems to be one of those things that must have some validity and I don't think anybody knows. My feeling is that I doubt whether it explains the enormous disparity between the concordant trait we find and the concordant trait you would expect if it was simply a single gene genetic disease. But, I just don't know. I have to start off with the caveat that I did for fear of a counter attack such as you've just made.

J. C. CRESTO: I have two questions. Dr. Pyke, have you some other studies about insulin deficiency in your twins? And, Dr. Kumar, have you correlated your twincs C-peptide deficiency with risk?

D. KUMAR: I must emphasize that all of our twins are distributed through-out the United States. Some of the co-twins are across the border. We have some twins in England and some of them are in Brussels, so we use international transport service to get samples to us. We have not done any functional studies, because of this limitation of distance. When we, there-fore, mention C-peptide data, I use the C-peptide data from a collaborative study done in America, so called early treatment of diabetic retinopathy which is done in about 22 centers. The C-peptide data is from that study, not from the twins. I want to emphasize that.

D. PYKE: We have studied the insulin secretion of the twins before they became diabetic and we have found, as other people do, that it tends to decline, the first phase particularly, but we found a good deal of variation. We don't find the apparently straight line decline that other people do. This may be simply that we're looking at them before they have got to the last 1% of their secreting capacity. Our attempts at predicting when a twin will get diabetes are not very good.

G. GRODSKY: I wonder about this first phase insulin release being interpreted as a decrease in mass. I would think that if you had 100% of all your cells still intact, which I'm not saying you do, but if you did and had a defect in first phase release that would show up as less insulin under that peak. If you have, say, an 80% or 90% loss of beta cell mass then you still get a first phase that was depleted. I think the way you distinguish it is what happens in the second phase, because if you really lost 80% mass you'd lose both first and second phase. So, I think a loss in first phase insulin per se does not mean that you have dropped off where you only have 10% of the insulin content, I mean 10% of the beta cells remaining. It can occur with any defect in terminal release of insulin even though you may have all the cells still there.

The question I wanted to ask Dr. Pyke is since I tend to think the lesions started in the beta cells, maybe it's appropriate to ask the question, the challenging question, that actually since you show the increase in T lymphocytes maybe it is still an immunological phenomenon rather than a biological insult or environmental insult and that these people are only differing, maybe, in their environmental pattern in how they have been damaged by that increase in immunological change. So, it is possible that your data also supports equally that we have an immunologic original problem and the individuals differ only in how they recognize that problem.

One question to Dr. Hoet. In your protein deficient diets what were the extra calories made up by? Carbohydrate or lipid?

J. HOET: Carbohydrate, so that they had only 8% of protein instead of 20%.

G. GRODSKY: Okay, so the lipids were normal.

J. HOET: Right. So that they had enough carbohydrates.

D. PYKE: Dr. Grodsky, if I've got this right, you're suggesting that there is an immunological attack which does not have metabolic consequences.

G. GRODSKY: Yes, essentially.

D. PYKE: I think in part you're right, but some of these twins who have not yet gone on to develop diabetes, and in most cases we think won't, have shown metabolic abnormalities, minor ones, as well as immunological ones. So, my guess is that the immunological markers are probably the most sensitive ones, but that they are accompanied by metabolic change if the immunological disturbance is at all severe. It's only in some cases, but that's only a guess.

F. SCOTT: Dr. Hoet, in light of what Dr. Gleichmann was telling us about Streptozotocin inducing T-cell changes or changes in the T-helper cells possibly, is it possible that your changes are due to the Streptozotocin you give the mothers and hence the mother somehow transferring this immunologically to the infant?

J. HOET: It might be possible, but there have been other experiments where Streptozotocin was given before pregnancy so that really there was no real influence of Streptozotocin being given before pregnancy and the same results were obtained.

F. SCOTT: So, basically, then what you have done is you imposed a protein deficiency on the effects of Streptozotocin.

J. HOET: Oh, I am sorry. That needs clarification. These are three different experiments, diabetes is one, moderate and severe, and the other one is without any diabetes and just plain protein deficiency.

C. HOWARD: I have a question for Dr. Pyke. You did not go very much into the NIDD, but there have been some studies in which patients who were insulin dependent, older age patients, overweight patients, were put on very strict calorie reduction and found to lose many of the signs and symptoms of diabetes fairly rapidly. The question raised then is can that delay the onset of diabetes? Have similar studies been done when you have the concordance of the older diabetic twin to indicate whether there would be the actual concordance within that short time period or whether by intervention that onset could be delayed?

D. PYKE: I've got no information on that in the twins, but just two points. Quite a lot of diabetics respond to diet and weight losing. I would submit two things. One is that a lot of diabetics, non-insulin dependent diabetics in Britain, are not overweight. Of course, a lot are, but a lot are not. And, the second point is that they respond to treatment before, in many cases, they have in fact lost weight. I think a lot of it is simply carbohydrate restriction. And, to go back to twins, we find this concordance even when the two twins are a non-insulin dependent pair of different weights, one is overweight, one is not. When one differes from the other by more than 7 kilograms, they're still concordant. So, I think you can probably abolish the manifestations of diabetes. My suggestion is that these people are still diabetic and that if they went back onto a full diet with or without regaining weight, the manifestation would return.

C. HOWARD: Dr. Hoet, I am intrigued by the slow virus aspect that is possibly causing the pathological damage. We did get the antibody to the intracisternal associated particle and we examined some of them and we do develop the amyloidotic lesion. We found it in some of them, but not in others. There seemed to be no correlation with those that became diabetic and those who were not. We also looked at some baboons, an unrelated species in this case, for which we have no information that they do develop diabetes, and again some were positive and some were not, at least by our testing techniques. I'm puzzled by it. I just simply offer it as a comment, because I don't know exactly where it's going to fit in. Certainly, the slow virus theory is one that I think should be examined.

J. HOET: It may very well depend upon what type slow virus. I think there is some indication for this.

VI.   TREATMENT OF PREDIABETES

DIABETOGENICITY OF VARIOUS PROTEIN SOURCES IN THE DIET

OF THE DIABETES-PRONE BB RAT

¶Fraser W. Scott, Ghulam Sarwar and Heather E. Cloutier

Nutrition Research Division, Food Directorate, Health Protection Branch
Health & Welfare Canada

Insulin dependent diabetes mellitus (IDDM) has a wide geographic distribution ranging from 0.8/100,000 in Japan to 9 in Canada, 14.7 in the U.S.A. to 28.6 in Finland. As well, there is discordance in identical twins, and it has been suggested we are in the midst of an "epidemic" of IDDM which cannot be explained easily in terms of genetics alone (1). Other epidemiological data, as well as studies in animals, suggest environmental factors may be important in determining the expression of this presumed autoimmune disease in genetically predisposed individuals. (2).

It is conceivable that diet may play an important role in expression of IDDM (3-5). Studies in the BB rat, which spontaneously develops a form of (autoimmune) insulin-dependent diabetes, have suggested that the source of dietary protein may be particularly important. It has been found that BB rats fed diets containing hydrolysed lactalbumin or a mixture of amino acids have a greatly reduced incidence of diabetes and possible insulitis when compared to BB rats fed certain less degraded protein sources (3,4). This is in keeping with the delayed appearance and dampening of symptoms of the SLE-like (autoimmune) syndrome in NZB/W F_1 mice which were fed a synthetic amino acid diet (6).

In order to test the effect of different sources of dietary protein on the expression of BB rat diabetes and some of the associated T lymphocyte population abnormalities, we have fed defined diets containing various sources of protein. Some of these have been supplemented to make all diets adequate in essential amino acids required for rat growth. The diets were also closely balanced with respect to other nutrients and fiber. Some of the plant protein sources we used are known to be associated with "antinutrients" such as trypsin inhibitors, glucosinolates, phytic acid and various mitogenic substances (7). In order to minimize the effects of these factors, we have either selected varieties low in known inhibitors or have autoclaved the protein preparations. Using this approach, we have been able to study the effects of different protein structure rather than quality on the expression of autoimmune diabetes in the BB rat.

The authors would like to thank Dr. P. Thibert and Mr. J. Souligny for maintaining the Health Protection Branch BB rat colony, Mrs. Z. Zawidzka for hematology analyses, Mr. R. Peace for preparing the autoclaved, lyophilized kidney bean preparation, Mr. C. Deslogues for animal care work and Mr. H. Botting for the amino acid analyses.

MATERIALS AND METHODS

120 Male, diabetes-prone, BB rats from 29 litters of the Health Protection Branch colony were randomly distributed into individual, stainless steel, wire-bottom cages to prevent coprophagy and facilitate individual measurements; body weight, food and water consumption and urine glucose were monitored weekly. Animals were considered diabetic when the following were observed: polyuria, polydipsia, weight loss (or failure to gain weight), urine glucose $\geq$ 2+ using Testape (Eli Lilly and Co., Indianapolis, Indiana) and fasting blood glucose 200 mg/dL. Diabetics were usually killed within 24 hours of discovery. Pancreases from all rats were fixed in Bouin's solution and paraffin-embedded sections were processed and stained with hemotoxyln and eosin. Coded samples were graded for the presence of lymphocytic infiltration of islets. Subjective rating was carried out using a scale ranging from 1 to 5, where 1 denoted absence of inflammation and 5 indicated major displacement of islet tissue by inflammatory infiltrate and destruction of most beta cells. The asymptomatic rats which remained at the end of the experiment were killed by exsanguination while under light halothane anesthesia (3% in O_2). Any of these animals which had fasting blood glucose of 200 mg/dL or higher as well as signs of insulitis were considered to be diabetic. Blood was collected into tubes containing anticoagulant or into serum separation tubes (Becton-Dickinson). Hematological characteristics were determined using a Coulter Model S blood Cell analyser. In selected asymptomatic animals, spleen, thymus and peripheral blood lymphocytes (PBL) were prepared using Ficoll gradients and blastogenic response to concanavalin A (Con A) and T cell subset distribution were determined. Free amino acids in pooled sera from 5 asymptomatic rats without insulitis from each diet group were measured using high pressure liquid chromatography. Statistical significance of differences was evaluated using Fisher's exact test, analysis of variance or variance or student's unpaired t test.

EXPERIMENTAL DIETS AND ANIMAL FEEDING

The test animals were fed isonitrogenous and isocaloric experimental diets based on the AIN-76 formulation (8) from weaning (21 days) to 162 ± 8 days of age; the dams of these rats were fed Purina Laboratory chow 5001. Diets were mixed every 2-3 weeks in batches of 14 Kg in large stainless steel mixing bowls and were stored refrigerated. The ingredients listed in Table 1 were obtained from the following suppliers (percent protein given in brackets): Casein (90.6%), ANRC Reference Protein, Humko Sheffield Chemicals, Kraft Co., Madison WI; Rapeseed flour (low glucosinolate; 58.8%), kindly provided by Dr. J.D. Jones, Food Research Centre, Agriculture Canada, Ottawa; Peanut meal (39.4%), Teklad Test Diets, Madison, WI; Kidney beans (25.7%), Great Canadian Bean Co., Ailsa Craig, Ontario (soaked in tap water for 18 h, drained and autoclaved at 121°C for 30 minutes, colled, lyophilized and ground to 35 mesh); Fish meal (59.9%), Sea Crest with ethoxyquin, Fish Reduction Ltd., Wood's Harbour, Nova Scotia; Wheat gluten flour (80.3%), Grain Process Enterprises Ltd., Scarborough, Ontario; Mazola corn oil; Corn starch was from Best Food Services, Montreal, Quebec; AIN-76 vitamin and mineral mixes, choline bitartrate and DL-methionine were purchased from ICN Biochemicals, amino acids were from Sigma Chemical Co.

RESULTS

BB rats fed rapeseed flour, peanut meal and kidney beans did not gain weight at the same rate as rats fed the control casein diet (Fig. 1A). This was due mainly to less food consumption in these groups and not to decreased food efficiency (Fig. 1B), suggesting the effect on body weight was due to a palatability problem but not ruling out the presence of residual anti-nutritional factors.

TABLE I

COMPOSITION OF DEFINED DIETS ON A PERCENT BASIS

NAME OF DIET	Casein (Control)	Rapeseed Flour	Peanut Meal	Kidney Beans	Fish Meal	Wheat Gluten
INGREDIENT						
Casein	22.1	0	0	0	0	0
Rapeseed flour	0	34.0	0	0	0	0
Peanut meal	0	0	50.7	0	0	0
Kidney beans	0	0	0	77.7	0	0
Fish meal	0	0	0	0	33.4	0
Wheat gluten	0	0	0	0	0	24.9
Corn oil	5.0	3.0	3.0	3.5	3.3	5.0
Corn starch	62.90	55.00	35.24	13.37	54.30	59.77
Cellulose fibre	5.0	3.3	2.0	0.4	4.3	5.0
AIN-76* Mineral mix	3.5	3.5	3.5	3.5	3.5	3.5
AIN-76A* Vitamin mix	1.0	1.0	1.0	1.0	1.0	1.0
DL-Methionine	0.3	0	2.4	0.33	0	0.01
Choline bitartrate	0.2	0.2	0.2	0.2	0.2	0.2
L-Lysine-HCL	0	0	1.9	0	0	0.54
L-Threonine	0	0	0.06	0	0	0.08

*All diets are based on the American Institute of Nutrition (AIN) recommended diet for nutritional studies in rats and mice (8).

The only instance in which diabetes incidence was different from the casein-fed (control) group was in animals fed wheat gluten as the sole protein source (P = 0.06, Table 2). It should be pointed out that the wheat gluten-fed animals were nearly identical to the casein-fed, control group in final body weight, food consumption and food efficiency.

Compared to the casein-fed group, age at onset differed only in animals fed rapeseed flour diets, which delayed appearance of diabetes from 88 to 150 days in the small number of animals which became diabetic. The control group had the highest number of rats remaining asymptomatic without insulitis and this difference was significant (P < 0.05) when compared to groups fed the kidney bean or wheat gluten-based diets.

Spleen/body weight ratios were increased in rats fed the peanut meal or kidney bean diets but were decreased in those fed fish meal or wheat gluten. Similar increases in kidney/body weight ratios were seen in the peanut meal and kidney bean groups, suggesting a more generalized effect of these diets, possibly related to residual antinutrients.

A major problem in studies of nutrition/immune system relationships is to differentiate general metabolic effects from specific interactions. For example, the peanut meal diet decreased the WBC and RBC counts as well as red cell distribution width while increasing MCV, spleen/BW and kidneys/BW ratios suggesting an overall inhibitory effect not seen in any of the other diet groups. This general inhibitory effect was also associated with the lowest diabetes incidence.

The fish meal diet also produced overall changes, which appeared not to be associated with increased diabetes incidence, such as decreased spleen/BW ratio, blood urea nitrogen, hemoglobin, MCV as well as increased kidney/BW ratios and red cell distribution width.

By contrast, although the kidney bean diet increased spleen/BW and kidneys /BW ratios and both cholesterol and triglyceride levels were significantly lower than the casein-fed rats, there were no significant changes in hematological parameters and again the diabetes incidence was low.

Apart from the increase in kidneys/BW ratio and somewhat decreased weight gain (due to reduced food intake), the rapeseed flour diet had few effects on metabolic or hematological parameters. This diet was associated with a low diabetes incidence but also had a relatively high number of asymptomatic rats with insulitis.

Cholesterol levels were lower on all diets compared to the casein diet but this was likely a reflection of the cholesterolemic nature of defined casein diets (9).

Although the wheat gluten diet was relatively diabetogenic, it too was associated with only minor decreases in blood urea nitrogen and spleen/BW ratio. All other parameters were similar to the casein-fed group.

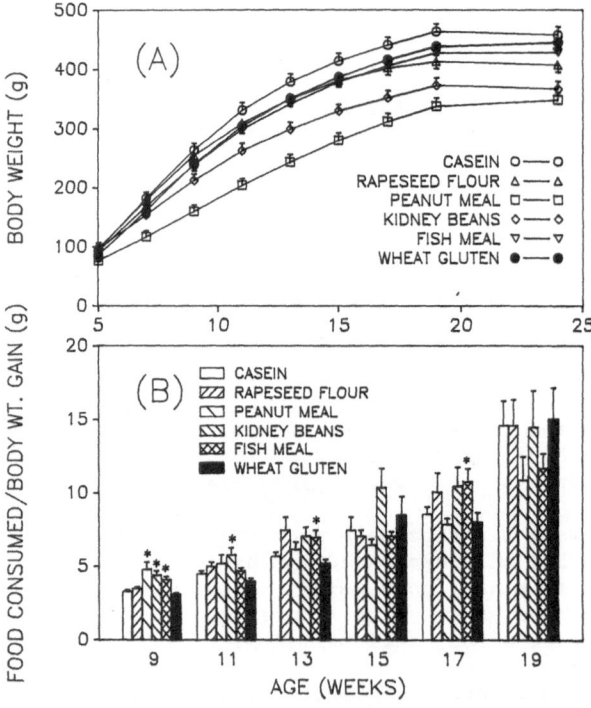

Fig. 1.   (A) Body weights (Mean ± SEM) of all BB rats which remained asymptomatic until 162 ± 8 days of age in each of the six diet groups. (B) Food efficiency (Mean ± SEM) was calculated from weekly food consumption/weekly weight gain.

TABLE 2

EFFECT OF DEFINED DIETS CONTAINING VARIOUS PROTEIN SOURCES ON DIABETES EXPRESSION AND METABOLISM

	Casein (Control)	Rapeseed Flour	Peanut Meal	Kidney Beans	Fish Meal	Wheat Gluten
Rats/Group	20	20	20	20	20	20
Number of Diabetic Rats	2	3	1	3	3	8*
Age at Onset (Days)	88 ± 25[†]	150 ± 22*	112	115 ± 21	112 ± 14	107 ± 29
Asymptomatic Rats with Insulitis	2	7	5	8*	3	4
Asymptomatic Rats without Insulitis	15[‡]	10	14	7*§	14	8*
Body Weight at Kill (g)[¶]	458 ± 59	396 ± 65*	351 ± 47*	351 ± 50*	429 ± 36	455 ± 55
	(17)	(17)	(19)	(15)	(17)	(12)
Spleen/Body Wt x 10^3	1.91 ± 0.42	1.70 ± 0.32	2.52 ± 0.76*	2.26 ± 0.24*	1.62 ± 0.39*	1.60 ± 0.22*
Kidneys/Body Wt x 10^3	5.94 ± 0.67	6.80 ± 1.00*	8.84 ± 0.82*	6.63 ± 0.64*	6.50 ± 0.54*	6.02 ± 0.57
Glucose (mg/dL)[¶]	152 ± 37	138 ± 36	142 ± 31	139 ± 25	138 ± 23	167 ± 33
Cholesterol (mg/dL)[¶]	146 ± 26	105 ± 33*	107 ± 20*	70 ± 9*	88 ± 16*	115 ± 18*
Triglycerides (mg/dL)[¶]	154 ± 67	118 ± 32	116 ± 39	82 ± 17*	128 ± 32	132 ± 63
Urea Nitrogen (mmol Urea-N/L)	5.83 ± 1.23	6.71 ± 3.56	5.47 ± 1.03	6.73 ± 1.83	4.65 ± 1.08*	4.90 ± 1.03*
White Blood Cell Count (x 10^9 cells/L)	3.89 ± 1.51	3.46 ± 1.78	2.77 ± 1.41*	3.05 ± 1.34	3.89 ± 1.42	3.73 ± 1.41
Red Blood Cell Count (x 10^{12} cells/L)	7.39 ± 0.64	7.80 ± 0.64	6.44 ± 0.80*	7.35 ± 0.49	7.43 ± 1.12	7.25 ± 0.70
Hemoglobin (mmol/L)	2.02 ± 0.15	2.07 ± 0.19	1.96 ± 0.19	2.03 ± 0.12	1.83 ± 0.31*	1.96 ± 0.12
Hematocrit (V RBC/V whole blood)	0.38 ± 0.03	0.39 ± 0.03	0.37 ± 0.01	0.38 ± 0.02	0.35 ± 0.06	0.37 ± 0.03
Red Cell Distribution Width (%)	15.4 ± 1.7	16.6 ± 2.5	13.9 ± 2.2*	14.4 ± 1.3	23.5 ± 9.8*	15.5 ± 2.4
Mean Corpuscular Volume (fL)	51.1 ± 2.1	50.1 ± 2.4	57.7 ± 3.6*	52.4 ± 2.3	46.6 ± 3.3*	51.1 ± 2.8

*Significantly different casein-fed (control) diet, P<0.05 (In the case of casein vs. wheat gluten-fed diabetics, P=0.06).
† All values are mean ± S.D.
‡ One rat died accidentally, no sign of disease.
§ Two rats cut themselves on the metal feed cups and bled to death at day 160, 165; disease-free at necropsy.
¶ These and all subsequent values from all remaining asymptomatic rats at 162 ± 8 days of age; number of rats in brackets.
¶ S.I. Units: Glucose mg/dL x 0.0555=mmol/L; Cholesterol mg/dL x 0.0259=mmol/L; Triglycerides mg/dL x 0.0113=mmol/L.

Note: As a result of a re-assessment of pacreatic sections and considering certain blood chemistry values, 3 rats which were previously categorized as asymptomatic at the end of the experiment were diagnosed as diabetic. Thus, the diabetes incidence reported for groups fed rapeseed flour and wheat gluten is slightly higher, 15 vs 5% and 40 vs 35%, than reported in a previous abstract (Fed. Proc. 46:588, 1987). Other values in these two groups have been corrected accordingly.

From Table 3, there were essentially no diet-related differences in serum amino acid levels, confirming the adequacy of amino acid levels in all diets.

With the exception of a slight increase in OX8+ thymus cells in rats fed the peanut meal diet, there were no diet-related changes in % W3/13+ (total T) cells, W3/25+ (helper/inducer) or OX8+ (cytotoxic/suppressor) cells in PBL, thymus or spleen cells (Table 4). Similarly, there were no significant differences in response to Con A by either thymus or spleen mononuclear cells.

TABLE 3

EFFECT OF DIETS ON BLOOD AMINO ACID PROFILE (μ M/dL).

	Casein (Control)	Rapeseed Flour	Peanut Meal	Kidney Beans	Fish Meal	Wheat Gluten	Pooled cv (%)
Arginine	15.7*	22.9	22.0	22.1	17.8	19.0	14.4
Histidine	7.2	8.4	8.3	9.6	6.7	7.0	14.0
Isoleucine	14.2	15.5	15.1	15.2	10.9	14.8	12.0
Leucine	21.7	24.4	24.9	23.1	17.1	22.9	12.6
Lysine	33.0	40.6	35.5	35.9	30.7	36.0	9.4
Methionine	7.7	8.1	7.6	7.6	7.3	6.7	6.3
Phenylalanine	9.8	11.2	11.1	11.1	14.4	9.7	15.2
Threonine	37.5	36.9	35.2	77.9†	24.2	34.3	45.6
Tryptophan	9.6	11.4	11.4	10.5	9.4	13.8	14.6
Valine	24.1	27.2	27.7	28.0	19.3	26.9	13.1
Alanine	42.7	51.1	53.6	60.5	51.0	42.7	13.5
Asparagine	5.2	5.8	6.2	5.8	4.8	4.7	11.2
Aspartic Acid	2.8	2.2	2.5	2.2	ND	1.5	21.5
Cystine	1.6	1.5	1.3	1.3	ND	1.2	11.9
Glutamic Acid	17.2	11.7	15.3	13.5	10.5	11.1	19.9
Glutamine	47.7	53.4	56.8	54.0	44.0	52.2	9.1
Glycine	33.5	44.7	38.9	50.4	51.7	35.7	18.0
Proline	21.2	23.9	25.0	25.3	22.9	23.9	6.3
Serine	27.9	32.4	33.9	46.4	30.7	30.0	19.7
Tyrosine	17.0	16.0	13.5	19.1	11.5	13.3	18.5
Citrulline	5.5	6.8	5.6	5.9	4.2	5.2	15.4
Ornithine	14.2	8.6	6.1	8.8	3.5	8.1	43.2
Taurine	32.8	33.7	31.7	30.4	26.3	26.3	10.6

*Mean of two determinations on pooled samples of serum from 5 asymptomatic, diabetes-prone, BB rats without insulitis.
†Significantly different from casein-fed control, P<0.05.
ND=not detected.

TABLE IV

CELLS BOUND BY ANTI–RAT (T CELL) MONOCLONAL ANTIBODIES AND RESPONSE TO CONCANAVALIN A OF LYMPHOID CELLS FROM BB RATS FED DIFFERENT PROTEIN SOURCE

	Casein (Control)	Rapeseed Flour	Peanut Meal	Kidney Beans	Fish Meal	Wheat Gluten
Number of rats	7	5	5	6	6	6
PBL W3/13+ (%)*	44 ± 6[†]	41 ± 4	29 ± 4	36 ± 6	33 ± 4	45 ± 6
PBL W3/25+ (%)[‡]	27 ± 4	25 ± 4	27 ± 5	31 ± 4	23 ± 1	26 ± 5
PBL OX8+ (%)[§]	24 ± 3	23 ± 2	22 ± 3	23 ± 3	26 ± 3	27 ± 1
W3/25÷OX8	1.2 ± 0.2	1.1 ± 0.2	1.5 ± 0.4	1.6 ± 0.5	0.9 ± 0.1	1.0 ± 0.2
Thymus W3/13+ (%)	69 ± 4	65 ± 8	64 ± 4	68 ± 4	75 ± 3	79 ± 7
Thymus W3/25+ (%)	56 ± 2	57 ± 5	58 ± 2	59 ± 3	58 ± 1	53 ± 3
Thymus OX8+ (%)	59 ± 1	64 ± 3	67 ± 1[ᴨ]	62 ± 2	63 ± 2	60 ± 1
W3/25÷OX8	1.0 ± 0.1	0.9 ± 0.1	0.9 ± 0.1	1.0 ± 0.1	0.9 ± 0.1	0.9 ± 0.1
Spleen W3/13+ (%)	41 ± 7	33 ± 5	41 ± 7	35 ± 2	37 ± 7	47 ± 8
Spleen W3/25+ (%)	21 ± 5	16 ± 1	18 ± 2	20 ± 3	16 ± 3	22 ± 8
Spleen OX8+ (%)	26 ± 2	25 ± 2	26 ± 3	23 ± 2	25 ± 3	29 ± 2
W3/25÷OX8	0.9 ± 0.2	0.7 ± 0.1	0.7 ± 0.1	0.9 ± 0.2	0.8 ± 0.3	0.7 ± 0.2
Thymus Con A, 1.25[¶] (cpm)	7302 ± 1151	7402 ± 998	9349 ± 3646	7930 ± 2248	5986 ± 2449	8379 ± 1990
Thymus Con A, 2.5 (cpm)	10395 ± 1754	9586 ± 922	10282 ± 4422	9425 ± 2446	5931 ± 2048	10702 ± 2201
Thymus Con A, 5.0 (cpm)	9961 ± 1673	10004 ± 2232	10842 ± 5972	9889 ± 2619	6309 ± 2635	10021 ± 3460
Spleen Con A, 1.25 (cpm)	11416 ± 3791	18504 ± 8173	17397 ± 7164	42782 ± 21737	17813 ± 6513	11931 ± 7450
Spleen Con A, 2.5 (cpm)	25749 ± 6976	40283 ± 15952	32631 ± 9719	68060 ± 26934	30811 ± 8948	21023 ± 10471
Spleen Con A, 5.0 (cpm)	30071 ± 7573	53570 ± 19830	36656 ± 12283	81930 ± 31045	37528 ± 11047	25594 ± 10794

*W3/13 is a monoclonal antibody which recognizes a sialoglycoprotein on rat thymocytes, T cells, plasma cells, polymorphs and brain.
[†] All values are mean ± SEM.
[‡] W3/25 is a monoclonal which recognizes T helper/inducer cells (also thymocytes and macrophages).
[§] OX8 monoclonal antibody binds to T suppressor/cytotoxic cells (also thymocytes and most NK cells).
[ᴨ] Significantly different from control, casein-fed rats, P<0.01.
[¶] Micrograms/microtiter plate well.

DISCUSSION

Since the source of dietary protein may be important in the genesis of BB rat diabetes, we examined different protein sources with a view to varying the protein and polypeptide structures presented via the oral route to the animal. Deficiencies in single amino acid levels may influence the immune system, so we supplemented the diets to ensure that all groups received similar amounts of essential amino acids. The data in Table 3 suggest this maneuover was successful.

The results of this experiment indicate that when wheat gluten was the sole source of protein in the diet, diabetes incidence was higher than that observed in casein-fed BB rats. This may be related to the recent finding that a large percentage of newly diagnosed humans with IDDM before 2 years of age had antibodies against gliadin, the active protein component involved in celiac disease (10).

Although the different protein sources in some instances affected certain metabolic parameters and red cell characteristics, producing in the case of peanut meal a general "metabolic inhibition" which may have been immunosuppressive, these alterations were not associated with an increased incidence of diabetes compared to control, casein-fed BB rats. Since animals on the rapeseed flour, peanut meal and kidney bean diets did not gain as much weight as the casein-fed rats, caloric restriction could have masked possible diabetogenic effects of these protein sources. This was not the case when comparing the wheat gluten-fed group to the casein-fed controls where rate of growth, body weight and food consumption were nearly identical. Therefore, in the absence of caloric restriction or differences in dietary amino acid content, it appears that the protein structure of wheat gluten (or some associated component of wheat gluten flour) produced a higher incidence of diabetes.

In general, none of these metabolic or disease-related differences was associated with significant alterations in (i) distribution of regulatory T cell subsets from PBL, spleen or thymus or (ii) response of mononuclear cells of spleen or thymus to Con A. This may simply mean that the diet/ diabetes interaction is related more to other areas of the immune response such as the gut-associated lymphoid tissues and their role in oral tolerance or to direct protection of the target beta cells in some manner.

The relative hypercholesterolemia in casein-fed BB rats could have conceivably affected both humoral and cellular immune responses but there was no indication of such an interaction on either the T cell subset distribution or Con A response in the cells of the organs we examined.

CONCLUSION

Proteins in wheat gluten (or associated ingredients) may be diabetogenic when fed as the sole protein source to weanling, diabetes-prone BB rats up to approximately 170 days of age. Compared to wheat gluten, more animals on the casein-based (control) diet remained asymptomatic with no signs of lymphocytic infiltration of the pancreatic islets. The mechanism involved in these interactions is not known but altered distribution of T regulatory cell subsets or response of spleen or thymus cells to Con A seem not to be involved.

REFERENCES

1. Krolewski, A.S., Warram, J.H., Rand, L.I., Kahn, C.R., 1987, Epidemiologic approach to the etiology of Type I diabetes mellitus and its complications. N Engl J Med 317: 1390-98.

2. LaPorte, R.E., Dorman, J.S., Orchard, T.J., Becker, D.J., Drash, A.L., Tajima, N., Ekoe, J-M., Tuomilehto,J., Rewers, M., Zimmet, P., Karp, M., Mohan, V., Lee, H.K., 1987, Preventing insulin-dependent diabetes mellitus: the environmental challenge. Brit Med J 295: 479-81.

3. Scott, F.W., Daneman, D., Martin, J.M., 1988, Evidence for a critical role of diet in the development of insulin-dependent diabetes mellitus. Diabetes Res (In Press).

4. Scott, F.W., 1988, Dietary initiators and modifiers of BB rat diabetes: A summary and working hypothesis. In: Lessons from Animal Diabetes II, Shafrir, E. and Renold, A.E., Eds., John Libbey & Co., London.

5. Borch-Johnsen, K. Mandrup-Poulsen, T. Zauchau-Christiansen, B., Joner, G., Christy, M., Kastrup, K., Nerup, J., 1984, Relationship between breast-feeding and incidence rates of insulin-dependent diabetes mellitus. Lancet ii: 1083-86.

6. Batsford, S., Schwerdtfeger, M. Rohrbach, R., Cambiaso, C., Kluthe, R., 1984, Synthetic amino acid diet prolongs survival in autoimmune murine disease. Clin Nephrol 21: 60-63.

7. Gupta, Y.P., 1987, Anti-nutritional and toxic factors in food legumes: A review. Plant Foods for Human Nutrition 37: 201-28.

8. Bieri, J.G., Stroewsand, G.S., Briggs, G.M., Phillips, R.W., Woodard, J.C., Knapka, J.J., 1977, Report of the American Institute of Nutrition ad hoc committee on standards for nutritional studies. J Nutrit 107: 1340-48.

9. Park, M.-S. C., Kudchodkar, B.J., Liepa, G.U., 1987, Effects of dietary animal and plant proteins on the cholesterol metabolism in immature and mature rats. J Nutr 117: 30-35.

10. Catassi, C., Guerrieri, A., Bartolotta, E., Coppa, G.V., Giorgi, P.L., 1987, Antigliadin antibodies at onset of diabetes in children. Lancet ii: 158.

EFFECT OF ALPHA-INHIBITORS ON BLOOD GLUCOSE AND INSULIN LEVELS

¶Laube, H., Federlin, K., Hillebrand, I.

Department of Internal Medicine
University of Giessen, FRG

Modification and delay of carbohydrate absorption is a highly effective mechanism in treating postprandial hyperglycemia in diabetes mellitus. Slowing down and lowering blood sugar rise reduces the unwanted and dangerous process of protein glycation, which contributes to the extent and onset of diabetic late complications (1).

Changes in dynamics of carbohydrate absorption can be achieved by changes in dietary composition, dietary additives (fibers) and by various chemical substances, such as alpha-glucosidase-inhibitors.

Alpha-Glucosidase inhibitors are a group of chemical compounds effective against pancreatic alpha-amylase by blocking the luminal hydrolysis of starch and by specific competitive, dosage dependent and reversible inhibition of brushborder disaccharidases, in particular maltase and sucrase (2). There is, however, no interference of alpha-glucosidases with the active transport of glucose and the facilitated transport of fructose.

We have investigated two of these compounds in several groups of Type II diabetics and healthy volunteers: Acarbose, a pseudo-tetrasaccharide with a molecular weight of 645, produced by an Actinoplanes strain and Miglitol (N-Hydroxyethyl-1-desoxynojirimycin), a product of streptomyces and piperidin derivatives (3).

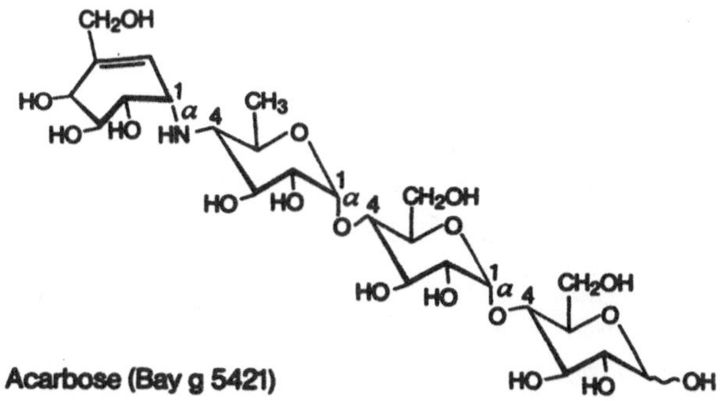

Acarbose (Bay g 5421)

Figure 1.   Molecular structure of ACARBOSE

MATERIAL AND METHODS

<u>Group A</u>:   10 dieting obese non-insulin-dependent diabetics, aged 53-79 years, were randomized and divided in 2 groups, that were not significantly different in either age, body weight, height or duration of diabetes.

The study lasted for a total period of 10 weeks, during which time all patients received 1 tablet, taken with meals, 3 times daily. Following a placebo period of 2 weeks, acarbose (3 x 100 mg) was given to half of the patients for the next 4 weeks. For the final 4 weeks they again received placebo and were then finally switched to acarbose for the remaining 4 weeks of the test period.

At the end of each period all patients were submitted to an hourly blood sugar test, lasting from 8 to 20 hours. During this test day, all patients received 5 diabetic-diet meals.

<u>Group B</u>: A long-term study was carried out with 24 sulphonylurea-treated diabetics over a period of 12 months. Acarbose or placebo was given for 6 months.

At 4-weekly intervals, body weight, blood glucose, urinary sugar, $HB-A_1$, cholesterol and triglycerides and fasting insulin were checked.

<u>Group C</u>: Miglitol, 3 x 50 mg, was given to 6 healthy volunteers in a double-blind cross-over study. There was a 7 day washout period between the two phases. The mean age of the volunteers was 26 years, the body weight did not exceed Broca index 0.93.

Blood sugar was measured enzymatically with the hexokinase method (Boehringer test combination). The serum insulin determination was performed as a triple assay with the radio-immunoassay (Behring-Werke, FRG). The fraction of glycated hemoglobins ($HB-A_1$) was determined by means of microcolumns (Fa. Panchem, FRG).

<u>Statistics</u>: For statistical evaluation mean values and standard deviations were used. In addition covariance analysis and the calculation of the areas under the blood glucose and serum insulin curves were applied.

RESULTS

<u>Group A</u>: The average blood sugar profile in all diabetic patients taking acarbose was markedly lower compared to control periods, when only placebo

BAY m 1099
N-Hydroxyethyl-1-desoxynojirimycin

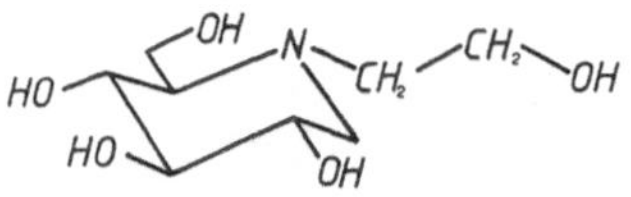

$C_8 H_{17} NO_5$
Mol. Weight 207,2

1,5-dideoxy-1,5-[(2-hydroxyethyl)imino]-D-glucitol

Figure 2.   MOLECULAR STRUCTURE AND MOLECULAR WEIGHT OF MIGLITOL.

288

was given (Fig. 1). The total blood sugar average following acarbose therapy was .221.1 mg% compared to 250.3 mg% in controls. While fasting blood glucose was only 15-20 mg% lower following acarbose, a striking difference was observed 1 hour after breakfast (38 mg%) and 2 hours after dinner (55 mg%). The difference of the average of the whole blood-glucose profile (area) was 21.1 mg% (p = 0.09).

The urinary glucose concentration was reduced by acarbose from 4.68 to 2.33 g/12 hours. No effect was seen with regard to body weight, serum-cholesterol and triglycerides.

Group B: Following acarbose, the mean daily blood glucose was significantly reduced (157 ± 31 mg% vs 223 ± 51 mg%). The maximum effect, however, was not reached before the end of the 2 months of treatment (Fig. 2). At the same time, the urinary glucose excretion fell significantly from 13 ± 6g/24h to 2 g/24 h. Over a period of 6 months glycated hemoglobin (HB-A$_1$) was reduced from 12.4 to 9.1% (Fig. 3). Fasting insulin, blood lipids and body weight did not exhibit any significant differences for the period with or without acarbose. When acarbose was stopped, blood glucose rose significantly again within 4 weeks.

Group C: Miglitol, at a dosage of 3 x 50 mg/daily suppressed the postprandial blood glucose and insulin rise in healthy volunteers significantly (p < 0.001-0.007). This effect was more pronounced after breakfast (73.8 mg%; ±1S:68.3-79.8) and lunch (81.9 mg%; ±1S:71.1-92.1) than after dinner (96.0 mg%); ±1S:85.5-107.7), when compared to placebo (98.5 mg%; ±1S:81.0-119.7 vs 111.7 mg%; ±1S:94.5-132.1 vs 113.2 mg%; ±1S:95.5-134.1

The area under the curve (AUC) however, was not significantly affected by miglitol.

Side effects: In group A and B, taking acarbose, considerable side effects, such as flatulence or mild diarrhea were reported up to 80% only in the first 4 weeks. They subsided thereafter and did not recur again during the rest of the experimental period. The extent of acarbose-induced side effects was concentration dependent.

Similar side effects were seen while taking miglitol.

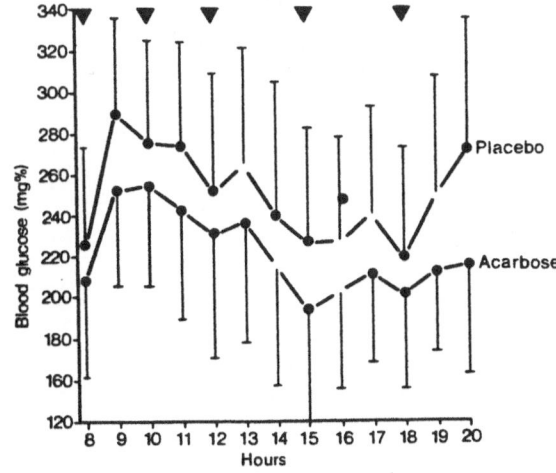

Figure 3. Blood sugar profile in Type II diabetic patients treated with acarbose and placebo (5).

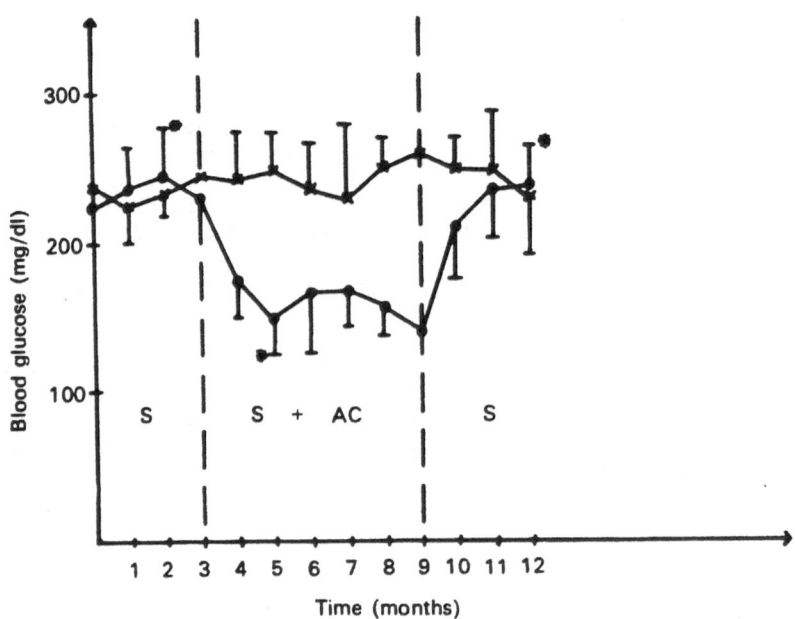

Figure 4. Mean daily blood glucose values in sulfonylurea-treated diabetics (8).

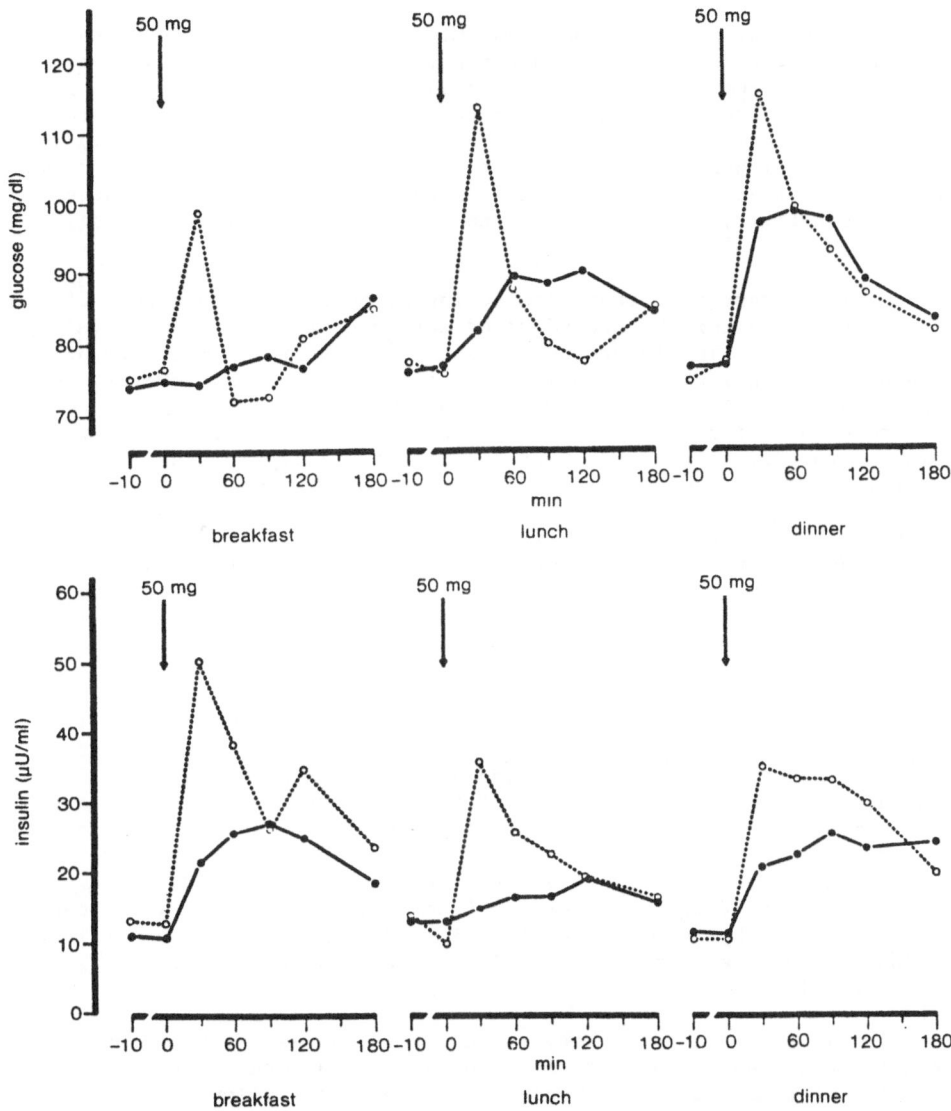

Figure 5. Mean blood glucose values and serum insulin levels in
healthy volunteers during treatment with Miglitol or
placebo (2).

DISCUSSION

Both glucosidase inhibitors, Acarbose and Miglitol, are similarly effective in lowering postprandial blood glucose in obese volunteers and non-insulin dependent Type II diabetics. Specific differences were not observed in regard to duration or type of efficiency or clinical side effects. There was no decrease of efficiency as long as both compounds were taken regularly. Hypoglycemic reactions never did appear.

Glucosidase inhibitors Acarbose and Miglitol act externally in the lumen or the surface of the small intestine, the brush border, and not internally in the organism. They cause a delay of glucose absorption and have primarily no effects on insulin secretion. A reduction of postprandial hyperglycemia, however, is consequently accompanied by a significantly decreased insulin release. This is important, not only because of its potential protective effect of β-cell function but also in view of an increasing insulin senstivity and a possible atherogenic effect of hyperinsulinemia (4).

Since glucosidase inhibitors are acting as competive inhibitors of enzymes, responsible for the breakdown of carbohydrates after each meal, fasting blood glucose levels are not affected by a short term treatment with Acarbose or Miglitol. Following long term application, however, increasing insulin sensitivity might be one of the causes for lower fasting blood glucose in sulfonyl-urea-treated diabetics. Similar effects were seen following metformin, however, accompanied by potentially more serious side effects (5).

Along with a marked lowering of the daily blood sugar profile, there is also a significant decrease of urinary glucose excretion and improvement of glycated hemoglobin. Glucosidase inhibitors are therefore preferred for the treatment of obese hyperglycemic-hyperinsulinemic patients but may also be used to smoothen the unwanted blood glucose fluctuations in insulin dependent diabetics (6).

The overall aim of a therapy with glucosidase inhibitors is a shift of carbohydrate digestion from the upper to the lower intestine, in order to delay glucose absorption. Clinical side effects such as flatulence, diarrhea and abdominal distress are signs of carbohydrate maldigestion and consequent fermentation in the gut (7). This is caused by an overspill of non-hydrolysed carbohydrates into the colon, due to a surplus of carbohydrates in the food and an absolute or relative overdosage of glucosidase inhibitors. There is also a wide range of tolerance from patient to patient. It can be effectively reduced by metronidazol (8). An individual titration of glucosidase-inhibitors in each patient appears to be helpful in reducing side effects initially.

Nearly all side effects, however, tend to disappear spontaneously within a few weeks due to an alteration of enzyme pattern in the intestine, changes of bacterial growth and subjective acceptance following long term application of glucosidase inhibitors (9).

Glucosidase inhibitors seem to be promising new compounds for the treatment of postprandial hyperglycemia in all types of diabetes mellitus. Obese Type II diabetics, however, will benefit preferably by the reduction of hyperinsulinemia.

The decrease of urinary glucose loss and the reduction of glycated hemoglobin might also contribute to a reduction of diabetes specific complications.

REFERENCES

1. Laube, H., Pfeiffer, E.F., 1978, Insulin secretion and the role of nutritional factors. In: Advances in Modern Nutrition. Katzen & Mahler, Eds., Hemisphere Publishing Corp. Vol. 2: 395.

2. Schmidt, D.D., Frommer, W., Junge, B., Muller, L., Wingender, W., Truscheit, E., 1982, Alpha-glucosidase inhibitors of microbial origin. Proc. First Int. Symp. Acarbose.

3. Hillebrand, I., Boehme, K. Graefe, K., Wehling, K., 1986, The effect of new alpha-glucosidase inhibitors (Bay m 1099 and Bay o 1248) on meal-stimulated increase in glucose and insulin levels in man. Klin Wschr 64: 393.

4. Laube, H., 1983, The clinical importance of delayed intestinal carbohydrate absorption. In: Delaying absorption as a therapeutic principle in metabolic diseases. Theime Verl. Creutzfeld/Folsch, eds., 136.

5. Schwedes, U., Petzold, R., Hillebrand, I., Schoffling, K., 1980, Comparison of metformin and acarbose treatment in non-insulin dependent diabetics. La clin dietolog 7: 450.

6. Federlin, K.F., Mehlburger, L, Hillebrand, I., Laube, H., 1987, The effect of new alpha-glucosidase inhibitors on blood glucose in healthy volunteers and in Type II diabetics. Acta diabetol. lat.24: 213.

7. Caspary, W.F., Lembcke, B., Creutzfeld, W., 1982, Inhibition of human intestinal a-glucoside hydrolase activity by acarbose and clinical consequences. Proc. First Int. Symp. Acarbose, Excerpta Medica, Int. Congr. Ser. 594: 27.

8. Lembcke, B., Folsch, U.R., Caspary, W.F., Creutzfeldt, W., 1982, Influence of metronidazol on intestinal side effects of acarbose. Proc. First Int. Symp., Acarbose. Excerpta Medica Int. Congr. Series 594: 236.

9. Sachse, G., Maser, Laube, H., Federlin, K., 1982, Effect of long-term acarbose therapy on the metabolic situation of sulfonylurea-treated diabetics. Proc. First Int. Symp. Acarbose. Excerpta Medica Int. Congr. Series 594: 5.

10. Laube, H., Aubell, R., Schmitz, H., Federlin, K., 1982, Acarbose, an effective therapy in lowering postprandial hyperglycemia in obese patients with Type II diabetes mellitus. Proc. First Int. Symp. Acarbose. Excerpta Medica, Int. Congr. Ser. 594: 344.

DISCUSSION

W. ROBISON: I have two questions for Dr. Scott here. First, with respect ·
to the Vitamin E deficient diets, did you compensate in those diets for
an oxidation of Vitamin A in the liver? It's been indicated by several
investigators that when you give a Vitamin E deficient diet you actually
decrease the storage of Vitamin A due to oxidation, and so in a Vitamin E
deficient animal you have a lack of some of the Vitamin A, maybe even to
the point of deficiency of Vitamin A in addition to the deficiency of
Vitamin E.

F. SCOTT: I should be clear about that, that it was not a Vitamin E
deficient diet. It was a low trace Vitamin E diet. It was not deficient.

W. ROBISON: Okay, that's clear then. And, then the other question
regarding the effect of sex hormones on the advent of diabetes. Are
there any indications that any of these diets change the level of sex
hormones?

F. SCOTT: We used both sexes and there are no sex differences as far
as we can tell, and we haven't looked at the sex hormones.

R. RODRIGUEZ: With the animal model described yesterday by Foglia, that
is the large total pancreatectomized rats in which diabetes appear after
one or two months of the operation. Giving different diets to the animals
immediately after total pancreatectomy he was able to show that if you
give the food every few minutes instead of three or four portions a day,
you have a higher incidence of diabetes and also with a higher protein
diet you have smaller incidence of diabetes.

More or less the same thing happens when you have an inhibition of the
alpha glucosidase in the diet. For instance, giving acarbose to the
animals after partial pancreatectomy because of the lower hyperglycemia
in the acarbose treated animals the incidence of diabetes was quite low.

F. SCOTT: A paper in 1947 looked at the effects of preventing alloxan
diabetes in animals with diets and found some very interesting things,
particularly, a high coconut oil diet prevented the mortality and morbidity usually associated with alloxan. He fed them several diets,
actually, and also found that a high protein diet protected the animals
against morbidity and mortality.

J. BARBOSA: I have a comment about Dr. Laube's paper. Well, certainly
an interesting enzyme inhibitor, but I'd be very concerned about multiple
possible complications, especially in long term treatments. It seems to
me that starting someone on these inhibitors is almost like putting someone
on a low carbohydrate diet. Do you have any data on lipids in these people?

H. LAUBE: The lipids and the cholesterol will not be lowered by acarbose
treatment.

J. BARBOSA: How long - what is the longest period of time that you have studied?

H. LAUBE: The longest treatment was six to a maximum of nine months. There were extensive studies done on the effect of acarbose on the absorption of various other substances like Digoxin or Tetracycline, but so far this has no effect. To the contrary, Guar do have an influence on the reabsorption kinetics of certain medication.

R. HERNANDEZ: Dr. Scott, you showed that by feeding the animals with lactoalbumin you have about 2% of diabetes. Can we consider that a protective agent? And, if so, by which mechanism?

F. SCOTT: Yes, I believe that what we're seeing is when we feed certain types of protein they seem to inhibit expression of the disease and when we feed a hydrolyzed source of amino acid that also protects, as does a synthetic amino acid diet. They do seem to be protective.

R. CAMERINI-DAVALOS: Dr. Laube, I was surprised with your comment that the longest a patient has been on treatment was for nine months.

H. LAUBE: Patients have been on acarbose for several years. I was just reporting about our personal studies.

R. CAMERINI-DAVALOS: You said acarbose will not stop or delay the beginning of overt diabetes. I'm not so sure about that, because more and more of us believe that the minimal hyperglycemia of prediabetes is a "diabetogenic factor". I wonder if you have some data to make that statement. I am really asking if you know anybody that has been on acarbose in that period where there is minimal hyperglycemia, but not really overt diabetes?

H. LAUBE: As you know, acarbose is not yet on the market. However, it is one of the best medications used in the last 10 years. Nearly 500 studies were done on patients with very little hyperglycemia or with a latent diabetes and with obese patients.

R. CAMERINI-DAVALOS: But, have you or anybody else been able to see a delay of the progression of diabetes?

H. LAUBE: In animals it was reported that delay occurred, but this depends on the amount you give. And, this might be different in different individuals. You should not block the carbohydrate digestion totally.. You can do this by an acarbose concentration high enough, but the side effects increase rapidly, particularly flatulence.

F. SCOTT: We take care each time to make sure the diets are isocaloric. If some of them don't have enough essential amino acids for the rat, we add them to those diets. And, we have measured the blood amino acids in all those diets and they're all exactly the same basically. So, there are no differences in amino acids. There are no amino acid deficiencies.

J. HOET: Dr. Scott, did you measure the number of beta cells in each of the diets, because there have been studies indicating multiplication of the beta cells in relation with the type of diet and especially with high protein diet.

F. SCOTT: It has been reported that functional demands imposed by diet on insulin secretion can increase beta cell mass in rodents and dietary protein has been linked to hypertrophy and hyperplasia of beta cells. By contrast, rats fed with diets containing partially hydrolyzed protein or elemental diets have been reported to show pancreatic hypoplasia.

KIDNEY DISEASE IN KK MICE: EFFECT OF GLYBURIDE

¶R.A. Camerini-Davalos[+] and A.S. Reddi[++]

[+]Department of Medicine, New York Medical College
Metropolitan Hospital Research Center, New York, New York
[++]Department of Medicine, UMDNJ - New Jersey Medical School, Newark, N.J.

In previous publications (1,2) and in the present volume, we reported that the KK mouse represents an ideal animal model for the study of kidney disease in Type II diabetes. We report here the effect of early and late glyburide (a second generation oral hypoglycemic compound) treatment on glucose metabolism and its relationship to glomerulosclerosis in KK mice.

MATERIALS AND METHODS

Animals: Both male and female KK mice were used in the study. They were divided into two groups. One group of mice was treated with glyburide from 20 to 100 days of age. These mice were sacrificed at 40, 50, 70 and 100 days of age (treatment period of 20,30,50 and 80 days, respectively). The other group of mice was treated with glyburide from 60 to 360 days of age and sacrificed at 120, 180, 270 and 360 days (treatment period of 60, 120, 210 and 300 days, respectively).

Glyburide was dissolved in 0.9% saline containing 5% acacia and was given (0.5 mg/kg) by oral intubation once a day, 7 days a week. Control mice received 0.9 saline (0.1 ml/10g).

Biochemical Studies: In an acute experiment, glyburide in concentrations of 0.125, 0.25, and 0.5 mg/kg (0.1 ml/10g) was given by oral intubation to mice fasted for 18 hr. Blood was drawn after 2hr. from the orbital plexus into capillary tubes. Twenty microliters of blood were transferred into Unopettes (BD Co., Rutherford, N.J.) containing NaF as a diluent. The remaining blood was centrifuged at 2000 x rpm and serum was collected and stored at -25° C for the determination of insulin.

In another acute experiment, the KK mice were fasted for 2 hr. They were arbitrarily divided into three groups. Group I received 0.9% saline (0.1 ml/10g). Groups II and III received 0.5 and 2.5 mg/kg (0.1 ml/10g) of glyburide, respectively. Blood was drawn at 0,1,2,3, and 4 hr. of treatment.

Oral glucose tolerance tests were performed in both saline and glyburide-treated KK mice at the time of sacrifice. The test was performed in

This work was supported in part by the Diabetes Research Fund, New York, New York and the Michael J. Bilotto Research Fund of Hope for Diabetics Foundation, New York, New York.

mice fasted for 18 hr. After collecting blood at 0 min., the mice were given 3g/kg of glucose by oral intubation using a gastric catheter, and subsequent samples were collected at 30, 60, and 120 min.

Blood sugar was determined by the ferricyanide method of Hoffman on the Technicon Autoanalyzer. The glucose area under the curve was calculated by the method of Chiles and Tzagournis (3). Serum immunoreactive insulin (IRI) levels were determined by the double antibody technique of Oppermann et al (4). Glucosuria and proteinuria were tested in mice of all age groups using N-multistix (Ames Co., Elkhart, Ind.).

Glucosyltransferase activity in renal cortical homogenates was determined using collagen as substrate and UDP-U-^{14}C-glucose as an acceptor, as described by Velasco et al (5).

Histologic Studies: For light microscopy studies, the mice were sacrificed by decapitation, kidneys excised, and portion of the kidney was fixed in 10% neutral formalin. The tissues were embedded in paraffin and sections 2-3 u thick were cut. They were stained in periodic acid-Schiff (PAS), hematoxylin and eosin, chromotrope silver methenamine and Congo red. Histologic evaluation of glomeruli was done in a blind fashion based on the following working classification (100 ± 20 glomeruli counted).

Not significant	(0)	No changes
		Few obsolescent glomeruli
		Diffuse glomerulosclerosis
		grade I
Mild	(m)	Diffuse glomerulosclerosis
		grade II
Severe	(s)	Diffuse and nodular
		Diffuse and nodular and/or
		deposits (exudative).

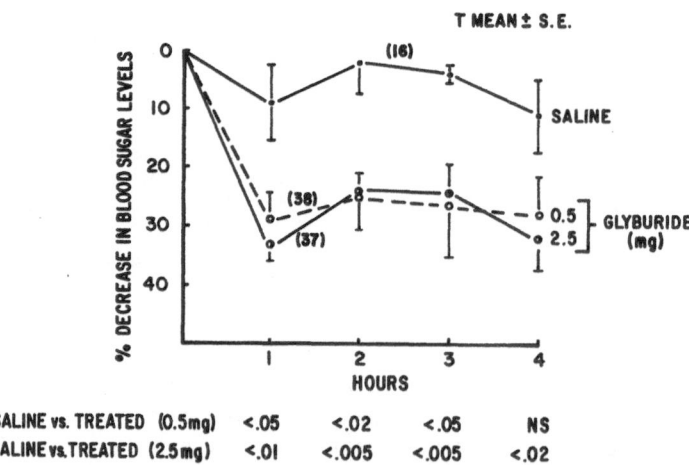

Figure 1.   Effect of saline and glyburide on blood sugar levels in KK mice after 2 hr. fast. Numbers in parentheses represent number of animals.

TABLE I

EFFECT OF ORAL GLYBURIDE TREATMENT ON CHANGES IN BLOOD SUGAR
AND SERUM IMMUNOREACTIVE INSULIN (IRI) LEVELS IN KK MICE
FASTED FOR 18 HR. (VALUES SHOWN ARE MEANS ± S.E.M.)

Dose (mg/kg)	% decrease in blood sugar levels 2 hr after drug	% increase in IRI levels 2 hr after drug
0.125	13 ± 4 (5)	61 ± 12 (5)
0.25	36 ± 4 (10)	246 ± 91 (7)
0.50	37 ± 4 (9)	328 ± 62 (6)

Statistical Analysis: All data are expressed as means ± S.E.M. Student's t-test was used to calculate the significance between means and P values above 0.05 were considered non significant.

RESULTS

Blood sugars and insulin levels: The effect of different concentrations of oral glyburide treatment on blood sugar and serum IRI levels in mice

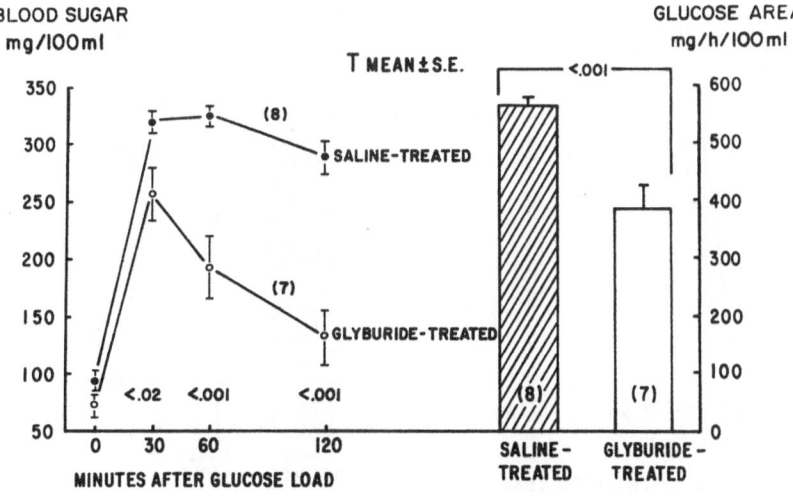

Figure 2. Oral glucose tolerance tests and glucose area levels in saline- and glyburide-treated KK mice aged 4–12 months of age. In "responders," no glomerulosclerosis was present. Numbers in parentheses represent number of mice.

fasted for 18 hr. is shown in Table I. A dose-related decrease in blood
sugars and an increase in serum IRI levels was observed in mice 2 hr. after
drug treatment.

Figure 1 shows the effect of saline and glyburide treatment (0.5 and
2.5 mg/kg) on blood sugar levels in mice for 2 hr. No appreciable decrease
in blood sugar levels in saline-treated mice was observed. However, a sig-
nigicant decrease in blood sugar levels was found in mice treated with both
doses of drug up to 3 hr. After 4 hr. of treatment, the blood sugar levels
were significantly decreased in mice treated only with 2.5 mg/kg. No significant difference in blood sugar levels was found between mice treated
either with 0.5 or 2.5 mg of glyburide.

Oral glucose tolerance tests: Figures 2 and 3 show the oral glucose tolerance curves and glucose area levels in a representative number of saline
and drug-treated animals. In some drug-treated mice, the tolerance to glu-
close was significantly improved, when compared to age matched saline-
treated mice ("responders") (Figure 2). In other mice, no effect of glyburide treatment on blood sugar levels was found ("non-responders") (Figure 3).

Glucosyltransferase activity: The effect of saline and glyburide treatment
on glucosyltransferase activity in the renal cortical homogenates of KK mice
is shown in Figure 4. The enzyme activity in normal control Swiss albino
mice is also plotted for comparison. GLyburide treatment caused a significant decrease in glucosyltransferase activity in KK mice at 40, 50 and 70
days of age. However, no effect of glyburide on enzyme activity was found
at 100 days of age. There was no difference in enzyme activity between
Swiss albino mice and glyburide-treated KK mice at all age periods.

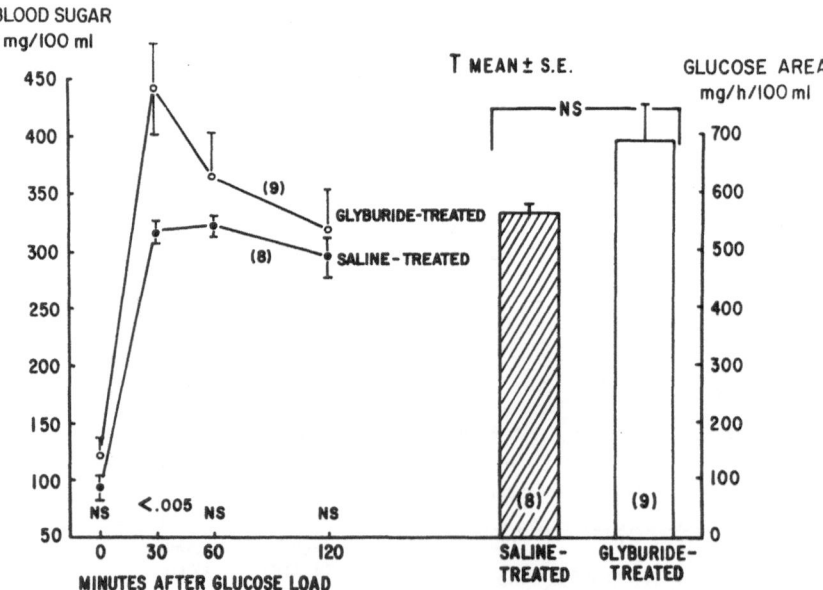

Figure 3. Oral glucose tolerance tests and glucose area levels in
saline- and glyburide-treated KK mice of 4-12 months of
age. Both mild and severe forms of glomerulosclerosis were
present in 90% of "non-responders." Numbers in parentheses
indicate number of mice.

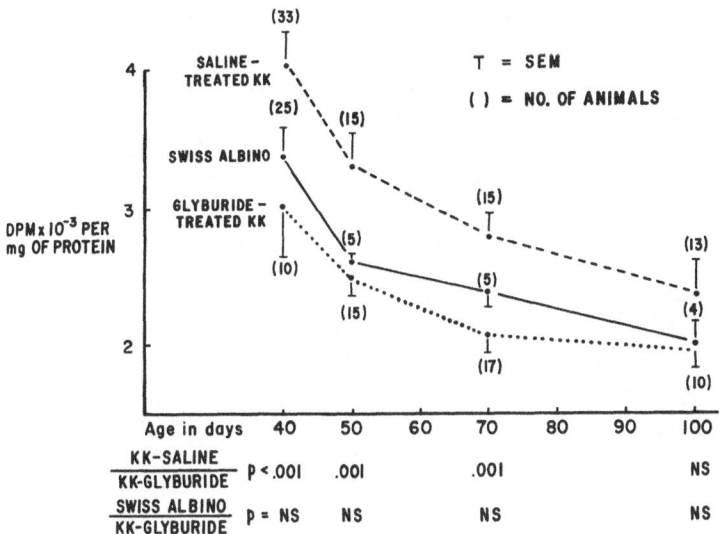

Figure 4. Effect of glyburide treatment on renal glucosyltransferase activity in KK mice. For comparison, the enzyme activity in normal control Swiss albino (SA) mice is shown.

Glomerulosclerosis: The effect of glyburide on the prevalence of mild and severe forms of glomerulosclerosis is shown in Figure 5. After 2 and 4 months of treatment, the mice showed only 17% of mild glomerulosclerosis when compared to 42% in saline-treated mice. In mice treated for 7 and 10 months, 47% and 33% of mild glomerulosclerosis was found in comparison with 45% and 9% in saline-treated mice. The severe form of glomerulosclerosis was found only in one out of six (17%), none out of 12 (0%) and none out of 17 (0%) mice after 2, 4, and 7 months of glyburide treatment. After 10

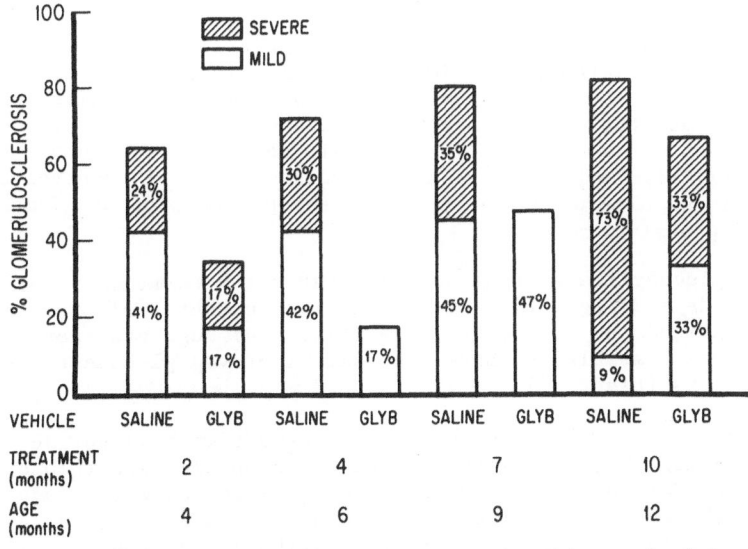

Figure 5. Effect of prolonged treatment of saline and glyburide on the prevalence of mild and severe forms of glomerulosclerosis in KK mice.

months of glyburide treatment, only one mouse (33%) showed the severe form of glomerulosclerosis.

Glucosuria was not present either in saline or drug-treated KK mice of all age groups. In saline-treated mice, proteinuria was present at the level of +2 and +3. In mice with improved glucose tolerance by glyburide, only trace amounts of proteinuria could be detected.

Mice with early treatment from 20 days of age had no glomerulosclerosis or proteinuria when sacrificed at 100 days of age.

Blood glucose and glomerulosclerosis: Figure 3 shows the blood glucose levels of those mice that did not show improvement in their glucose tolerance despite glyburide treatment. Of the nine mice, eight (89%) had glomerulosclerosis and proteinuria when sacrificed. None of the seven mice with significant improvement in their glucose tolerance had either glomerulosclerosis or proteinuria (Figure 2).

DISCUSSION

Glyburide, a second generation sulfonylurea compound, has been found to increase insulin secretion and reduce blood glucose levels in both animals and human beings with Type II diabetes mellitus. We have also observed similar changes in our KK mice.

The treatment of mice with glyburide did not result in improved tolerance to glucose in all of them. Some mice showed improved tolerance, while some did not respond to the drug. The cause for the lack of effect of glyburide in the latter group of mice is not known. However, the possibility of a secondary failure due to chronic treatment of the drug cannot be excluded.

The chronic treatment of glyburide was found to delay the progression of glomerulosclerosis in KK mice. It is of interest to note that the severe form of glomerulosclerosis was reduced to the mild form in all age groups of treated mice. This is particularly striking in mice treated for 4 to 7 months.

The delay in the progression of glomerulosclerosis in drug-treated mice appears to be related to the improvement in blood sugar levels. This is supported by data shown in Figure 2. In these mice no glomerulosclerosis was present and their tolerance to glucose was improved. By contrast, the mice which showed no improvement in their tolerance to glucose had glomerulosclerosis (Figure 3). These data suggest that early control of blood sugar levels in KK mice delays or prevents the progression of glomerulosclerosis and proteinuria.

Although glucosyltransferase activity was not determined in mice treated from 60 to 360 days of age, the available evidence that early treatment with glyburide normalized the enzyme activity (Figure 4) suggests that a similar normalization was possible in those mice with improved glucose tolerance and glomerulosclerosis (Figure 2).

In conclusion, the data suggest that treatment with glyburide is effective in delaying the progression of genetic diabetic glomerulosclerosis in some KK mice. This delay in progressin of glomerulosclerosis appears to be related to the early control of blood sugar levels. Preliminary data suggest that at least part of the effect of glyburide on the genetic diabetic glomerulosclerosis is also due to its effect on some of the enzymes involved in the synthesis or removal of basement membrane or basement membrane-like glycoprotein.

REFERENCES

1. Camerini-Davalos, R.A., Oppermann, W., Mittl, R., and Ehrenreich,T., Studies of vascular and other lesions in KK mice. Diabetologia 6: 324-329.

2. Reddi, A.S., Oppermann, W., Velasco, C.A., Strugat , L.H., and Camerini-Davalos, R.A., 1980, Diabetes mellitus in the KK mouse: Similarities and differences between genetic and other types of diabetes. In Secondary Diabetes: The spectrum of the diabetic syndromes, Podolsky, S. and Viswanathan, M., Eds., New York, Raven Press: 455-469.

3. Chiles, R., and Tzagournis, M., 1970, Excessive serum insulin response to oral glucose in obesity and mild diabetes. Study of 501 patients. Diabetes 19: 458-464.

4. Oppermann, W., Mehtalia, S.D., Sodero, E.C., Cole, H.S., and Camerini-Davalos, R.A., 1969, A sensitive micromethod for the simultaneous determination of insulin and growth hormone by double antibody precipitation. Clin. Biochem. 2: 341-348.

5. Velasco, C.A., Oppermann, W., Marine, N., and Camerini-Davalos, R.A., 1974, Effect of genetic diabetes on kidney glucosyltransferase. Horm Metab Res 6: 427.

KIDNEY DISEASE IN KK MICE: EFFECT OF GLIPIZIDE

¶A.S. Reddi[+], C.A. Velasco[++], M.Y. Khan[+],
J.M.B. Bloodworth[+++], Jr. and R.A. Camerini-Davalos[++]

[+]Department of Medicine, UMDNJ-New Jersey Medical School, Newark, N.J.
[++]Department of Medicine, New York Medical College
Metropolitan Hospital Research Center, New York, New York
[+++]Department of Pathology, University of Wisconsin Medical School
Madison, Wis.

We previously demonstrated that glomerulosclerosis and proteinuria
can be prevented by control of blood glucose levels either by insulin or
glyburide in genetically diabetic KK mice (1,2). Also, we demonstrated
that poor control of glucose despite treatment with glyburide did not
prevent glomerulosclerosis in a subset of KK mice (2). This reinforces
the impact of glycemic control in the prevention of diabetic nephropathy.
The purpose of the present study is two-fold: 1) to evaluate the efficacy
of another second generation sulfonylurea compound, glipizide, in
controlling blood glucose levels in KK mice; and 2) to investigate the
relationship between glucose control and structural, biochemical and
functional characteristics of kidney disease in KK mice.

MATERIALS AND METHODS

Animals: A total of 40 male and female littermates of KK mice from our
colony were used in the study. They were divided into two groups. One
group (N = 20) of mice was treated with glipizide, 1 mg/kg, from 20
to 180 days of age. The second group of mice received an equal amount
of saline. Both glipizide and saline (0.1 ml/10 g) were given daily
six days a week via a gastric catheter. All mice were fed Purina mouse
chow ad lib and given free access to tap water. Both groups of mice
were weighed 3-4 times a week.

Glipizide was supplied by Pfizer Research Labs (Groton, CT). It
was dissolved initially in a few drops of N NaOH and made to a final
volume with normal saline.

Oral glucose tolerance tests: These tests were done 1 week prior to
sacrifice and were completed between 10 a.m. and 12 noon. After
collecting blood from the orbital plexus at 0 minutes, the mice were
given glucose (1.5 g/kg) by gavage, and subsequent samples of blood
for glucose were obtained at 30, 60 and 120 minutes. Blood glucose
was determined by glucose oxidase method (Sigma).

Supported in part by the Diabetes Research Fund, New York, the
Michael J. Bilotto Research Fund of HOPE for Diabetes Foundation, New
York, the Veterans Administration Research Fund, Washington, D.C., the
Southern Wisconsin Diabetes Association, and Pfizer Pharmaceutical,
New York.

Glycosylated hemoglobin Al: Total glycosylated hemoglobin Al was determined by the procedure of Chen et al. (3).

Determinations of glucosyltransferase and N-acetyl-B-glucosaminidase activities: The activities of these two enzymes were assayed in renal cortical homogenates and serum as described previously (4).

Light microscopy studies: Mid coronal section of the kidney was fixed in 10% neutral formalin, embedded in paraffin and sections 1-2 u were cut. They were stained in periodic acid-Schiff (PAS), hematoxylin and eosin, silver methenamine and Congo red. All glomeruli were evaluated in a double blind fashion. Sclerosis was defined as an increase in mesangial cells with demonstrable increase in mesangial matrix. The presence of more than 2 mesangial cells in a given glomerular tuft with or without accentuation of matrix was considered pathologic. The degree of involvement was graded as mild (1+) when less than 25% of glomeruli showed such change, moderate (2+) when 25 to 50% glomeruli involved and severe (4+) when more than 50% glomeruli involved.

Electron microscopy studies: A portion of the cortex was fixed in 2.5% glutaraldehyde in 0.1M cacodylate buffer and their post-fixed in 1% osmium tetroxide. Blocks were prepared and sectioned with a Sorrall Porter Blum Ultramicrotome - MT2. Grids were stained with uranyl acetate and lead citrate and examined on a Philips EM 300.

Photographs of the glomerular capillaries were made with a magnification of 20,500. Glomerular basement membrane (GBM) width was measured on MOP-3 (Zeiss). At least 7-12 capillaries were evaluated from each animal. Repeat measurements fell within 98% of the first measurements.

Proteinuria: Three days prior to sacrifice, all mice were individually placed in metabolic cages, and urine was collected for 24 hours. It was centrifuged at 1000g for 5 minutes and the sediment discarded. Protein in the urine was determined by the method of Lowry et al. (5).

Statistical Analysis: All data are expressed as means $\pm$ S.E.M. student's t-test for unpaired samples was used to calculate the significance between means, and P values greater than 0.05 were considered non-significant.

RESULTS

The effect of different doses of glipizide on blood glucose levels in nonfasted KK mice is shown in Fig. 1. As evident, all doses of glipizide were effective in lowering blood glucose levels up to 8 hours; however, only the dose of 1 mg/kg was found to be effective up to 18 hours. After 24 hours, the blood glucose levels returned to base line values.

Based upon glycosylated HbA_1 and oral glucose tolerance, glipizide-treated mice were divided into "responders" (N = 10) and "non-responders" (N = 9), as shown in Figs. 2 and 3. It is evident from these figures that the areas under the glucose curves were significantly lower in "responders" and higher in "non-responders".

Table 1 shows general information on "responders". No difference in body weight was observed; however, a significant decrease in kidney weight was found in this group of glipizide-treated KK mice.

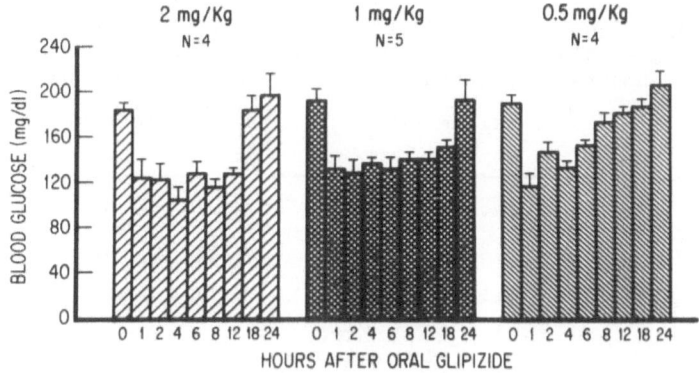

Fig. 1. Effect of various doses of glipizide on blood glucose levels in nonfasted KK mice.

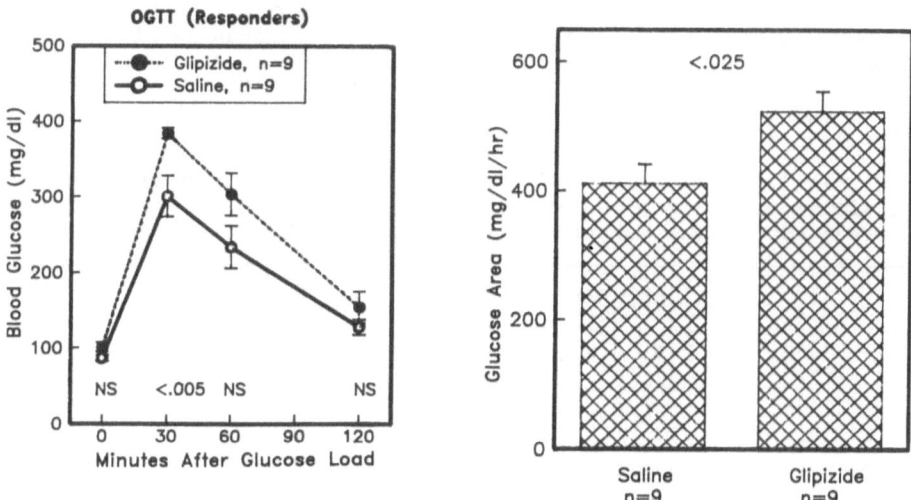

Fig. 2. Oral glucose tolerance tests (OGTT) and glucose areas in saline and glipizide-treated ("responders") KK mice.

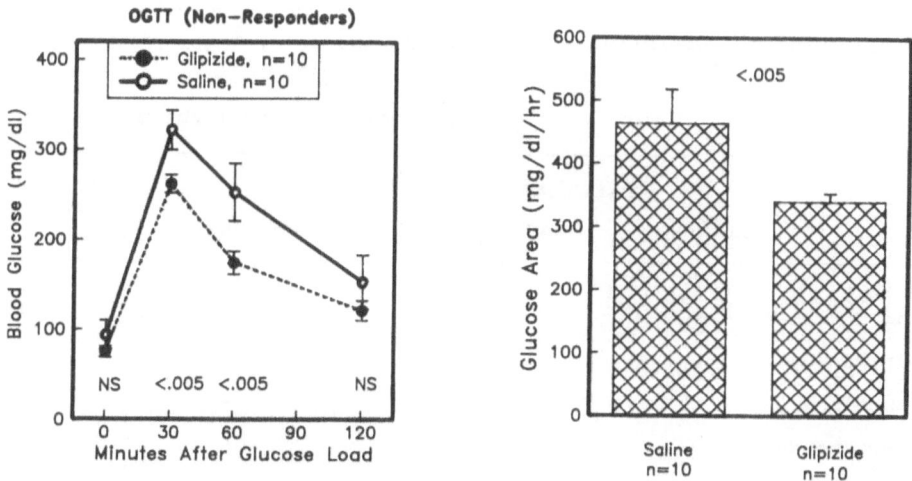

Fig. 3. Oral glucose tolerance tests (OGTT) and glucose areas in saline and glipizide-treated ("non-responders") KK mice.

Table 1. Body weight, kidney weight and glycosylated hemoglobin A_1 (HBA_1) in saline and glipizide-treated ("responders") KK mice. Values shown at means $\pm$ SEM. Numbers in parentheses represent number of animals.

	Saline (10)	Glipizide (10)	P
Body wt. (g)	32.10 ± 0.71	30.90 ± 2.00	NS
Kidney wt. (g)	0.414 ± 0.008	0.347 ± 0.03	<0.01
Glycosylated HbA_1 (%)	5.22 ± 0.73	3.73 ± 0.48	<0.025

Glucosyltransferase and N-acetyl-B-glucosaminidase activities in renal cortical homogenates and serum in "responders" are shown in Table 2. As evident, no difference in glucosyltransferase activity either in the kidney or serum was found between the two groups of mice. However, the kidney N-acetyl-B-glucosaminidase activity was significantly higher in "responders", but no difference in serum enzyme was found.

Table 2. Glucosyltransferase and N-acetyl-B-glucosaminidase activities in the kidney and serum of saline and glipizide-treated KK mice. Values shown are means $\pm$ SEM. Numbers in parentheses indicate numbers of animals

Mice	Glucosyltransferase		N-acetyl-β-glucosaminidase	
	Kidney*	Serum**	Kidney[1]	Serum[2]
Saline (10)	791 ± 38	676 ± 38	4843 ± 194	59 ± 2
Glipizide (10)	889 ± 22	648 ± 41	$5614 + 262$	58 ± 1
P	NS	NS	<0.01	NS

*DPM/mg protein; **DPM/ml/min.; [1]nmol PNP/mg protein; [2]nmol PNP/ml/min.

Table 3. Number of mice with glomerulosclerosis by light microscopy.

Mice	Histology grading*			Total No. of mice
	Mild (+)	Moderate (2+)	Severe (4+)	
Saline	7	2	9	18
Glipizide				19
Responders	3	7	–	
Non-responders	–	–	9	

* Periodic acid-Shiff stain

The presence of glomerulosclerosis in saline and glipizide-treated mice is shown in Table 3. About 50% of saline-treated mice had severe glomerulosclerosis. In "responders", no kidney showed severe glomerulosclerosis; however, the majority of these mice had only moderate glomerulosclerosis. By contrast, "non-responders" had only severe form of glomerulosclerosis.

Table 4. Proteinuria and glomerular basement membrane (GBM) width in control (saline) mice and "responders". Values shown are means $\pm$ SEM.

Mice	No.	Proteinuria (mg/d)	GBM Width (Å)
Saline	9	19.44 $\pm$ 5.44	1162 $\pm$ 113
Glipizide	9	4.12 $\pm$ 2.75	671 $\pm$ 120
P		< 0.02	< 0.01

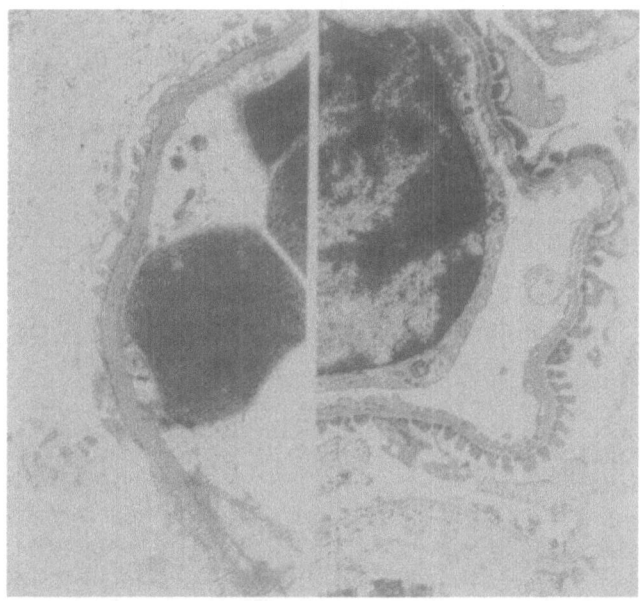

Fig. 4. Electron micrograph showing the glomerular basement membrane in saline (left) and glipizide-treated ("responders") KK mice. x 20,500.

Proteinuria and GBM width in saline and glipizide-treated ("responders") mice are shown in Table 4. As evident, both were significantly lower in "responders". Improvement in GBM width is clearly evident as shown in Fig. 4.

Table 5 gives information on "non-responders". No differences either in body weight, kidney weight, glycosylated HbA_1, proteinuria or kidney and serum enzyme activities were found between controls and "non-responders".

Table 5. Body weight, kidney weight, glycosylated HbA, proteinuria and kidney or serum enzyme activities in control (saline) mice and "non-responders". Values shown are means $\pm$ SEM.

Treatment	No.	Body wt. (g)	Kidney wt. (g)	Glyco.HbA$_1$ (%)	Proteinuria (mg/d)	Glucosyltransferase		N-acetyl-β-glucosaminidase	
						Kidney (DPM/mg protein)	Serum[1] (DPM/mg protein)	Kidney (nmol PNP/mgprotein)	Serum* (nmol PNP/mgprotein)
Saline	9	33.00 $\pm$ 1.00	0.346 $\pm$ 0.015	4.90 $\pm$ 0.31	8.83 $\pm$ 2.11	595 $\pm$ 42	638 $\pm$ 22	4665 $\pm$ 149	80 $\pm$ 3
Glipizide	9	30.88 $\pm$ 0.87	0.318 $\pm$ 0.007	5.04 $\pm$ 0.17	4.21 $\pm$ 1.31	643 $\pm$ 56	602 $\pm$ 15	4585 $\pm$ 267	86 $\pm$ 1

[1]DPM/ml/min; *nmol PNP/ml/min.

DISCUSSION

The present study demonstrates that glipizide treatment improved glucose tolerance only in 50% of KK mice. In these mice, glycosylated HbA$_1$ was found to be lower than in controls. This suggests that chronic glipizide treatment in Type II diabetic KK mice improved glucose metabolism in half of the treated mice. The reason for the failure in improving glucose metabolism in the remaining 50% of glipizide-treated mice remains unclear.

Control of hyperglycemia in "responders" seems to be responsible for less glomerulosclerosis, reduced GBM width and proteinuria, since no improvement either in glomerulopathy or proteinuria was found in "non-responders". These data confirm our previous observations that good glycemic control is associated with less glomerulosclerosis and proteinuria in KK mice (1,2)

Renal hypertrophy has been described in newly diagnosed Type I (insulin-dependent) diabetic subjects and in streptozotocin diabetic rats (6-8). This increase in kidney size may provide an increase in filtering surface area causing elevation in glomerular filtration rate, thus predisposing to glomerulopathy (8). Good blood glucose control by insulin in diabetic rats returns kidney size to normal (8). Our study shows about 13% decrease in kidney weight in "responders". Whether this decrease in kidney size is associated with less glomerulopathy and proteinuria remains speculative at this time. To our knowledge, this is the only study to show the beneficial effect of an oral hypoglycemic agent on kidney size in Type II diabetic animals and more work is needed to confirm this finding.

Glucosyltransferase, an enzyme involved in the synthesis of the disaccharide unit of the glycoprotein of the basement membrane collagen and other collagens, was found to be elevated in renal cortical homogenates of alloxan and streptozotocin-induced diabetic rats (6-8) and animals with spontaneous hereditary diabetes (6-8). Also, the activity of this enzyme was found to be elevated in glomeruli from long-term streptozotocin diabetic rats (4). This increase in glucosyltransferase activity is attributed to an increase in renal collagen synthesis in diabetic animals. In addition, enzymes involved in glycoprotein catabolism such as B-galactosidase and N-acetyl-B-glucosaminidase activities were found to be decreased in diabetic animals (6-8). This suggests that increased synthesis followed by decreased removal are responsible for enhanced deposition of basement membrane glycoprotein seen in the diabetic kidney. In the present study, the renal glucosyltransferase was not affected, but the N-acetyl-B-glucosaminidase was significantly increased in "responders", indicating enhanced removal of glycoprotein from the kidney. This is consistent with decreased accumulation of mesangial matrix and reduced GBM width in glomeruli from "responders".

In summary, the results of the present study suggest that early glipizide treatment causes improvement in glucose metabolism only in 50% of KK mice and this improvement is associated with less glomerulopathy and proteinuria. Increased degradation of glycoprotein seems partly responsible for improvement in glomerulosclerosis. Control of hyperglycemia is, therefore, indicated in diabetic subjects to prevent kidney complications.

Acknowledgements: We thank Mr. P.R. Reddy, Dr. Sarita Dhuper and Karen Killary for their technical assistance.

REFERENCES

1. Reddi, A.S., Velasco, C.A., Wehner, H., and Camerini-Davalos, R.A., 1988, The effect of early insulin therapy on diabetic glomerulo-sclerosis (GS) and proteinuria in KK mice. FASEB 2 (6): A1593 (abstract).

2. Reddi, A.S., Opperman, W., Patel, D.G., Ehrenreich, T., and Camerini-Davalos, R.A., 1978, Diabetic microangiopathy in KK mice. III. Effect of prolonged glyburide treatment on glomerulosclerosis. Exp. Mol. Pathol. 29: 92-101.

3. Chen, J., Freeman, G., Zarco, R., and Halbert, S., 1982, A standardized system for the determination of hemoglobin A_1 using a computerized photometer. J. Clin. Lab. Automat. 2: 183-90.

4. Reddi, A.S., 1985, Metabolism of glomerular basement membrane in normal, hypophysectomized and growth hormone-treated diabetic rats. Exp. Mol. Pathol. 43: 196-208.

5. Lowry, O.H., Rosenbrough, N.J., Farr, A.L., and Randall, P.J., 1951, Protein measurement with the Folin Phenol reagent. J. Biol. Chem. 193: 265-75.

6. Reddi, A.S., 1978, Diabetic microangiopathy. I. Current status of the chemistry and metabolism of the glomerular basement membrane. Metabolism 207: 107-24.

7. Reddi, A.S., and Camerini-Davalos, R.A., 1982, Metabolism of glomerular basement membrane in diabetes mellitus. In Diabetes, 1982, Mngola, E.N., Ed. Amsterdam, Excerpta Medica 1983: 449-57.

8. Reddi, A.S., and Camerini-Davalos, R.A.: Diabetic nephropathy: An update (submitted).

EFFECT OF GLICLAZIDE ON NON-INSULIN DEPENDENT DIABETES MELLITUS

¶B.J. Wajchenberg, A.T.M. Santomaruo, J.J. Cherem, D.A.C. Malerbi,
A. Giurno Filho, A.C. Lerario and D. Giannella Neto

Diabetes Section, Endocrine Division and Laboratory of Medical Research
(LIM n 25), Hospital das Clinicas, Sao Paulo, Brazil

The hyperglycemia of non-insulin dependent diabetes mellitus (NIDDM) has been attributed to both glucose overproduction by the liver and glucose under-utilization by peripheral tissues caused by deficient insulin secretion and resistance to insulin action. There is recent evidence that the induction of insulin deficiency creates insulin resistance (1). Several mechanisms have been postulated for the chronic "hypoglycemic" effects of sulfonylurea therapy in NIDDM. In relation to gliclazide (GCZ), there are studies indicating an effect on insulin secretion (2,3,4) and an extra-pancreatic action related to potentiation of the bioeffects of insulin (5,6). In the present study we examined the effects of chronic GCZ therapy on basal insulin levels, glucose and non-glucose (arginine) stimulated insulin responses (Study I), hepatic glucose production rate, peripheral tissue sensitivity to insulin and on red blood cells (RBC) insulin binding (Study II).

MATERIAL AND METHODS

Fourteen non-obese NIDDM men, 48-66 years of age, were studied before and after 3 months of GCZ treatment (80-160 mg/day): Study I. Five patients with fasting plasma glucose (FPG) above 200 mg/dl were submitted to an oral glucose tolerance test (75g), an IV glucose tolerance test (0.3 g/Kg injected in 1 min.) and an arginine test (given as an IV bolus of 5 g). All tests were repeated after 3 months of therapy. The insulin response to arginine was studied at two different plasma glucose levels and the effect of GCZ on beta cell sensitivity after arginine pulses was evaluated when steady state glucose levels were reached:

Study II. Nine NIDDM males were arbitrarily divided into 2 groups: those with FPG > 200 mg/dl (patients 6-10 and those with FPG < 200 mg/dl (patients 11-14). All patients (except two) were within 10% of ideal body weight according to the Metropolitan Life Insurance Tables. At the start of the study and after 3 months on GCZ, basal glucose turnover was determined by the continuous infusion technique as previously described (6). Glucose turnover was measured in a similar fashion, 1 week later, when peripheral sensitivity to insulin was evaluated during the steady-state of a constant IV infusion of glucose (6 mg/Kg/min) and insulin (0.8 mU/Kg/min)

This study was supported by a grant from Institut of Recherches Internationales, Neuilly-sur-Seine, France.

(6). The insulin-receptor binding studies were performed in RBCs according to a technique already described (7).

The statistical analysis was performed by a Student's t test for paired and unpaired observations, defining the significance of the difference between the group means.

RESULTS

Study I. Clinical data: Body weights did not change significantly after 3 months of GCZ treatment. FPG fell significantly from 277 ± 16 mg/dl (mean ± SEM) to 133 ± 9 mg/dl (p < 0.005) and the corresponding glycosylated hemoglobin levels from 13.9 mg/dl (p < 0.005) and the corresponding glycosylated hemoglobin levels from 13.9 ± 2.2 to 7.9 ± 0.8% (p < 0.05), respectively. The results are shown in Figure 1. The mean plasma glucose and insulin responses to IVGTT before and after GCZ are illustrated in Figure 2. The mean glucose and insulin levels of the arginine tests are indicated in Figure 3.

Study II. As in the first study the patient's body weight did not change significantly after the three months of GCZ. FPG fell from 288 ± 23 to 143 ± 25 mg/dl (p < 0.005) and from 153 ± 11 to 125 ± 11 mg/dl (p < 0.05) in the groups with FPG > 200 and < 200 mg/dl respectively. The glycosylated hemoglobin values decreased from 15.1 ± 1.3 to 8.9 ± 0.7% (p < 0.05) and from 10.0 ± 0.6 to 8.9 = 0.8% (NS), respectively.

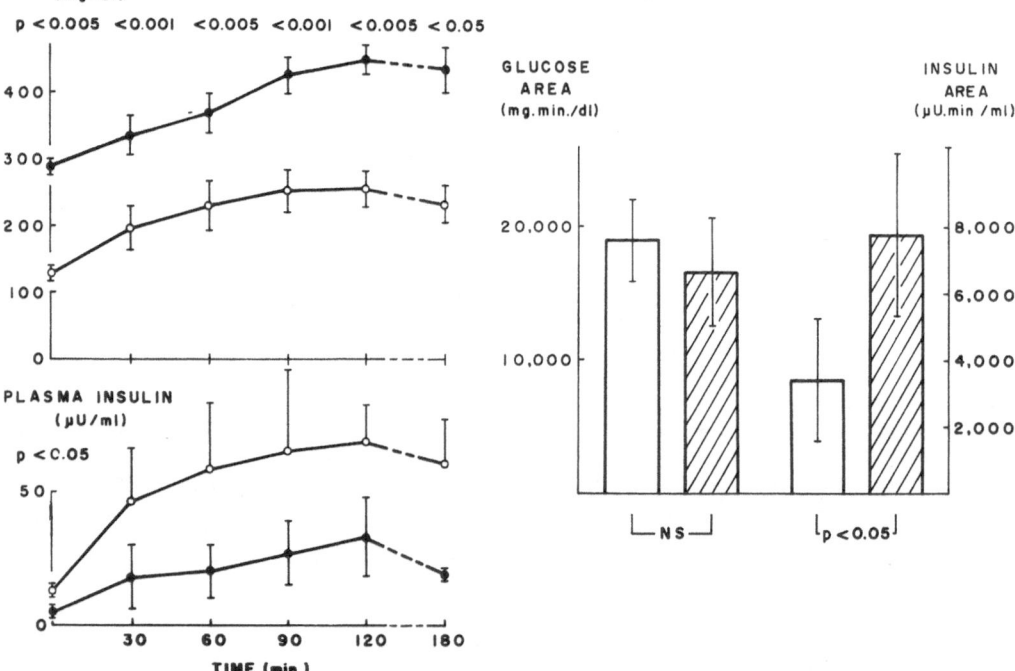

Figure 1. Plasma glucose and insulin levels (mean ± SEM) during a 75 g oral GTT in 5 NIDDM patients before (closed circles) and after (open circles) gliclazide therapy. Columns and bars indicate the mean ± SEM of the incremental total glucose and insulin areas during the oral GTT before (open columns) and after (hatched columns) gliclazide.

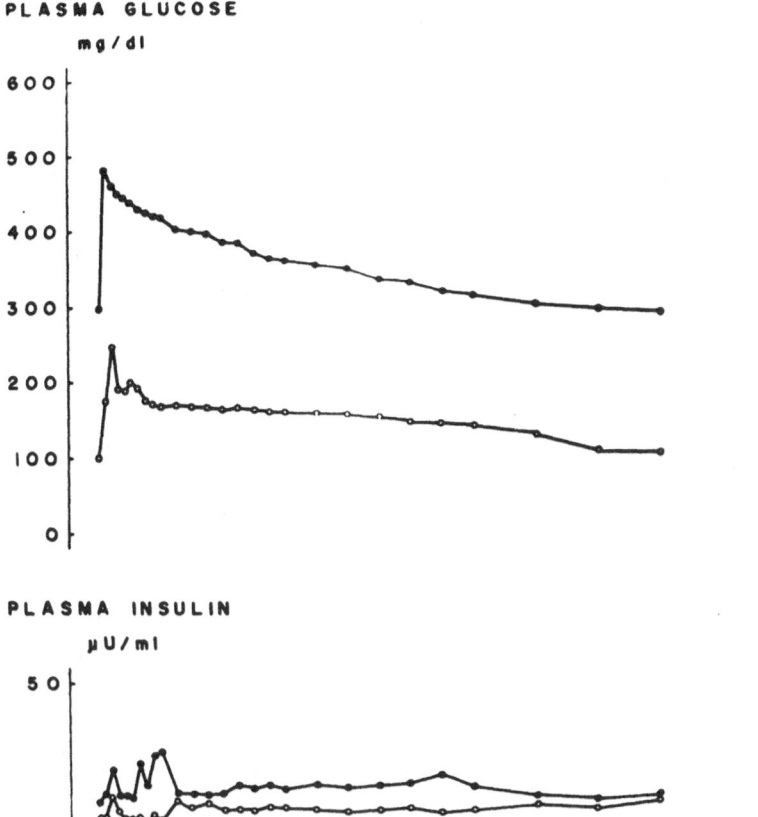

Figure 2. Mean plasma glucose and insulin levels in 5 NIDDM in response to IVGTT before (closed circles) and after (open circles) gliclazide treatment.

a) Basal plasma glucose metabolism (Figure 4). Plasma glucose and in-sulin levels were stable during the 90 to 150 min interval in all experiments and the height of the columns indicated in Figure 4 represent the mean of the 7 samples collected from 90 to 150 min of the tracer infusion. There was a significant correlation between FPG during the tracer infusions and HGP when all data (before and after GCZ) were combined ($r = 0.90$; $p < 0.001$). After GCZ, there was a significant correlation between the fall in HGP and the percent fall in FPG ($r = 0.71$; $p < 0.05$). In the patients with FPG < 200 mg/dl before therapy, the percent rise in fasting insulin after GCZ pre-sented a highly significant correlation with the fall in HGP ($r = 0.94$; $p < 0.01$).

b) Glucose metabolism during the glucose + insulin infusion (Figure 5). There were no significant differences in the steady-state plasma in-sulin (SSPI) attained within or among groups of patients during the 2 study periods, confirming that we were assessing the ability of the patients to dispose of a glucose load under identical insulin stimulus. Thus, the overall degree of insulin resistance, as measured by the height of the steady-state plasma glucose (SSPG) level during the infusion, was signifi-cantly greater before than after GCZ treatment in the 2 groups of patients. Although the SSPG was significantly different in the untreated state, it became similar after GCZ when both groups of patients were compared.

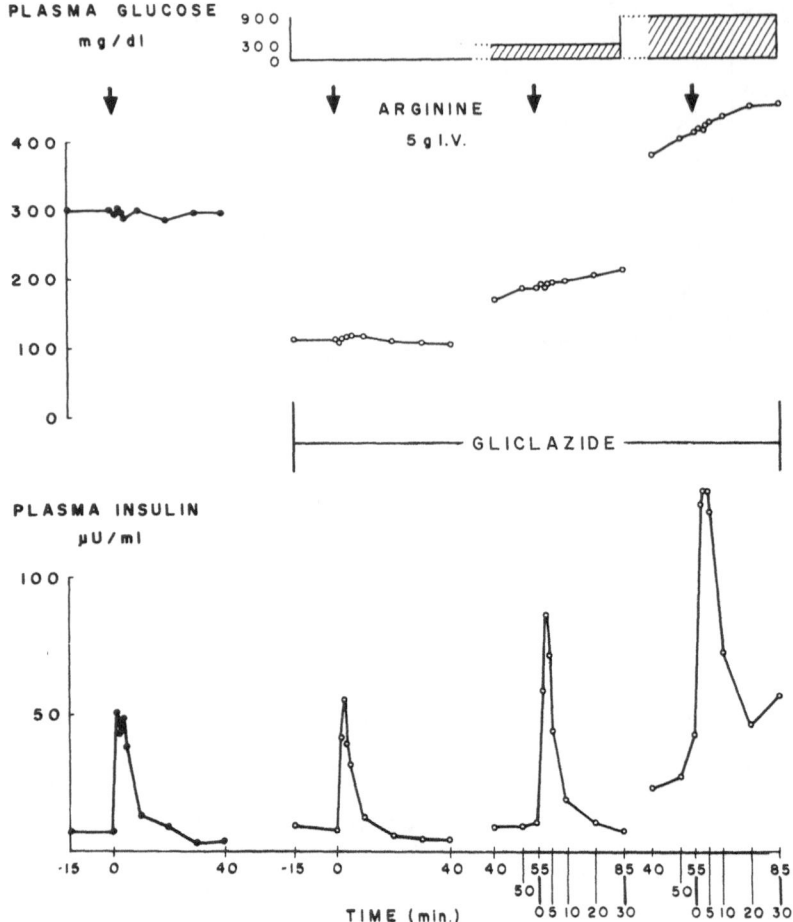

Figure 3. Mean glucose and insulin responses to arginine infusion in 5 NIDDM before (closed circles) and after (open circles) gliclazide treatment in the basal state and during stepwise glucose infusion of 300 and 900 mg/min.

During the pretreatment study, our patients could be classified into 2 groups: those with FPG > 200 mg/dl, presenting resistance to the suppression of HGP by insulin, clearly indicated by comparing HGP during the basal (Figure 4) and glucose-insulin infusion (Figure 5) studies, and patients with FPG < 200 mg/dl showing not only significantly lower basal HGP than the IR (Figure 4) but also the ability to suppress HGP with exogenous insulin infusion. On the other hand, the CL_G was not significantly different before treatment between the groups, indicating similar insulin-mediated glucose uptake by peripheral tissues. After GCZ treatment, with the fall in FPG there was a significant enhancement of insulin effectiveness at both the level of the liver (significant reduction HGP) and peripheral tissues (increase in DL_G) in the IR patients. In the IS patients, the hypoglycemic effect of GCZ was accompanied by a significant improvement in Cl_G without a significant change in the degree of suppression of HGP by insulin, almost complete before treatment.

c) RBC insulin receptor studies – The parameters of insulin-receptor interaction are indicated in Table I. The mean specific 125-I-insulin binding at tracer concentration ($\%B_o$) and the mean number of receptors per cell (N) were not significantly different from the normal mean values for men, before GCZ. After GCZ, the $\%B_o$ decreased significantly ($p < 0.05$) but not the mean N in the IR, without significant changes in either K_e (affinity constant at low receptor occupancy) or K_f (affinity constant at high receptor occupancy). In the IS patients, neither $\%B_o$ or number of receptors changed significantly nor were there changes in the affinity constants after GCZ treatment.

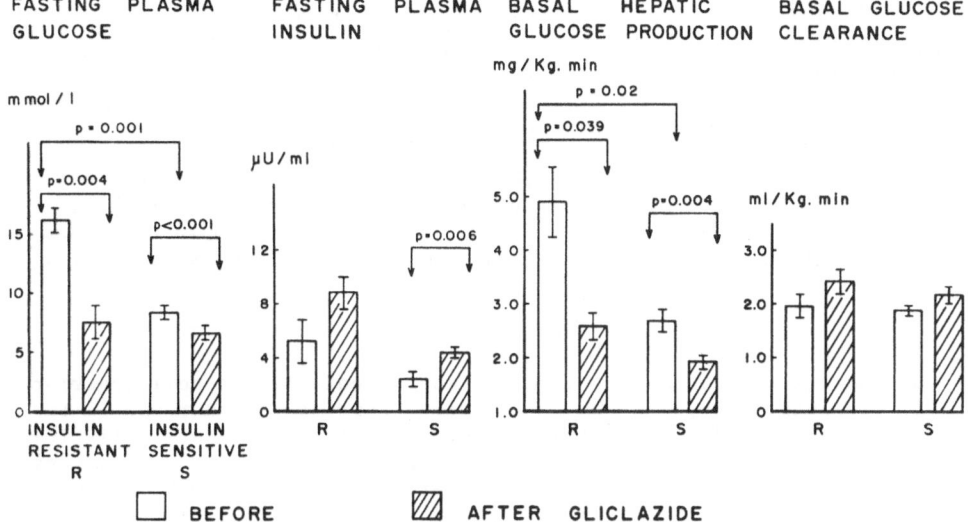

Figure 4. Comparison of mean ± SEM basal glucose metabolism parameters of insulin resistant (n=5) and sensitive (n=4) NIDDM patients before (open bars) and after (hatched bars) gliclazide therapy (from reference 8).

TABLE I

RBC INSULIN RECEPTOR PARAMETERS (MEAN ± SEM) IN 9 DIABETIC MALES (STUDY II) BEFORE (PRE) and AFTER (POST) GLICLAZIDE

	THERAPY $\%B_o$		N/CELL		$K_e (10^8 M^{-1})$		$K_f (10^8 M^{-1})$	
	PRE	POST	PRE	POST	PRE	POST	PRE	POST
INSULIN RESISTANT (N=5)	9.14 ± 0.92	6.38 ± 0.15	59.4 ± 6.8	43.8 ± 6.0	2.21 ± 0.21	1.97 ± 0.20	0.34 ± 0.09	0.35 ± 0.005
INSULIN SENSITIVE (N=4)	7.80 ± 0.47	7.02 ± 0.76	58.0 ± 5.9	57.5 ± 3.2	2.00 ± 0.18	1.77 ± 0.24	0.35 ± 0.07	0.41 ± 0.06
NORMAL MALES (N=10)	9.22 ± 0.50		63.9 ± 3.0		2.17 ± 0.13		0.29 ± 0.03	

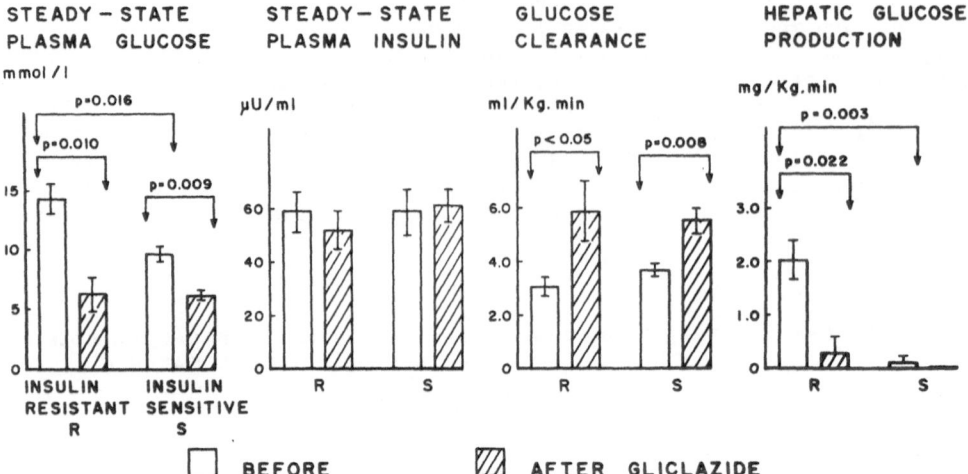

Figure 5.   Comparison of mean ± SEM glucose metabolism parameters during glucose-insulin infusion of insulin resistant (n = 5)
and sensitive (n = 4) NIDDM patients before (open bars) and
after (hatched bars) gliclazide therapy (from reference 8).

DISCUSSION

     Our results are consistent with an improvement in beta cell function
of NIDDM patients on chronic GCZ treatment.   There was an increase in fasting insulin levels and a reduction in FPG, suggesting that beta cells increase insulin secretion at lower plasma glucose levels.   These increments
in basal insulin levels, related to the pretreatment FPG, may be an important mechanism by which GCZ exerts its hypoglycemic action.   In addition,
there was an increase in the incremental insulin area after the oral glucose load despite the same glycemic stimulus (reflected by the same incremental glucose area) in the presence of an improvement in insulin action
at target tissues after GCZ (Figure 1).   Accordingly, the insulinogenic index, at all times of sampling, was significantly greater after sulfonylurea.
Our finding that the decline in FPG during GCZ therapy was correlated with
the fall in HGP suggests that the glucose-lowering effect of the drug in
fasting state is mediated by inhibition of glucose production.   The uniform
increase in fasting plasma insulin in all subjects in which HGP was measured
and the highly significant correlation between the rise in fasting insulin
levels and the fall in basal HGP in the IS subjects points to the importance
of the enhanced insulin secretion as the mechanism by which GCZ lowers HGP.
Further, blood glucose and plasma insulin responses to meals in patients on
GCZ have persistent lower blood glucose accompanied by sustained elevations
of plasma insulin (4).   Regarding the effects of GCZ on the dynamics of insulin secretion, there was a slight correction of the early 2nd phase insulin
response (10-20 min) (Figure 2).   Since the 2nd phase insulin release is pro-
portionate to the steady-state glucose concentration preceeding the glucose
challenge, its improvement after the significant reduction in FPG is sug-
gestive that GCZ increased beta cell sensitivity to the glucose stimulus at
the 2nd phase insulin release (8).   In relation to the non-glucose secretagogue arginine, the apparently normal insulin response in the untreated diabetics (8) similar to that obtained when their plasma glucose was near normal levels after GCZ seems to be maintained, at least in part, by the elevated plasma glucose levels seen before treatment.   However, the increased
basal insulin levels and responsiveness to arginine when the sulfonylurea-
treated subjects were tested at the same mean PG levels as before GCZ sug-

gested that there was an improvement of the beta-cell sensitivity to the non-glucose stimulus which was masked by the decrease in plasma glucose during GCZ treatment. Thus, GCZ enhances the beta-cell response to an aminoacid as well as to glucose. The results from Study II also indicate that the chronic hypoglycemic action of GCZ in non-obese or slightly obese men with NIDDM is associated with an improvement in insulin action, suggesting that GCZ potentiates the effects of endogenous and exogenous insulin on target tissues. Our data clearly show that 3 months of GCZ therapy improved glycemic control in NIDDM with fasting hyperglycemia enhancing insulin effectiveness at the level of the liver and peripheral tissues. Basal HGP was suppressed and both hepatic sensitivity to insulin and insulin-stimulated glucose disposal were increased in the two groups of patients with FPG > 200 mg/dl (IR) and < 200 mg/dl (IS). Furthermore, considering that HGP is more sensitive than glucose disposal to changes in insulin, the small, although significant, changes in peripheral insulin levels during chronic sulfonylurea therapy are probably associated with a larger effect on HGP than on glucose disposal, as observed in our patients under GCZ.

Finally, our data failed to demonstrate enhanced insulin binding to RBCs after GCZ, as previously shown in a similar study by Ward et al (6).

REFERENCES

1. Garvey, W.T., Olefsky, J.M., Griffin, J., Hamman, R.F. and Kolterman, O.G., 1985, The effect of insulin treatment on insulin secretion and insulin action in Type II diabetes mellitus. Diabetes 34: 222-234.

2. Chiasson, J-L., Bergman, R.N., Verdy, M., Hamet, P. and De Lean, A., 1987, Study of the effect of gliclazide on secretion and action of insulin in normal and Type II diabetic humans. IDF Bull. 32: 9-11.

3. Matthews, D., Hosker, J. and Turner, R., 1987, Effects of gliclazide on insulin secretion indiced by glucose and aminoacids. IDF Bull 32: 12-15.

4. Wajchenberg, B.L., Nery, M. Leme, C.E., Silveira, A.A., Fioratti, P. and Germek, O.A., 1980, Effect of prolonged gliclazide treatment on blood glucose and plasma insulin responses in obese patients with maturity-onset diabetes. Clin Pharmacol Therap 27: 375-378.

5. Wajchenberg, B.L., Malerbi, D.A., Giurno Filho, A., Giannella, Neto, D., Cherem, J.J., and Lerario, A.C., 1987, Effect of gliclazide treatment on red blood cell insulin receptors, hepatic glucose production and peripheral glucose utilization in non-insulin-dependent diabetes mellitus. IDF Bul 32: 16-21.

6. Ward, G., Harrison, L.C., Proietto, J., Aitken, P. and Nankervis, A., 1985, Gliclazide therapy is associated with potentiation of postbinding insulin action in obese non-insulin-dependent diabetic sugjects. Diabetes 34: 241-245.

7. Judzewitsch, O.G., Pfeifer, M.A., Best, J.D., Beard, A.C., Halter, J.B. and Porte, Jr., D., 1982, Chronic chlorpropamide therapy of non-insulin dependent diabetes augments basal and stimulated insulin secretion by increasing islet sensitivity to glucose. J Clin Endocrinol Metab, 55: 321-328.

8. Pfeifer, M.A., Halter, J.B. and Porte, Jr., D., 1981, Insulin secretion in Diabetes mellitus. Am J Med, 79: 579-588.

PLASMA ACTIVITY OF THE ENZYME N-ACETIL-BETA-GLUCOSAMINIDASE
IN HEALTHY AND DIABETIC SUBJECTS:
EFFECTS OF TREATMENT WITH A SULFONYLUREA DRUG

¶Giraudo, J.R., Fugante, M., Blaque Quadri, J.,
Reyes, G., and Duran Saucedo, N.*

*Instituto Modelo de Diabetes Endocrinologia y Nutricion
Cordoba, Argentina

The pathophysiological mechanism of diabetic microangiopathy is based on experimental and clinical evidence. The complex sequence of events which determine the vascular lesion is not entirely elucidated. Some of the mechanisms involved, both quantitatively and qualitatively in the alteration process have been demonstrated.

The pathophysiological basis of microangiopathy is an increased thickness of the capillary basement membrane, which can result from either an increased synthesis or a reduced degree of degradation of the above.

Regarding the synthesis of the basement membrane, it is known that its main component is Type IV collagen. This Type IV collagen is composed of hydroxyproline, hydroxylysine and glycosylated hydroxylysine in the form of a disaccharide glucosylgalactosyl-hydroxylysine. The latter is synthesized by means of a post-translational modification which requires the catalytic intervention of 4 intracellular enzymes: glucosyl-transferase, galactosyl-transferase, lysylhydroxylase and prolylhydroxylase (1).

Experimental studies involving the glomerular basement membrane have demonstrated the increased activity of these enzymes, which in term reflect the increased synthesis of the basement membrane, therefore establishing a positive relationship with microangiopathy (2).

The opposite process, i.e. degradation of the basement membrane is mediated by glycosidase enzymes which release glycosaminoglycans, glycolipids and glycoproteins. Together with other hydroxylases responsible for the degradation of glycoproteins and mucopolysaccharides, the lysosomal enzymes which have been the subject of most study are N-acetyl-beta glucosaminidase (NABG), beta-glucuromidase and beta-galactosidase. In the diabetic patient, the plasma levels of these enzymes are increased (2,3). This rise could reflect a limiting biochemical reaction on excessive deposits of mucopolysaccharides and glycoproteins, which are related to the pathophysiology of the microangiopathy (8). Another interpretation could be that it reflects a decreased degradation of these products in the basement membrane, therefore leading to plasma accumulation of such enzymes (1). Another interpretation could be that it reflects a decreased degradation of these products in the basement membrane, therefore leading to plasma accumulation of such enzymes (1).

A positive relationship has been established between the increased plasma levels of these enzymes and the severity of hyperglycemia and presence of microangiopathy.

Considering these previous studies, the aim of this study was to establish the plasma activity of NABG in healthy subjects (non diabetics) and in controlled and uncontrolled diabetic patients both with and without documented microangiopathy. The potential effects of an oral hypoglycemic treatment (gliclazide) on the enzyme activity were then evaluated.

MATERIAL AND METHODS

295 patients were included in the trial and were divided into groups as follows:

Group 1. 56 subjects (healthy, non diabetics) with no family history of diabetes, normal oral glucose tolerance test or normal fasting and postprandial blood glucose and normal glycosylated hemoglobin. The mean age was 44 years, 32 were female and 24 male. Mean BMI (weight/height^2) was 24.5 in women (normal range 19-24) and 26.8 in men (normal range 20-25). No documented endocrine or metabolic pathology existed.

Group 2. 32 patients (controlled diabetics without documented complications). 18 women (12 NIDD and 6IDD) and 14 men (9 NIDD and 5 IDD). Mean BMI was 24.3 in women and 26.2 in men. Diabetes was considered controlled if the mean of the previous two fasting and post prandial blood glucose determinations was less than 180 mg and if glycosylated hemoglobin was less than 10.5%. The mean age was 45 years.

Group 2b. 56 diabetic patients (controlled but having documented retinal and/or renal complications). 36 were female (20 NIDD and 16 IDD) and 20 male (12 MIDD and 8 IDD). Mean age was 43 years. Mean BMI was 25 in women and 26.6 in men.

Group 2c. 34 diabetic patients (uncontrolled without complications) with mean blood glucose greater than 180 mg and glycosylated hemoglobin greater than 10.5%. 20 were female (13 NIDD and 7 IDD) and 14 male (11 NIDD and 3 IDD).
Mean age was 45.5 years. Mean BMI was 24.3 in women and 26 in men.

Group 2d. 45 diabetic patients (uncontrolled with documented complications). 32 were female (20 NIDD and 12 IDD) and 13 male (8 NIDD and 5 IDD). Mean age 43.5 years. Mean BMI was 23.9 in women and 25.8 in men.

Group 3. 82 diabetic patients who received gliclazide for 6 months at a dose of 160-240 mg/day.

Patients were divided into 4 sub-groups as follows:

Subgroup I: 20 controlled diabetics without documented complications, previously treated with another oral hypoglycemic drug or with insulin, until the initial examination. In the first case, gliclazide was substituted for the oral hypoglycemic agent, and in the second case, it was associated with insulin. 11 were female (7 NIDD and 4 IDD) and 9 male (5 NIDD and 4 IDD). Mean age was 46.5 years. Mean BMI was 24.3 in women and 26.2 in men. Mean duration of diabetes was 4.8 years.

Subgroup II: 23 controlled diabetics with documented complications. Treatment protocol was similar to that of the previous group. 15 were female (10 NIDD and 5 IDD) and 8 male (5 NIDD and 3 IDD). Mean age was

42.8 years. Mean BMI was 24 in women and 25.8 in men. Mean duration of diabetes was 9.5 years.

Subgroup III: 20 uncontrolled diabetics without documented complications. Treatment protocol was similar to that of the previous group, but poor diabetic control was demonstrated at three consecutive controls at intervals of one month. Poor diabetic control was attributed to non compliance with diet and therapy. 11 were female (8 NIDD and 3 IDD), 9 were male (4 NIDD and 5 IDD) with a mean age of 42 years. Mean BMI was 24.8 in women and 26.3 in men. Mean duration of diabetes was 5.5 years.

Subgroup IV: 19 uncontrolled diabetics with documented complications. Treatment protocol was similar to that of previous groups. 9 were female (6 NIDD and 3 IDD) and 10 were male (5 NIDD and 5 IDD) with a mean age of 47 years. Mean BMI was 25.2 in women and 26.8 in men. Mean duration of diabetes was 11 years.

All patients included in group 3 were subjected to biochemical control including at least 2 fasting and 2 post prandial blood glucose determinations, glycosylated hemoglobin, lipid profile and monthly evaluation of the enzyme activity of NABG, during the 6 month treatment with gliclazide. Enzyme activity changes over time with gliclazide were evaluated by calculating the differential mean between pre and post treatment values.

METHODS

Blood glucose was determined on capillary blood using Haemoglucotest strips and a reflectometer and also on venous plasma.

The evaluation of the plasma enzyme activity was performed using the technique of Walker et al. (4). Both p-nitrophenol standard (10 to 50 nmol) and samples were examined together, results were expressed as nmol of p-nitrophenol/ml/min.

Glycosylated hemoglobin was determined using the DiabeTest a_1 Kit micro columns supplied by Chemar Laboratories of "Industria Argentina." Normal values for the laboratory fluctuate between 5 and 8.6%.

The retinal vasculature was evaluated by means of fluorescein angiography. Renal function was evaluated by blood urea, blood creatinine, 24 h. urinary protein excretion and creatinine clearance measurements.

RESULTS

Data obtained are summarized in Tables I and II.

GROUP 1 (NON DIABETIC SUBJECTS)

Mean plasma enzyme activity of NABG was 12.58 ± 0.52 (± SEM) in the 56 healthy subjects. These values were considered abnormal and were used for comparison with those of the other groups.

GROUP 2 (CONTROLLED DIABETICS WITHOUT COMPLICATIONS)

Mean plasma enzyme activity of NABG was 13.28 ± 0.35 in the 32 patients. Compared to group 1 (control group) values, there was no statistically significant difference (p NS > 0.05).

GROUP 2b (CONTROLLED DIABETICS WITH COMPLICATIONS)

TABLE I

NABG ACTIVITY IN BOTH DIABETIC AND NON-DIABETIC PATIENTS,
EITHER CONTROLLED OR NOT, WITH OR WITHOUT COMPLICATIONS
P: COMPARISON BETWEEN MEAN VALUES AND HEALTHY GROUP.

GROUP	No	AGE	SEX		BODY MASS INDEX		TYPE OF DIABETES		DURA-TION	NABG	P
			F	M	F	M	I	II			
I HEALTHY	56	44	32	24	24.5	26.8	-	-	-	12.68 ±0.52	-
2a CDNC	32	46	18	14	24.3	26.2	11	21	6	13.28 ±0.35	NS
2b CDWC	56	43	36	20	25.0	26.6	24	32	9,5	21.70 ±0.76	< 0.001
2c UDNC	34	45.6	20	14	25.2	26.0	10	24	6.3	23.97 ±1.46	< 0.001
2d UDWC	45	43.5	32	13	25.9	26.8	17	28	11	24.79 ±0.87	< 0.001

TABLE II

NABG ACTIVITY BEFORE AND AFTER A 6 MONTH TREATMENT WITH GLICLAZIDE
*DIFFERENTIAL MEAN WITH RESPECT TO BASELINE VALUES

GROUP 3 SUBGROUPS	NABG BASELINE	No	AGE	SEX		BODY MASS INDEX		TYPE OF DIABETES		DURA-TION	NABG* 6 MONTHS	P
				F	M	F	M	I	II			
I CDNC	13.30 ±0.52	20	46.5	11	9	24.3	26.2	8	12	4.8	-3.30 ±1.71	< 0.02
II CDWC	21.70 ±0.76	23	42.8	15	8	24.0	25.8	8	15	9.5	-3.87 ±1.34	<0.02
III UDNC	24.00 ±1.46	20	42.0	11	9	24.8	26.3	8	12	5.5	0.30 ±1.83	NS
IV UDWC	25.00 ±0.90	19	47.0	9	10	26.2	26.8	8	11	11.0	3.13 ±1.67	NS

Mean NABG value was 21.70 ± 0.75 in the 56 patients.   Comparison with normal values: p ≤ 0.001.

GROUP 2C (UNCONTROLLED DIABETICS WITHOUT COMPLICATIONS)

Mean NABG value was 23.97 ± 1.45 in the 34 patients.   Comparison with normal values: p < 0.001.

GROUP 2D (UNCONTROLLED DIABETICS WITH COMPLICATIONS)

Mean NABG value was 24.79 ± 0.87 in the 45 patients.   Comparison with normal values: p < 0.001.

GROUP 3 (GLICLAZIDE TREATED DIABETICS) (TABLE II)

Subgroup I: (Controlled without complications) (N 20)
The differential mean between pre and post-treatment mean values was calculated. In all cases, we observed a decrease in enzyme activity, with a mean fall of -3.30 ± 1.71 (p < 0.02).

Subgroup II: (Controlled with complications) (N 23)
The differential mean fall was -3.87 ± 1.34 (p < 0.02).

Subgroup III: (Controlled with complications) (N20)
Differential mean: 0.32 ± 1.83 (p NS).

Subgroup IV: (Uncontrolled with complications) (N 19)
Differential mean: 3.13 ± 1.67 (p NS).

For the controlled and uncontrolled groups treated with gliclazide, statistical analysis was carried out using a test for paired series, while the other groups were analysed using a test for independent series.

DISCUSSION

1) NABG plasma activity values observed in the healthy subjects (control group) were statistically similar to those obtained by other authors using the same Walker et al. method (4).

2) Considering the statistical analysis of results obtained in the diabetic groups, we can conclude:

    a) In all uncontrolled diabetics, with or without retinal complications, a significant increase in plasma enzyme activity was observed with respect to normal values. Thus, reinforcing the idea that a positive relationship between hyperglycemia and enzyme value exist. Other authors have reported similar results (4-5-6).

    b) In the diabetic groups with reasonably good metabolic control, enzyme activity was significantly greater in those with documented microangiopathy. That is to say, once hyperglycemia - which is a known enzyme increasing factor - was eliminated, microangiopathy itself was associated with an increased plasma NABG. This rise reflects the decrease in the degradation process of the capillary basement membrane, which consequently thickens, sometimes association with an increased synthesis as suggested by Camerini-Davalos et al. (4) who demonstrated that the muscle NABG enzyme activity concomitantly decreased. Such inversely proportional tissular and plasma values had already been reported by other authors (7).

c) Treatment with Gliclazide of the various diabetic groups studied, clearly demonstrated that this hypoglycemic drug significantly reduced the plasma enzyme activity, whether or not the diabetes was insulin-dependent and with or without documented complications. However, only in cases where reasonably good glycemic control was maintained, Gliclazide does not seem to be effective in uncontrolled diabetes.

Plasma NABG activity fell when blood glucose was controlled with diet and insulin (7). Camerini-Davalos et al. observed that in chemical diabetes, glipizide reduced the high plasma enzyme activity levels, with a concomitant increase in those of the muscle and a decrease in the basement membrane thickness (4).

Data obtained from the present study suggest on the one hand that NABG plasma activity is a biochemical index of the degree of glycemic control in diabetes, and on the other hand, and independent of the above mentioned, an index of the existence of microvascular complications in the controlled diabetic patient.

Gliclazide treatment is capable of reducing the activity of this lysosomal enzyme in controlled Type I and II diabetes, but not in uncontrolled diabetes, where hyperglycemia masks or cancels out the drug effect.

Our investigations indicate that the determination of the levels of the enzyme involved in the degradative process of the capillary basement membrane, can be used as a measure of the existence, worsening or improvement of microangiopathy.

Thus, the results obtained show that gliclazide treatment could retard the mechanisms of synthesis and activate the basement membrane degradation in insulin-dependent or non insulin-dependent diabetes, thus potentially delaying the onset or worsening of diabetic microangiopathy. Such an hypothesis requires further long-term and prospective investigation.

REFERENCES

1. Kefalides, N.A., 1973, Structure and biosynthesis of basement membranes. Int Rev Connect Tissue Res 6: 63-104.

2. Velasco, C., Oppermann, W., Marine, N., Camerini-Davalos, R.A., 1974, Effect of genetic diabetes on kidney glucosyltransferase. Horm Metab Res 6: 427.

3. Belfiore, F., Vecchio, L.L., Napoli, E., 1973, Serum enzymes in diabetes mellitus. Clin Chem 19: 447-452.

4. Camerini-Davalos, R.A., Velasco, C., Glasser, M., 1986, Enzyme activities as a predictor of diabetic vasculopathy. Am J of Med 80: 574-581.

5. Fushimi, H., Tarui, S., 1976, Retina, tear and serum B-N-acetyl-glucosaminidase activities in diabetic patients. Clin Chem Acta 71: 1-8.

6. Perdichizzi, G, Cucinotta, D., Saitta, A., Cavalieri, A., Squadrito, G., 1983, Serum and urinary activities of beta-N-acetylglucosaminidase and beta-glucuronidase in diabetic patients. Acta Diabetol Lat 20: 257-264.

7. Camerini-Davalos, R.A., Velasco, C.A., Glasser, M., Bloodworth, J.M.B., Jr., 1983, Drug-induced reversal of early diabetic microangiopathy. N Engl J Med 309: 1551-1556.

8. Spiro, R.G., 1973, Biochemistry of the renal glomerular basement membrane and its alterations in diabetes mellitus. N Engl J Med 288: 1337-1342.

CONTINUOUS INSULIN TREATMENT IN THE CHINESE HAMSTER
A REVIEW

¶Gerold M. Grodsky

Metabolic Research Unit, University of California, San Francisco

Diabetes in the adult diabetic Chinese hamster is characterized by subnormal plasma and pancreatic insulin, impaired stimulated insulin secretion, and insulin resistance (1-3). In most regards this model resembles non-obese NIDDM reviewed in (2). Of particular interest is the observation that in young pre-diabetic animals, with little or no hyperglycemia, hyperinsulinemia is observed (4). Furthermore, perfused pancreata from 6-12 week animals respond normally to stimuli; impairment of insulin release is noted only by 17-21 weeks (1). Thus, there is a predictable onset of diabetes (to 95% in certain sublines).

It has been established that onset of diabetes is highly dependent on diet. Thus, diet restriction (4), isocaloric low fat diets (5), and diets low in saturated fats (6), when administered during the pre-diabetic period, ameliorate, or prevent, the onset and severity of the predicted diabetes. The effect of comparably administered insulin is reviewed in the report.

METHODS

Acute effect of insulin delivered by minipump. Details for loading of minipumps (Alza Corp., Palo Alto, CA) with insulin (10 U/kg/day), and their placement in Chinese hamsters at four one-week sequences, were described (2). Chinese hamsters were from normal (M) and diabetes (X) sublines (Upjohn Co., Kalamazoo, MI). Diabetics were defined as those animals with fed morning blood sugars of greater than 200 mg/dl, 11.1 mM. Methods for isolation and perfusion of pancreata, and insulin and glucose assays were given (2).

Chronic effects of insulin delivered by minipumps. Minipumps were loaded as above, but to deliver 6 U/kg/day (3). The concentration of insulin was changed each week to maintain the same dosage with respect to the young hamster's increasing body weight. Chinese hamster sublines, (M) and (X), were used as above. Insulin infusion was initiated at six weeks of age; any animal from the diabetic subline whose fed morning blood sugars exceeded 120 mg/dl, 6.7 mM was excluded from the study (3).

This work was supported by grants from NIH (DK01410) and by the Diabetes Research and Education Foundation.

329

Acute effects of insulin administered by minipump (2). When diabetic animals were administered continuous insulin (10 U/kg/day) for four weeks, blood and urinary glucose progressively dropped during the first two weeks, and were subsequently maintained at almost normal levels (2). Figure 1 shows the results when pancreas isolated at the end of this period were perfused with a stimulating concentration of glucose. Pancreas from diabetic animals pretreated with saline showed the expected impairment of diphasic insulin release. Pancreas of those animals, whose blood sugar had been normalized, demonstrated improved first phase release. This increase in the rapid component of insulin release could be expected to contribute to the improved glucose homeostasis in the intact animals, and was an early example of the phenomenon that reduction of hyperglycemia results in reversal of islet cell desensitization in human diabetes (7). In less severe diabetic hamsters, the same continuously administered insulin dosage caused progressive decline in blood sugar over the four weeks resulting in hypoglycemia and, in some cases, hypoglycemic death (2). These results in the Chinese hamster are also consistent with studies in human diabetes which indicate that a period of decreased hyperglycemia results in increased insulin sensitivity and decreased peripheral insulin resistance (7). It is emphasized that when the pancreata of these hypoglycemic animals were perfused, insulin secretion was impaired in both phases (2). Thus, if these observations in the Chinese hamster are applicable to human diabetes, lowering of the blood sugar can have the beneficial effects of improved insulin resistance and insulin secretion. However, chronic hypoglycemia is to be avoided, since it results in reduced capability of the pancreatic islets to release insulin in response to a stimulus. Possible mechanisms that could account for this secretion impairment after prolonged hypoglycemia were reviewed (2).

Effects of insulin administered by minipump on eventual onset and severity of diabetes (3). Figure 2 shows the eventual effects of four weeks of continuous insulin administration, starting at the critical period of approximately one week before detectable onset of hyperglycemia (age 6 weeks).

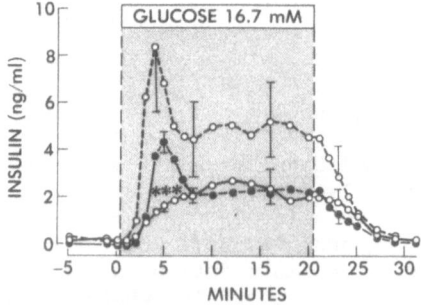

Figure 1. Effect of four weeks of insulin (10 U/kg) or saline treatment in vivo on subsequent in vitro pancreatic response to glucose. Pancreas from normal subline M, 0--0; pancreas from diabetic sublines X, given saline alone, 0——0,   , pancreas from diabetic sublines, X, given insulin, 0——0 data from (2).

In these experiments, the dose of 5 U insulin per kg/body weight per day was selected since the higher dose used in the acute studies caused hypoglycemia in mildly diabetic animals and would have been a serious overdose in euglycemic pre-diabetics. The dose employed was sufficient to double resting morning plasma insulin levels though no change in the morning blood sugar was detectable (3). As seen in Figure 2, after the initial growth spurt, terminating at 10-20 weeks body weights and food consumption in all

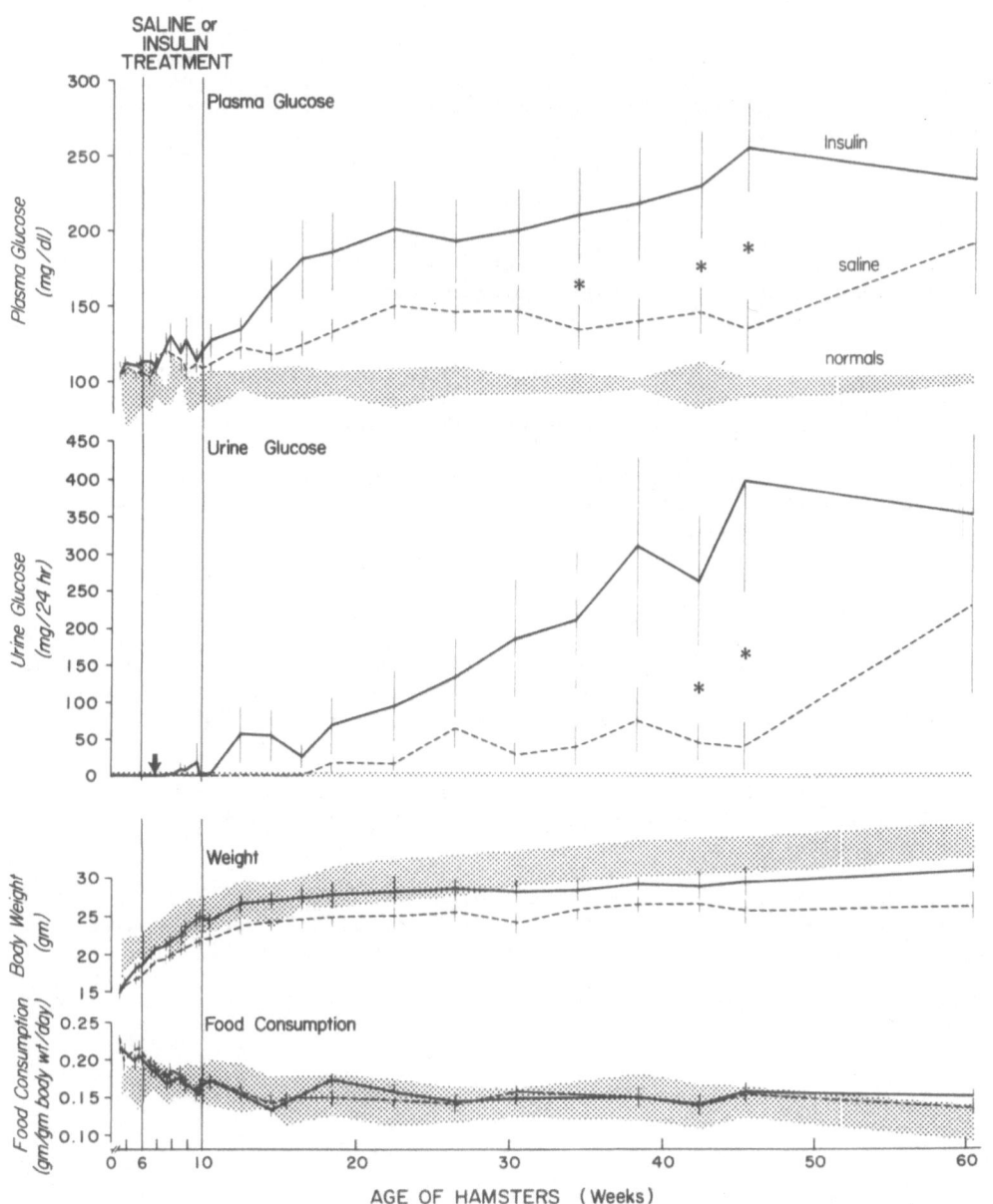

Figure 2. Effect of four weeks of insulin (5 U/kg), or saline, on non-fasting plasma and urine glucose, body weight and food consumption of genetically prediabetic Chinese hamsters.

animals were similar. This is a required control in the experimental design, since food consumption can affect the ultimate intensity of diabetes (4). Administration of insulin did not prevent the small (non-significant) rise in blood sugar through the four-week insulin treatment period as onset of diabetes began. The treatment did not postpone or prevent the onset of diabetes measured either as blood or urine sugar. In fact, with time, those animals which had received insulin, showed a significantly greater intensity of hyperglycemia and urine glucose. The data clearly show that, in this animal model for non-obese Type II diabetes, administration of insulin during the critical time of onset of diabetes does not prevent, and may actually exacerbate, the ultimate diabetic state. Thus, exogenous insulin does not "rest" and protect endogenous beta cells. Instead, it may cause relatively permanent enhancement of insulin resistance (increased fat cells?). Since food restriction during this same period was shown to ameliorate subsequent diabetes, it is perhaps not surprising, in retrospect, that increased fuel storage stimulated by insulin could cause opposite and deleterious effects.

REFERENCES

1. Frankel, B.J., Heldt, A.M., Gerritsen, G.C., Grodsky, G.M., 1984, Insulin, glucagon, and somatostatin release from the prediabetic Chinese hamster. Diabetologia 27: 387.

2. Frankel, G.J., Schmid, F.G., Grodsky, G.M., 1979, Effect of continuous insulin infusion with an implantable seven-day minipump in the diabetic Chinese hamster. Endocrinology 104: 1532.

3. Frankel, B.J., Grodsky, G.M., 1979, Effect of continuous low-dose insulin treatment on subsequent incidence of diabetes in genetically prediabetic Chinese hamsters. Diabetes 28: 544.

4. Gerritsen, G.C., 1982, The Chinese hamster as a model for the study of diabetes mellitus. Diabetes 21: 14.

5. Grodsky, G.M., Frankel, G.J., Gerich, J.E., Gerritsen, G.C., 1974, The diabetic Chinese hamster: in vitro insulin and glucagon release; the "chemical diabetic;" and the effect of diet on ketonuria. Diabetologia (Suppl.) 10: 521.

6. Gerritsen, G.C., Connel, M.A., Blanks, M.C., 1981, Effect of environmental factors including nutrition on genetically determined diabetes of Chinese hamsters. Proc. Nutr. Soc. 40: 237.

7. Unger, R.H., Grundy, S., 1985, Hyperglycaemia as an inducer as well as consequence of impaired islet cell function and insulin resistance: Implications for the management of diabetes. Diabetologia 28: 118.

KIDNEY DISEASE IN KK MICE: EFFECT OF INSULIN

¶R.A. Camerini-Davalos[+], A.S. Reddi[++], H. Wehner[*],
and C.A. Velasco[+]

[+]Department of Medicine, New York Medical College
Metropolitan Hospital Research Center, New York, New York
[++]Department of Medicine, UMDNJ-New Jersey Medical School, Newark, N.J.
[*]Institute of Pathology, University of Freiberg, West Germany

We reported that improvement in glucose metabolism with prolonged oral therapy is associated with prevention of glomerulosclerosis and proteinuria in KK mice. However, it is not known whether short-term insulin treatment with improvement in glucose metabolism would similarly prevent the development and progression of glomerulosclerosis in these KK mice. We provide evidence that good glycemic control by early insulin therapy improves both glomerulosclerosis and proteinuria in KK mice.

MATERIALS AND METHODS

Eighteen KK mice of both sexes were used in the study. They were divided into 2 groups. One group (N = 9) was injected subcutaneously into the nuchal area with Lente Pork insulin in the amount of 2.5 units/100g once a day in the morning hours from 20 to 41 days of age. The other group of mice (N = 9) received 0.9% saline and served as controls. Insulin was diluted in 0.9% saline containing 1% albumin.

Oral glucose tolerance tests were done in both groups of mice at 38 days of age. For 24 hr. urine collection, 5 mice from each group were placed individually in metabolic cages. Urine samples were collected at start of the experiment and subsequently 10 and 20 days after saline or insulin treatment. Protein was determined by the biuret method.

For light microscopy studies, a portion of the kidney (coronal section) was fixed in 10% neutral formalin, embedded in plexiglass, sections 0.5--1.0 u thick cut and stained in silver methenamine.

All data are expressed as means ± S.E.M. Student's t-test was applied to calculate the significance between means, and P values   0.05 were considered significant.

RESULTS

Figure 1 shows oral glucose tolerance tests in saline and insulin-

---

This work was supported in part by the Diabetes Research Fund, New York, New York and the Michael J. Bilotto Research Fund of Hope for Diabetics Foundation, New York, New York.

treated mice. No significant difference in fasting blood sugars was observed between the two groups of mice. However, the blood sugars were significantly lower at 30, 60 and 120 min. following glucose load in insulin-treated KK mice.

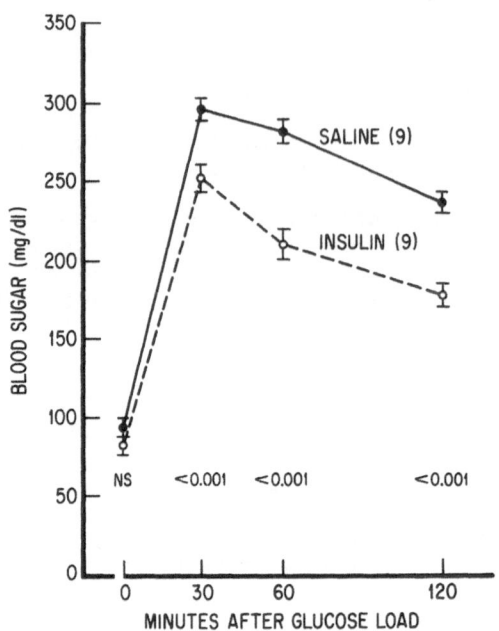

Figure 1. Oral glucose tolerance tests in saline and insulin-treated KK mice. Numbers in parentheses indicate number of animals.

RESULTS

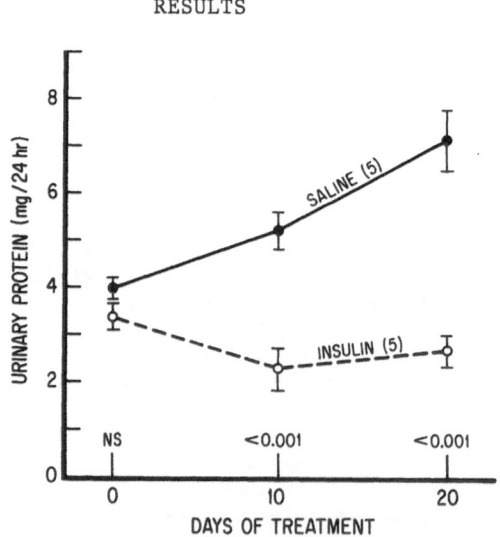

Figure 2. 24-hr. urine proteinuria in KK mice at start, 10 and 20 days after either saline or insulin treatment. Each point represents the mean ± SEM. Numbers in parentheses represent number of animals.

Twenty-four hr. urinary protein concentration is shown in Figure 2. In control mice, proteinuria gradually increased with duration of diabetes and insulin treatment prevented this increase in proteinuria.

Figures 3 and 4 represent glomeruli from control and insulin-treated KK mice. The glomerulus from the control mouse (Figure 3) shows marked increase in mesangial matrix with widening of the mesangial space when compared to the glomerulus from insulin-treated KK mouse (Figure 4), which shows less deposition of mesangial matrix without widening of the mesangial space.

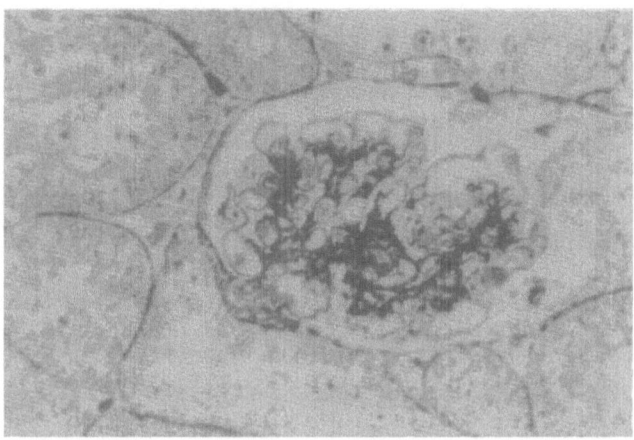

Figure 3. Representative glomerulus from saline-treated KK mouse (40 days of age). Note severe increase in mesangial matrix deposition. Silver methenamine X 1,000.

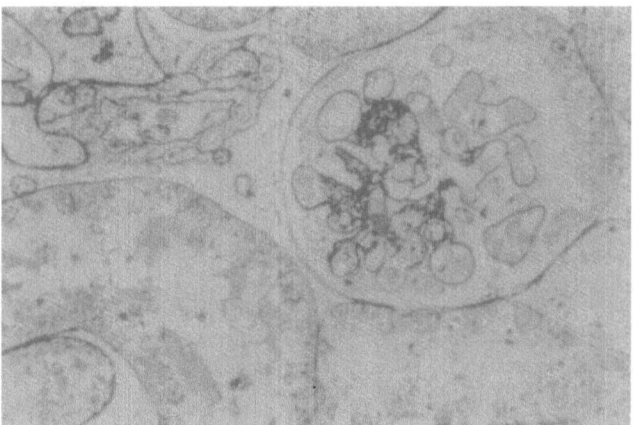

Figure 4. Representative glomerulus from insulin-treated KK mouse (40 days of age). Note improvement in the accumulation of mesangial matrix compared to the glomerulus in Figure 3. Silver methenamine X 1,000.

DISCUSSION

The pathogenesis of diabetic nephropathy is not clearly understood.

Hyperglycemia and/or insulin deficiency or defective insulin action seem to be responsible for kidney complications in diabetic human beings. Indeed, studies in animals have provided strong evidence in support of this hypothesis. Strict metabolic control is, therefore, advocated as a preventive and therapeutic measure in the management of diabetes and its complications. The results of the present study support the thesis that short-term insulin therapy with improved glycemic control can reduce proteinuria and prevent the development of glomerulosclerosis. The protective effect of insulin in glomerular changes has been reported in both spontaneous and drug-induced diabetic rats (1-6).

How good glycemic control prevents proteinuria and glomerulosclerosis remains conjectural. It is possible that glucose control improves systemic and glomerular hypertension, alters renal glycoprotein metabolism and affects enzymatic and nonenzymatic glycosylation reactions of glomerular and serum proteins. Our studies show that enzymes involved in renal glycoprotein synthesis and degradation are altered in diabetic kidneys and glycemic control improves these enzyme alterations. Preliminary results suggest that insulin treatment increases the activity of N-acetyl-B-glucosaminidase, an enzyme involved in glycoprotein degradation, in KK mice. Removal of glycoprotein material from the kidney seems partly responsible for less glomerulosclerosis seen in insulin-treated KK mice (7).

In summary, our data suggest that early insulin therapy with good glycemic control prevents glomerulosclerosis and reduced proteinuria in KK mice. Also, the data provide evidence that early treatment with good glucose control seems warranted in the prevention of diabetic nephropathy.

REFERENCES

1. Fox, C.J., Darby, S.C., Ireland, J.T., Sonksen, P.H., 1977, Blood glucose control and glomerular capillary basement membrane thickening in experimental diabetes. Br Med J 2: 605-607.

2. Tchobroutsky, G, 1979, Prevention and treatment of diabetic nephropathy. Adv Nephrol, 1979, 8: 63-86.

3. Wehner, H., Kosters, W., Strauch, M., Staudenmeir, M., 1980, Effect of islet transplantation on the glomerular changes in Streptozotocin-diabetic rats. Virchows Arch A Pathol Anat Histol 388: 137-154.

4. Mauer, S.M., Steffes, M.W., Brown, D.M., 1981, The kidney in diabetes. Am J Med 70: 603-612.

5. Rasch, R, 1981, Studies on the prevention of glomerulopathy in diabetic rats. Acta Endocrinol 97 (suppl. 242): 43-44.

6. Cohen, A.J., McGill, P.D., Rossetti, R.G., Guberski, D.L., Like, A.A., 1987, Glomerulopathy in spontaneously diabetic rat. Impact of glycemic control. Diabetes 36: 944-951.

7. Reddi, A.S., Bloodworth, J.M.B., Jr., Velasco, C.A., Camerini-Davalos, R.A., 1988, Possible prevention of diabetic nephropathy in KK mice by Glipizide. Diabetes 37 (Suppl. 1): 247a. (Abstract).

DISCUSSION

P. BENNETT: I'm not sure I quite understand why the Chinese hamsters given insulin developed hyperglycemia earlier.

G. GRODSKY: Well, it's easy because we really don't know the details of what goes on, only that one has to emphasize that it's during that critical growth period that an additional supply of fuels into the animals tissue seems to be extremely critical on what happens later. We don't know if that's down regulation at the receptor level or post receptor or what.

H. GLEICHMANN: Even in the NIDDM patients there are reports that early treatment with insulin helps the beta cell to recover faster and not to develop more hyperglycemia or insulin resistance.

SOME CHARACTERISTICS OF CHEMICALLY-INDUCED BETA-CELL LESIONS AS POSSIBLE CONTRIBUTING FACTORS IN DIABETES

¶Gerold M. Grodsky and Janice L. Bolaffi

Metabolic Research Unit, University of California, San Francisco

It is generally accepted that the prediabetic state in IDDM is characterized by a progressive attack on the B cells, resulting in eventual B-cell death, and overt diabetes. The immune system, viruses or toxic chemicals in the environment may be involved. However, little is known how: chemical agents, possibly arising from these sources, are lethal to the B cell; these effects are propagated; and eventually how the target B cell can be protected from such chemical attacks.

Streptozotocin (Sz) is a well-established diabetogenic agent with highly specific B-cell toxicity, both in vivo and in vitro. (Reviewed in 1--3). The present report will emphasize two characteristics of Sz's action on B cells that suggest its continued importance as a model substance for production of chemically induced B-cell lesions:

1) In addition to its well established immediate effects on the B cell to inhibit insulin secretion/synthesis, and induce plasma membrane changes (reviewed in 2--3), transient exposure to Sz also can cause a slow propagation of signal, leading to progressive B-cell destruction (3).

2) Toxicity of Sz can be completely prevented by nicotinamide and related nucleotides. A possible role of nucleotides to prevent other forms of diabetes is suggested (4-5), indicating they can have a broad positive effect on B-cell viability. In our systems, we find the natural nucleotide, thymidine, to be more protective than nicotinamide or methyl nicotinamide (2). Some of the studies with thymidine as a protective agent are summarized in this presentation.

METHODS

In Vitro Experiments.

Islets were isolated from pancreata of male rats (300-350 g) by collagenase, and continuously perifused for 24 hours as previously described (3). Perifusion conditions were controlled by a computer-programmable perifusion apparatus (APS-1000, Endotronics, Inc.). Perifusate consisted of a fully defined media, HB 104 (Hana Biologics, Alameda, CA) containing .7%

This work was supported by grants from NIH (DK 01410) and by the Diabetes Research and Education Foundation.

339

BSA with no insulin. Media was continuously gassed (5% CO_2/95% O_2) and perifused at flow rates of 6 ml/hr. Perifusate effluent and acid alcohol extracts of 0 and 24-hour islets were frozen for subsequent insulin assay. Net insulin production was determined as total recovered insulin in effluent media plus final islet content, minus original islet content, and reported as percent of initial content.

Islets were preincubated in a shaking incubator for 45 min in Krebs-Ringer, HEPES buffer, containing 2 mM glucose (2). In protection experiments, incubation was continued for 20 minutes in fresh buffer containing thymidine (20 mM). Sz, freshly dissolved in 1 mM citrate buffer, pH 4.5, was added to a final concentration of 2 mM. After 20-min incubation with Sz, with or without thymidine, islets were washed and transferred to the perifusion apparatus.

In experiments, employing as secretagogue, phorbol ester in the complete absence of glucose, or those involving measurement of NAD, islets were pre-treated as above, but subsequently stimulated in batch for one hour in KRB-HEPES media.

In other experiments, islets were cultured in RPMI-1640 + 10% FCS and antibiotics, as described (3). Media was changed daily over four days. Details for determination of islet cell number and volume were given (3).

NAD was measured by the method of Jacobson and Jacobson (2,). Islet extracts and media insulin were assayed by IRI, using rat insulin standards.

In Vivo Experiments

Streptozotocin-induced diabetes. Sz, dissolved in cold, 0.1 M citrate buffer, pH 4.5, was injected into the tail vein of lightly restrained animals at a dosage of 50 mg/kg body weight. The second set of animals were similarly treated, except that thymidine, 65 mg/animal) was injected i.p. at 90 and 30 minutes pre Sz, and 60 min post Sz. This dosage of thymidine was administered twice daily through day 16 and then discontinued. Urinary glucose, blood glucose, an body weight were monitored periodically over the subsequent 102 days. Animals were considered diabetic if urinary glucose values were plus 2 (Diastix test strips, Miles Labs, Elkart, IN) or if fasting plasma glucose exceeded 200 mg/dl (11.1 mM).

Spontaneously occurring diabetes. BB rats (Department of Pathology, University of Massachusetts, Worcester, MA) were injected twice daily with saline or thymidine from ages 34 to 104 days with the following thymidine dose per injection; 30 mg, days 34-41; 40 mg, days 42-48; 50 mg, days 49-104).

RESULTS

Figure 1 shows the characteristic release when islets were continuously perifused at 11 mM glucose for 24 hours. First phase insulin release in these experiments was not distinguished since all fractions were collected at 20-minute intervals. As previously reported (6), there was a progressive increase in insulin secretion during the first two to three hours of stimulation, a phenomenon that reflects time-dependent potentiation of the secretory mechanism. Subsequently, there was a spontaneous decrease in insulin release to a new steady state level of 10-20% of peak secretion, which is referred to as the desesnsitized phase. If islets were pretreated with Sz for 20 min prior to initiating stimulation, secretion was immediately inhibited, and inhibition was sustained throughout the 24-hour period. In contrast to normal islets, the Sz pretreated islets no longer responded to an added glucose stimulus at the 24th hour. Total insulin production was reduced by prior Sz from an increment of 67.8 down to 4.8% of initial islet content (Figure 1). Thus, Sz inhibits both secretion and net synthesis in this experimental system.

We previously observed that phorbal ester, is an effective secretagogue in the complete absence of glucose (2). Figure 2 shows that insulin secretion stimulated by phorbol ester alone, was also strongly inhibited by Sz. Thus, inhibition of insulin secretion by Sz is not restricted just to the effects of glucose or glucose-dependent secretagogues.

Figure 3 illustrates the effect of a one-hour preexposure of islets to Sz on the loss of islet cell volume during subsequent culture over four days. In this fully in vitro system, there was a progressive loss of islet cell volume during the experimental period to about 40% of initial values. Islet cell number also decreased to about 65% (3). In contrast, islets not exposed to Sz were maintained in culture with little loss of islet tissue. It is emphasized that the loss of cell mass was not simply the reflection of an early cell death followed by a progressive disappearance of cytoskeletal structure during prolonged culture. As we have previously shown (3), at each time period measured, the remaining islets, were fated for destruction, but were still "alive" in the sense that they continued to exclude trypan blue. Insulin secretion and production/islet was consistently inhibited throughout (3).

The naturally occurring nucleotide, thymidine, when added shortly before Sz, completely prevented Sz's inhibitory effects on glucose-stimulated insulin secretion (Figure 1). Secretion was restored to normal throughout

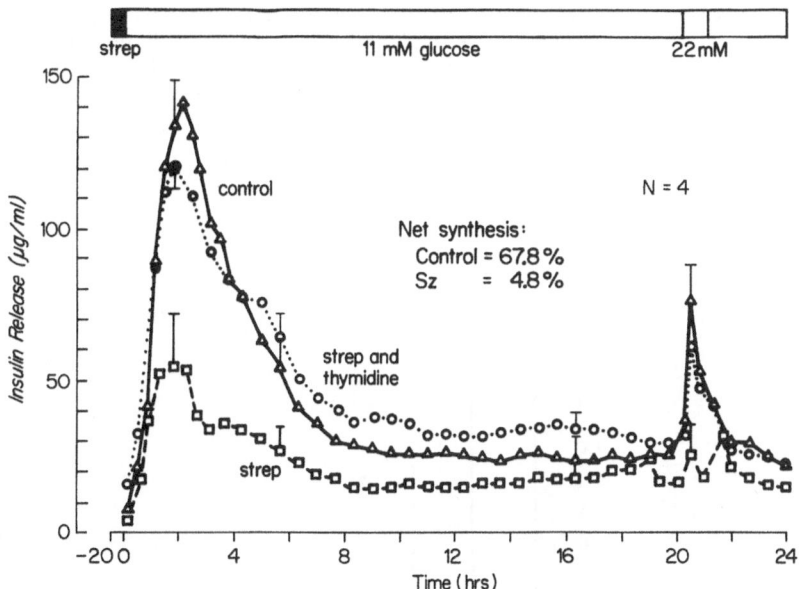

Figure 1. Effect of Sz, with and without thymidine, on insulin secretion and synthesis during continuous perifusion with glucose for 24 hours. Islets were pretreated with Sz in batch for 20 min, then perifused in HANA media. In other experiments, thymidine was present 20 min before and throughout the period of pretreatment with Sz. Δ———Δ , control, pretreatment with saline only; □— —□ pretreatment wth Sz, O········O pretreatment with Sz plus thymidine.

the 24-hour perifusion test period, including both the potentiation and de-sensitization phase. In other studies, islet response to glucose-forskolin, and to phorbol ester, were similarly normalized by thymidine (2).

Thymidine also prevented the characteristic rapid drop of islet cell NAD (Figure 4). At the doses used to block Sz action, thymidine, alone, had no direct effect on either insulin secretion or NAD levels, (Figure 4).

Thymidine, given two times daily, prevented Sz-induced diabetes in rats, (Figure 5). Approximately 70% of the animals in the thymidine-Sz group were normoglycemic for at least 70 days; half of the total group remained non-diabetic throughout the 111 days of the study. The other 30% expressed a rapid onset of hyperglycemia identical to the animals treated with Sz alone, and remained unprotected. Interestingly, some of the animals, with normal glucose levels in the first 70 days, slowly proceeded into hyperglycemia, indistinguishable from the animals treated with streptozotocin alone. These animals were considered to be partially protected, but subject to progressive impairment of glucose homeostasis. Urine sugars and body weights of individual animals paralleled the degree of protection reflected by the blood sugars (data not shown). Normal controls treated with thymidine over the same period remained euglycemic, had typical weight gain (increase of 212 grams), and showed no obvious ill effects of the thymidine treatment. The time of administration of thymidine prior to Sz was critical; in a group of five animals, administration of thymidine 140 and 80 minutes prior to Sz, instead of the 90 and 30 minutes used in the standard protocol, resulted in no protection.

In a pilot study, in which thymidine was injected twice daily to BB rats through the critical period of 34 to 104 days of age, neither the time of onset nor severity of hyperglycemia, were affected. In controls, and thymidine-treated animals, onset of hyperglycemia (glucose greater than 200 mg/dl, 11.1 mM) ranged between 73 and 104 days with no difference between the two groups. Final blood sugars averaged 302 ± 48 mg/dl, 16.8 ± .3 mM for controls and 283 ± 60 mg/dl, 15.7 ± .3 mM for the thymidine-treated animals.

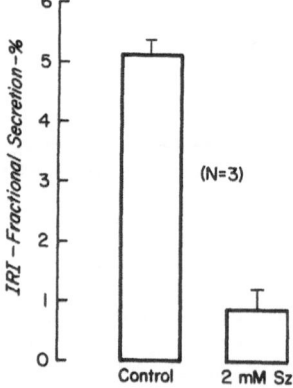

Figure 2. Effect of pretreatment by Sz to inhibit insulin secretion stimulated by phorbol ester, 10^{-7} M, in KRB-HEPES media containing no glucose. Data from (2).

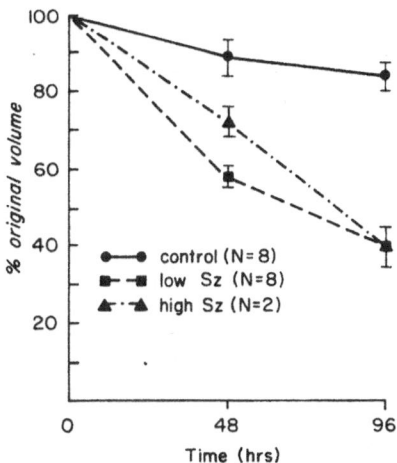

Figure 3. Relative changes in islet volume over four days
during culture of control and Sz-pretreated islets.
Sz was presented for one hour, followed by extensive
washing of islets, before initiating culture at 0 hr.
Figure from (3).

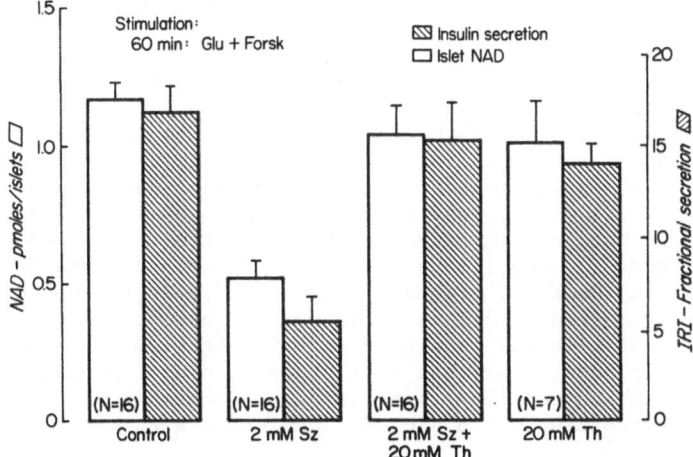

Figure 4. Effect of thymidine to protect against Sz-induced inhibition of insulin secretion and depletion of islet NAD. Islets were pretreated with Sz, or Sz and thymidine, and after
thorough washing, were stimulated in batch for one hour with
5 mM glucose and 25 uM forskolin in KRB-HEPES medium. Left
hand bar of each pair depicts islet NAD levels; right hand
bar depicts insulin secretion. Figure from (2).

343

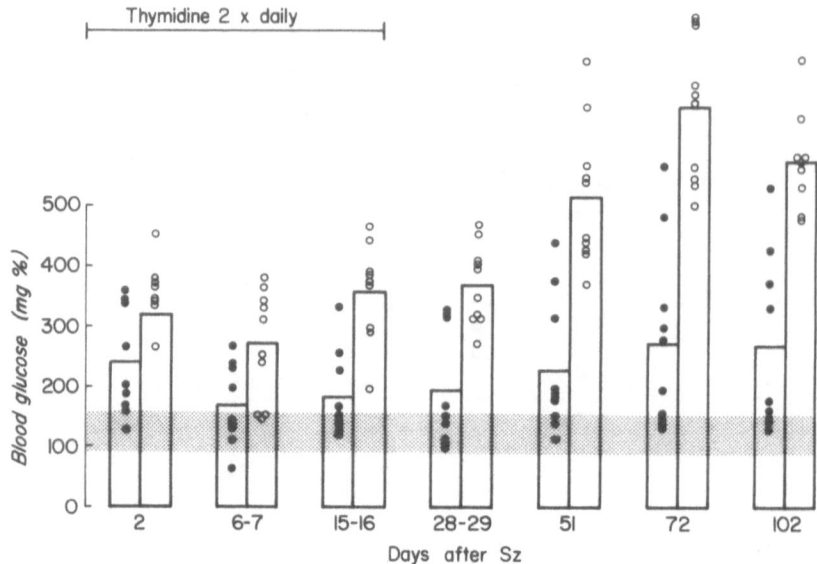

Figure 5. Effect thymidine to prevent hyperglycemia in rats
given a single diabetogenic dose of Sz. O SZ only,
● SZ + thymidine. Stippled area - range of fed blood
sugars in normal animals (5.4 to 8.8 mM).

DISCUSSION

The present studies illustrate two important features of Sz's action
on islet B cells that may have implications extending to other chemical
agents arising during B-cell attack by an altered immune system, virus,
toxic chemicals in the environment, etc.

The first feature is the time dependent killing of B cells which
continues long after the chemical has been removed. Our 24-hour perifusion experiments extend earlier observations by others indicating that
Sz causes a rapid and permanent inhibition of insulin secretion and total
insulin production. Early changes in plasma membrane function and structure (reviewed in 2,3) may account for the rapid impairment of insulin pro-
duction/secretion, but this impairment may not equate to cell death. As
previously reported (3), the islets were still capable of pumping trypan
blue. These islets, however, progressively "died" over a subsequent four
days in culture (measured as a loss of islet cell number and volume). Results are consistent with the possibility that islets may be lethally at-
tacked by brief exposure to Sz, but that there is a self-propagating killing of the cells which continues long after the chemical is removed, and
in an in vitro environment which excludes an immune attack.

This propagation of cell death over days or weeks after brief exposure to Sz has been observed in vivo as well, particularly when low doses
of Sz or new-born animals are used (Grodsky, unpublished observation, 7).
Our current observation that some of the animals partially protected
against Sz by thymidine may progress to severe diabetes after two months
of normal blood sugars may reflect the same phenomenon. The mechanism
by which transient injury by Sz could cause progressive injury to B cells

is unknown. Although a secondary immune attack could be a contributing factor in vivo, this cannot explain the results in our fully in vitro system. Sz is known to cause immediate, though transient, nicks in DNA, an increase in the DNA repair enzyme, poly (ADP-ribose) synthetase, and a decrease in the substrate, NAD (Reviewed in 2,3). Thus, changes in DNA, or gradual exhaustion of the DNA repair system, could deplete critical enzyme or substrate pools causing progressive cell death, However, NAD levels partially recover during culture of islets, suggesting that sustained NAD depletion is not the cause of progressive cell destruction (2). Evidence that Sz acts through free radical generation is inconclusive (reviewed in 2,3) but propagation of oxygen-radical formation in the lipid bilayers of beta cell membranes could occur. Recently, alkylation of cytosolic or membrane proteins has been implicated in Sz's action and this could also be a contributing factor (8).

This progression of beta cell death after a transient chemical attack is not restricted to the Sz model but may also extend to chemical mediators more closely associated with human diabetes. Thus, the exposure of islets to a mixture of lymphokines, in culture, causes an almost identical temporal pattern of progressive beta cell loss (Alex Rabinovitch, personal communication) as we (Figure 3) have observed with Sz. These data suggest that a useful approach to ameliorating an immune attack on beta cells in Type I diabetes could be by intervention at the level of the chemical mediators produced, or at their action on the target B cell.

Our current studies showing that the natural nucleotide, thymidine, can protect against Sz-induced B-cell toxicity emphasizes the well-established role that nicotinamide, and related nucleotides, have as protective agents on the beta cell. These agents are known to prevent the Sz-induced depletion of NAD, at least in part, by their action as inhibitors of poly (ADP)-ribose/synthetase (for example see Figure 4) (reviewed in 2,3).

The application of these nucleotides as protective agents for the beta cell also extends beyond the Sz model. Thus, nicotinamide can reduce the generation of diabetes in the partially pancreatectomized normal animal (4), and can partially prevent the spontaneous onset of diabetes in the NOD mouse (5). We were not able to prevent onset or intensity of diabetes in the BB rat with thymidine, similar to the lack of protection by nicotinamide observed by others (9). Possibly, there may be some unique differences between diabetes in these two animal models. Most interesting, though yet to be confirmed, is the report that nicotinamide extends the honeymoon period in the Type I human diabetic (10). The observation that nicotinamide can increase beta cell replication (measured by radioactive thymidine uptake) (11), suggests that these nucleotides may have positive effects on beta cell stability and regeneration.

Any clinical application of these agents, however, should be approached with caution since some may increase tumors in animals with reduced beta cell capacity or function. Although thymidine has been used as an anti-tumor agent, its tumor promoting characteristics in islet cells has not yet been studied. If thymidine is less tumorogenic than nicotinamide, it could prove useful in treatment of some forms of IDDM, precipitated by chemical, or immune attack.

REFERENCES

1. Wilson, G.L., Patton, N.J., McCord, J.M., Mullins, D.M., Mossman, B.T., 1984, Mechanism of streptozotocin- and alloxan-induced damage in rat B cells. Diabetologia 27: 587.

2. Bolaffi, J.L., Nagamatsu, S., Harris, J., Grodsky, G.M.. 1987, Protection by thymidine, an inhibitor of polyadenosine diphosphate ribosylation, of streptozotocin inhibition of insulin secretion. Endocrinology§ 120: 2117. § Figure from this article reproduced here with permission of The Endocrine Society.

3. Bolaffi, J.L., Nowlain, R.E., Cruz, L., Grodsky, G.M., 1986, Progressive damage of cultured pancreatic islets after single early exposure to streptozotocin. Diabetes§ 35: 1027. §Figure from this article reproduced here with permission of American Diabetes Association, Inc.

4. Yonemura, Y., Takashima, T., Miwa, K., Miyazaki, I., Yamamoto, H., Okamoto, H., 1984, Amelioration of diabetes mellitus in partially depancreatized rats by poly (ADP-ribose) synthetase inhibitors. Evidence of islet B-cell regulation. Diabetes 33: 401.

5. Yamada, K., Nonaka, K., Hanafusa, T., Miyazaki, A., Toyoshima, H., Tarui, S., 1982, Preventive and therapeutic effects of large-dose nicotinamide injections on diabetes associated with insulitis. An observation in non-obese diabetic (NOD) mice. Diabetes 31: 749.

6. Bolaffi, J.L., Heldt, A., Lewis, L.D., Grodsky, G.M., 1986, The third phase of in vitro insulin secretion; evidence for glucose insensitivity. Diabetes 35: 370.

7. Riley, W.J., McConnel, T.J., Maclaren, N.K., McLaughlin, J.V., Taylor, G., 1981, The diabetogenic effects of streptozotocin in mice are prolonged and inversely related to age. Diabetes 30: 718.

8. Wilson, G.L., Hartig, P.C., Patton, N.J., LeDoux, S.P., 1988, Mechanisms of nitrosourea-induced B-cell damage: activation of poly (ADP-ribose) synthetase and cellular distribution, Diabetes 37: 213.

9. Rossini, A.A., Mordes, J.P., Gallins, D.L., Like, A.A. 1983, Hormonal and environmental factors in the pathogenesis of BB rat diabetes. Metabolism (Suppl 1) 32:33.

10. Vague et al., 1987, Nicotinamide may extend remission phase in insulin-dependent diabetes. Lancet, 14: 619.

11. Sander, S., Andersson, A., 1986, Long-term effects of exposure of pancreatic islets to nicotinamide in vitro on DNA synthesis, metabolism and B-cell function. Diabetologia 29: 199.

EFFECTS OF IMMUNOSUPPRESSION WITH CYCLOSPORINE ON BETA CELL FUNCTION AND CLINICAL REMISSION IN VERY EARLY OVERT TYPE I DIABETES

¶J. Dupre and C.R. Stiller

University of Western Ontario, London, Ontario, Canada

The hypothesis that insulin-dependent diabetes mellitus (IDDM) in man results from destruction of the pancreatic beta cells by an autoimmune process was prompted by circumstantial evidence. The association of IDDM with markers of the major histocompatibility complex suggests that genetic factors are important in determining susceptibility to the disease, and indicates possible involvement of the immune system. Antibody-mediated and cell-mediated immunological phenomena are demonstrable in high-risk subjects in the pre-clinical phase, and in patients with early overt disease. The histology of the Islets of Langerhans was consistent with an inflammatory immune attack. The hypothesis was strengthened by recognition that IDDM can occur in animals as the result of an autoimmune attack on the pancreatic beta cells, and that the process in animals can be prevented by immunomodulatory interventions. On this background, and with growing experience of the use of immunosuppressive drugs in organ transplantation, clinical trials of immunotherapy early in the course of overt IDDM have been undertaken. This summary deals with the now substantial experience with Cyclosporine as the immunosuppressive agent.

Immunotherapy with Cyclosporine in Insulin-Dependent Diabetes Mellitus

Studies of endogenous secretion of insulin in patients receiving conventional insulin therapy for IDDM showed that beta cell function commonly increases from very low levels at the time of diagnosis to values in the low-normal range, spontaneously or as a result of administration of the insulin, with an optimum three or four months after diagnosis (1). This coincides with the nadir of insulin dosage, and of glycohemoglobin in the blood. Historical experience shows that remission of IDDM to a condition in which target metabolic control can be maintained without administration of insulin sometimes occurs, although the rate of such remissions at one year following diagnosis is < 10% in conventionally-treated patients (2). The rationale for studies with immunosuppressive agents in man was that benefit might accrue from suppression of the hypothetical autoimmune attack on the beta cells, with improvement of endogenous secretion of insulin, of metabolic control, and with an increase in the rate of clinical remissions. It is also possible that such effects might modify the long term course of the disease and its complications.

Definitions of Remission of Insulin-Dependent Diabetes Mellitus

The term "remission" has been used to describe the phase of amelioration of the diabetes in the early months after diagnosis, when the dose of

TABLE I

FREQUENCY OF EARLY REMISSION OF DIABETES,
ACCORDING TO SELECTED CHARACTERISTICS AT ENTRY

	ALL PATIENTS (N = 40)	PATIENTS NOT NEEDING INSULIN AT 4 Mo (N = 27)	PATIENTS NEEDING INSULIN AT 4 Mo (N = 13)
	no. of patients	*no. of patients (% in remission)*	
Duration of polyuria (days)			
<30	25	20 (80)	5 (20)
30–90	15	7 (47)	8 (53)
Weight loss (% of body weight)			
<5	18	18 (100)	0
5–10	15	8 (53)	7 (47)
>10	7	1 (14)	6 (86)
Ketoacidosis			
Without	29	24 (83)	5 (17)
With	11	3 (27)	8 (73)
Hemoglobin A_{1c} (%)			
<10	9	8 (89)	1 (11)
10–13	26	19 (73)	7 (27)
>13	5	0	5 (100)

insulin required diminishes temporarily, and when administration of insulin can be interrupted in some patients.

Open Studies with Cyclosporine in Insulin-Dependent Diabetes Mellitus

In the light of experience with Cyclosporine in organ transplantation, and of studies in the BB rat which demonstrated that this agent can prevent diabetes in this animal model, Cyclosporine was tested in pilot (open) clinical trials in recent-onset IDDM in man. In the first of these studies Cyclosporine was given in an initial dose of 10 mg/kg/day, with adjustment to maintain serum trough levels in the range 150-200 ng/ml (polyclonal RIA) in patients with IDDM of less than one year's duration. There was an unexpectedly high rate of remission to a non-insulin-receiving state (maintained target control of glycemia < 7.8 mmol/L ac meals), with 40% of patients in this condition at one year. Glucagon-stimulated C-peptide levels (CP) in the plasma rose and were maintained in the mean in the physiological range to 12 months of treatment. These effects appeared to be unprecedented since patients who entered the study with overt diabetes of more than two months duration showed no clinical response, entry of patients who had been receiving insulin through a longer interval was discontinued. The continuing experience, in which the great majority of the patients were aged nine years or more at the time of clinical diagnosis, was consistent with the initial report, and led to a number of conclusions regarding the characteristics of patients likely to respond to Cyclosporine. Non-insulin-receiving remission was more frequent in patients who had been on insulin therapy for not more than three weeks at entry. The chances of remission were greater in patients aged 16 years or more, at entry, than in younger patients. The outcome did not correlate with the CP level in the plasma at entry, or with the presence or absence of islet cell antibodies in the blood. It was also shown in the Canadian Open Study that interruption of treatment with Cyclosporine after one year in NIR (non-insulin receiving remission) patients, or after as long a period as 44 months, was followed by relapse of such remissions within a few weeks. The results of an open study with Cyclosporine in France were similar, in terms of clinical remissions as defined by the insulin treatment status. The clinical and biochemical adverse effects of Cyclosporine observed in these studies were not different from those in other experiences, and were reversible within weeks of discontinuation of the drug.

A further open study employing Cyclosporine in children with IDDM of recent onset has been reported. Cyclosporine dosage was adjusted so that the whole blood trough level was maintained at 150-350 ng/ml (polyclonal RIA). This regimen did not result in significant effects on kidney function. Most of the patients were entered within two months of onset of symptoms and within two weeks of the start of insulin therapy. Among 42 children aged seven to fifteen years, 67% were in non-insulin-receiving remission at four months, and 45% were in such remission at twelve months. Patients who remitted were characterized by a lesser degree of weight loss, a lower initial hemoglobin A1C level, and lower frequency of ketoacidosis on entry (Table I). The findings suggested that high rates of remission can be in-

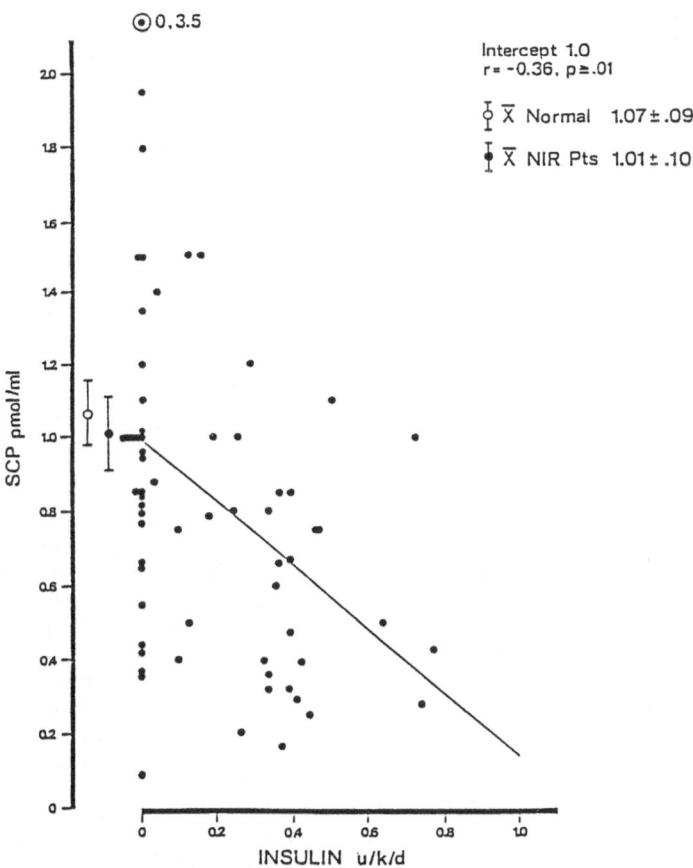

Figure 1. Plasma CP levels (SCP) and concurrent daily insulin dose in invididual patients tested at 3 months of Cs treatment. The solid symbol with bars indicates the mean ± SEM for all NIR patients. The open symbol with bars indicates the mean ± SEM in 22 normal subjects.

349

duced even in young children, when the intervention is made very soon after development of overt disease. It was also found that the response of CP in the plasma to stimulation of glucagon was higher in those who entered remission than in those who did not. There were no differences between remitting and non-remitting patients with respect to age, sex, HLA phenotype, the presence or absence of antibodies to insulin or islet cell antigens, or the blood levels of Cyclosporine.

Endocrine Metabolic Status in IDDM in Remission

Many patients in NIR remission as defined exhibit glucagon-stimulated CP levels in the blood within the normal range. Serial determinations of Glucagon-stimulated CP in all patients receiving Cyclosporine in the Canadian Open Study showed that patients in NIR remission exhibited a mean glucagon-stimulated CP value that was not different from normal, though the variance was wider in the diabetic subjects (Figure 1). The overlap of glucagon-stimulated CP values between patients who entered NIR remissions and those who did not was considerable.

These studies also show that the release of immunoreactive insulin and C-peptide into the blood is virtually absent during intravenous infusion of glucose in patients in NIR remission. On ingestion of glucose there were grossly obtunded increases of the levels of insulin and CP by comparison with those in normal subjects. However the responses of insulin and CP to ingestion of a standardized mixed meal (Sustacal) were substantially greater.

Thus it appears that patients in remission show an abnormality of response to glucose similar to that described in the pre-clinical phase of the disease in high-risk siblings of diabetic patients (3). Therefore it seems that patients in remission revert to a condition similar to that of those in the "immediately pre-clinical" phase of the disease. It is also pointed out that patients in NIR remission maintain normal range levels of immunoreactive insulin in the blood in the post-absorptive and fed states.

Findings in Randomized Control Trials with Cyclosporine

The first randomized control trial with Cyclosporine in IDDM was completed by a multicentre study group in France. In this trial 122 patients were randomized to treatment with Cyclosporine or placebo. The protocol required continued administration of insulin, with minimization of the dose as consistent with target control of glycemia, and blinding of the managers of the diabetes to the nature of the study drug. Cyclosporine was administered in pre-determined dosage, without adjustment on the basis of blood levels, initially at 7.5 mg/kg/day. The Cyclosporine was increased to 10 mg/kg after three months if the insulin dose exceeded 50% of that given. So-called "complete remission" was recognized when blood glucose levels were maintained < 7.8 mmol/L before meals, and < 11.1 mmol/L after meals, with glycohemoglobin levels = < 7.5% (upper limit of normal 5.8%) without administration of insulin. Partial remission was recognized when similar metabolic control was acheived with insulin dosage - < .25 U/kg/day. After six months, administration of cyclosporine was discontinued in patients who showed no remission, while patients in remission continued to take cyclosporine, the dose of which was decreased by 20% monthly, to reach 5 mg/kg/day before nine months. The "complete remission" rates at nine months were 24% in the Cyclosporine-treated groups and 6% in the placebo-treated group (p < 0.1). When the findings were examined in relation to the observed blood levels of Cyclosporine it was found that many Cyclosporine-patients had levels in the range considered to be subtherapeutic on the basis of experience in organ transplantation (< 300 ng/ml whole blood trough levels polyclonal RIA, Table II). At six and nine months the

TABLE II

INCIDENCE OF REMISSIONS ACCORDING TO INITIAL
CYCLOSPORIN BLOOD TROUGH LEVEL*

—	Placebo	CyA < 300 ng/ml	CyA ≥ 300 ng/ml
Complete remission			
6 mo	20·8"„ (11/53)	25·0"„ (3/12)	37·5"„ (12/32)
9 mo	6·8"„ (3/44)	16·7"„ (2/12)	37·0"„ (10/27)
Partial or complete remission			
6 mo	32·1"„ (17/52)	25·0"„ (3/12)	65·6"„ (21/32)
9 mo	15·9"„ (7/44)	25·0"„ (3/12)	55·6"„ (15/27)

*CyA = Cyclosporin. Mean of 5 determinations (days 7 and 15, months 1, 2, and 3), corresponding to cyclosporin dosage of 7·5 mg/kg per day. Patients who had cyclosporin determination on plasma and drop-out patients are not taken into account.

"complete" remission rate was 37% in patients with mean serum trough levels > 300 ng/ml through the first three months, compared to 20% and 7% respectively in the placebo-group patients. This study demonstrated that Cyclosporine can induce remissions of Type I diabetes. Observations on the insulin secretory status, and on the later clinical course of patients in remission in this study, were not presented. The administration of cyclosporine was associated with increases of serum creatinine levels, but no unexpected untoward effects were recorded.

PERCENTAGE OF PATIENTS NIR

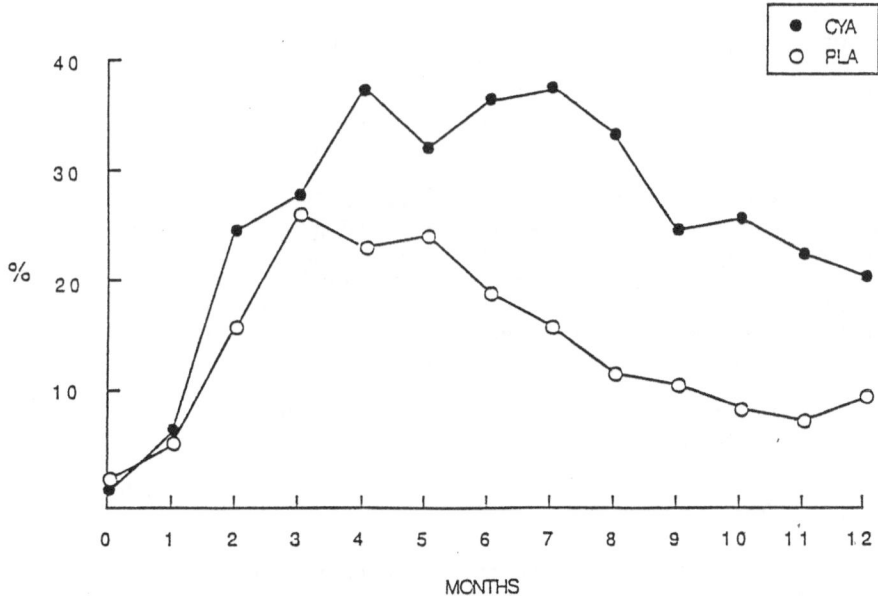

Figure 2. NIR remission rates in the cyclosporine and placebo-treated groups of patients at intervals through one year.

The Canadian-European Randomized Control Trial with Cyclosporine

In this study 188 patients with ketonuric IDDM were entered within 14 weeks of onset of symptoms, and with no more than six weeks of treatment with insulin. Patients ranged in age from nine years to 35 years, but 86% of patients were 16 years or older. The study was designed to examine the effects of Cyclosporine on remissions and on beta cell function through a period of one year. A clinical definition of non-insulin-receiving remission required target control of glycemia without administration of insulin (plasma glucose concentrations 7.8 mmol/L or less before breakfast, i.e. below the level diagnostic of diabetes). A compound definition of remission required either the non-insulin-receiving state as defined or a glucagon-stimulated C-peptide level in the plasma = > 0.6 nmol/L. The initial dose of Cyclosporine was 10 mg/kg/day, and this was adjusted to produce trough levels equivalent to 400-600 ng/ml of whole blood (polyclonal RIA). The dose of Cyclosporine was reduced if serum creatinine levels increased by more than 50 % of the entry value, or in response to other unacceptable adverse effects. Glycemic control was monitored by determinations of glycosylated hemoglobin levels, and beta cell function was assessed by determination of glucagon-stimulated CP levels in the plasma at three month intervals.

In this study the blood glycosylated hemoglobin levels were similar in the two treatment groups through the period of study, validating comparison of the remission rates. A highly significant increase in the rate of non-insulin-receiving (NIR) remission was observed in the cyclosporine-treated group. During the first three months of observation clinical remissions to the NIR state accumulated at similar rates in the two treatment groups, but from four months onwards the rate was higher in the Cylosporine-treated group (Figure 2). By six months NIR remission was present in 38% of cyclosporine-treated patients and 19% of placebo patients, and at 12 months the rates were 24% and 9% respectively. Multiple logistic regression analysis showed that these differences were statistically highly significant. Significant differences also existed between the rates of remission as described by the compound definition. It was further shown that a significantly greater increase in the response of plasma CP to stimulation with glucagon was present in cyclosporine-treated patients.

This trial confirmed the efficacy of cyclosporine in induction of clinical remissions in insulin-dependent diabetes mellitus, and showed for the first time that this is associated with enhancement of beta cell function. The results also indicated a striking relationship between the duration of diabetes at entry and the response to Cyclosporine (Table 3). Clinical remissions in the Cyclosporine-treated group were heavily concentrated among the 40% of patients who entered the study with less than two weeks of administration of insulin. The clinical and biochemical adverse effects of Cyclosporine in this trial were consistent with those reported in the open studies. Changes in calculated creatinine clearance agreed well with direct measurements of glomerular filtration rate in subsets of patients in the Cyclosporine and placebo groups, with mean reductions of calculated creatinine clearance of 20%, and of directly measured GFR of 21%, in the cyclosporine-treated group.

Magnitude and Significance of the Effect of Cyclosporine in Induction of Remissions of IDDM.

It may be noted that the rate of remission to the non-insulin-receiving state with satisfactory glycemic control was higher in the open studies than in the randomized control trials, at one year. While this may represent a "study effect" in the open condition, in the Canadian open study intensified Cyclosporinetherapy was used at the time of suspected relapse, and this was not the case in the randomized control trials, as a consequence of the blinding of investigators to treatment. It should also be noted that the relatively high remission rate in the Canadian open study may be related to the administration of an oral hypoglycemic agent in approximately 10% of the patients.

Safety of Immunosuppression with Cyclosporine in IDDM

The major concern with respect to toxicity of Cyclosporine remains its adverse effects on the kidney. The regimens employed in diabetes are similar to the longterm use of Cyclosporine in kidney tramsplantation. There is no definite evidence of progressive damage with cyclosporine in this experience. However recently it has been reporteed that histologic damage attributable to Cyclosporine in the transplanted kidney is related to the duration of treatment with the drug (5). In view of the importance of the question of nephrotoxicity, kidney biopsies were obtained from 17 volunteers taking part in the Canadian-European trial, and were evaluated together with 23 biopsies from other patients in studies using similar protocols in France and Canada. Some biopsies showed histopathologic changes associated with administration of cyclosporine, though not specifically attributable to the drug. The lesions assessed were glomerular obsolescence or segmental focal sclerosis, artiolopathy, tubular atrophy, and interstitial fibrosis, rated on 5-point scales. The median score for glomerular change was zero, but one biopsy showed abnormalities in more than 10% of glomeruli. The commonest finding was interstitial fibrosis, with a median score of "slight." The median score for tubular atrophy was "minimal-slight;" this abnormality was the only one that correlated with trough levels of Cyclosporine in the blood. Tubular atrophy showed a median score of "minimal" in biopsies from patients in whom the mean Cyclosporine trough levels had been less than the approximate median value for the studies. The findings suggested that an upper limit of 400 ng/ml whole blood (polyclonal RIA) for the 12-hour trough levels of cyclosporine should minimize the occurrence of structural damage. This is supported by findings in the recent open study with Cyclosporine in children in France, in which the upper limit of Cyclosporine level in the blood was 350 ng/ml (polyclonal RIA), and in which no definite functional or structural adverse effects on the kidney were observed. Preliminary experience in open studies of a remission induction regimen employing similar dosage of Cyclosporine, but with short-term administration of anti-inflammatory glucocorticoid (methylprednisolone 1.25 grams within three days of entry) suggests that this regimen too can induce remissions in the absence of demonstrable adverse effect on the kidney (6). Thus it appears that doses of Cyclosporine which are not demonstrably nephrotoxic can induce high rates of remission in IDDM.

Recognition and Management of Relapse of Clinical Remissions In IDDM

The occurrence of relapses of Cyclosporine-induced remissions during the first year after diagnosis of IDDM is clearly of concern with respect to the possible clinical applicability of such treatment. Although experience of the effects of immunosuppression in IDDM of recent onset has emphasized the importance of very early intervention by showing that clinical remissions of the disease are very rarely induced by treatments initiated more than a few weeks from the onset of symptoms, it has also been noted in open studies that secondary remissions can be induced by immunotherapeutic treatment of relapse inferred from loss of glycemic control at intervals up to many months after diagnosis. Thus in the Canadian open study exploratory trials of alternative immunotherapies with agents other than Cyclosporine, which were undertaken in NIR patients at intervals exceeding one year from entry, resulted in loss of glycemic control with the

TABLE III

OUTCOME		6 MONTHS		12-MONTHS[3]	
		SHORT[1] (n)	LONG (n)	SHORT (n)	LONG (n)
NIR OR C-PEP $\geq$ 0.6 NMOL/L	CY	71.1 (38)	38.2 (55)	39.5 (38)	28.3 (53)
	PLA	31.6 (38)	30.4 (56)	16.2 (37)	23.6 (55)
	P	.001	.39	.02	.58
	P diff[2]		.02		.15
NIR	CY	55.3 (38)	27.3 (55)	31.6 (38)	18.9 (53)
	PLA	13.2 (38)	23.2 (56)	2.7 (37)	14.5 (55)
	P	.001	.62	.001	.55
	P diff[2]		.003		.06

[1]SHORT = $\leq$ 6 weeks symptoms and $\leq$ 2 weeks insulin, to entry

[2]P value for difference in treatment effect between short duration and long duration subsets

[3]The minor discrepancies between numbers of subjects in the two response groups are accounted for by data falling outside predetermined time windows.

need to resume insulin treatment. However, on resumption of protocol therapy with Cyclosporine, NIR remissions were retrieved in 60% of cases (4). Furthermore preliminary experience with the experimental remission induction therapy employing Methylprednisolone and Cyclosporine described above has shown that remissions can be retrieved by this means in a proportion of cases (6). Further experience in the treatment of relapse of immunotherapeutically-induced remissions in IDDM is clearly important to possible advances in this approach to the disease.

Duration of Immunotherapy in IDDM

With respect to the duration of treatment, the available information strongly suggests that longterm immunomodulatory therapies will be necessary for maintenance of remissions in IDDM. This is indicated not only by the relatively short-term experience in experimental immunosuppression in IDDM of recent onset, with the demonstrable likelihood of relapse on interruption of therapy at intervals from one to four years from initiation of immunosuppression, but also by experience of segmental transplantation in discordant identical twins.

DISCUSSION

The efficacy of immunosuppression with Cyclosporine in enhancement and preservation of beta cell function and in induction of clinical remissions has been clearly demonstrated. It has been shown that these effects are most likely to occur in patients with very recent onset diabetes mellitus. Moreover, the insulin secretory capacity of patients in remission suggests that a substantial functional beta cell mass is preserved. These findings, which strongly support the autoimmune hypothesis for B cell damage in human diabetes, and the rationale for continuing exploration of immunomodulatory therapies can be considered as the first stage in this approach to effective intervention potentially capable of changing the course of the disease. The present objective of clinical research with this categorically experimental treatment is optimization of the remission induction therapy. The importance of prompt action early in the overt disease indicates the need for studies of other treatments that have proved effective in management of analogous "immunorejection" crises. Preliminary studies with high-dose glucocorticoid therapy (6) or with antibodies directed towards immunoreactive lymphocytes, have been presented (7). There is a need to test various therapies for maintenance of remissions, and to explore the recognition and treatment of relapse.

REFERENCES

1. Marner, B., Agner, T., Binder, C., Lernmark, A., Nerup, J., Mandrup-Oulsen, T., Walldorf, S., 1985, Increased reduction in fasting C-peptide is associated with islet cell antibodies in Type I (insulin-dependent) diabetic patients. Diabetologia 28: 875-880.

2. Drash, A.L., 1987, In: Clinical Care of the Diabetic Child, Year Book Medical Publications Inc., Chicago: 33-51.

3. Srikanta, S., Ganda, O.P., Eisenbarth, G.S., Soeldner, J.S., 1983, Islet-cell antibodies and beta-cell function in monozygotic triplets and twins initially discordant for Type I diabetes mellitus. N Engl J Med 308: 322-325.

4. Dupre, J., Stiller, C.R., Gent, M., Donner, A., Graffenried, B., Murphy, G., Heinrichs, D., Jenner, M.R., Keown, P.A., Laupacis, A., Mahon, J., Martell, R., Rodger, N.W., and Wolfe, B.M., 1988, Effects of Immuno-suppression with Cyclosporine in Insulin-Dependent Diabetes Mellitus of Recent Onset: The Canadian Open Study at 44 months. Transplantation Proceedings. Vol. XX, No. 3, Suppl. 4: 184-192.

5. Ruiz, P., Kolbech, P.C., Scroggs, M.W., Sanfilippo, F., 1988, Associations between Cyclosporine therapy and interstitial fibrosis in renal allograft biopsies. Transplantaion, 45: 91-95.

6. Dupre, J., Stiller, C.R., Gent, M., von Graffenried, B., Momah, C.I., Jenner, M., Wolfe, B.M., Mahon, J., Atkinson, P., 1988, Shortterm Methylprednisolone combined with nephrotoxic doses of cyclosporine induces high rates of remission in Type I diabetes. Proceedings International Confereence, Immunointervention in Autoimmune Diseases.

7. Assan, R., 1988, The Use of Cyclosporine in Adult Type I Diabetes. Proceedings International Conference, Immunointervention in Autoimmune Diseases.

IMMUNOMODULATION OF PRE-DIABETES IN BB RATS
FOR PREVENTION OF THE DISEASE

J.F. Markmann, A. Naji, C.F. Barker, and K.L. Brayman
Department of Surgery, University of Pennsylvania School of Medicine
Philadelphia. PA

The use of insulin therapy in the treatment of diabetes was naturally heralded as a cure for this otherwise lethal malady (1). It has now become apparent that, although insulin therapy avoids the acute morbidity and mortality associated with the disease, it allows those afflicted to develop a host of chronic debilitating complications. To eliminate such complications it seems likely that more refined treatment modalities and/or effective disease prevention strategies will be necessary, and that this will require further understanding the pathogenesis of insulin dependent diabetes mellitus (IDDM).

Perhaps the first step in elucidating the disease process was made in 1901. The histological observations made by Opie at this time indicated that specific destruction of the pancreatic islets of Langerhans was correlated with diabetes mellitus (2). With further studies, lymphocytic infiltration of the pancreatic islets became recognized as a pathognomonic finding for the insulin dependent form of diabetes mellitus (3). In the 1940's, the characteristic histological lesion of IDDM was identified and appropriately denoted insulitis, which can be translated literally as an inflammation of the islands.

A major advancement in understanding the pathogenesis of IDDM is the consensus, reached only within the last decade, that the disease results from an autoimmune response directed against the beta cells of the pancreatic islets (4). Findings supporting this assertion in reference to the human disease include the presence of anti-islet cell antibodies disease association with certain MHC alleles, and the fact that immunosuppression can attenuate or temporarily ablate the progression of beta cell loss (5).

Evidence implicating an autoimmune basis for the BB diabetes is even more compelling and has played a pivotal role in the general acceptance of the autoimmune etiology of human IDDM (6). As in the human disease, anti-islet cell auto antibodies and activated T lymphocytes (recognized by their class II positivity) are present and precede the onset of hyperglycemia. Another similarity to the human disease is that diabetic rats have a common allele at the rat MHC locus (RT1). Providing a basis for the later human trials was the finding that BB diabetes could be prevented by a variety of immunosuppressive protocols, including treatment with antilymphocyte serum (ALS), cyclosporin A (CsA) or monoclonal antibodies specific for lymphocyte determinants.

Interestingly, disease prevention is not limited to protocols that suppress the BB's immune system. In fact, diabetes can also be avoided by manipulation of pre-diabetic animals in ways that enhance their immune responsiveness. It is studies relying on this latter strategy which will be the focus of this chapter.

The consistent finding that diabetic BB rats are immunologically deficient naturally lead to consideration of the possibility that this aberration was a necessary predisposing factor for autoimmunity. It was hypothesized that the absence of normal immunoregulatory mechanisms in diabetic BB rats might produce an environment indifferent, if not conducive, to the initiation and propagation of an anti-beta cell autoimmune response. Recent results from a number of studies now lend support to this notion.

Genetic analyses, emplying breeding studies of BB diabetics with non diabetes prone animals indicate a strong association of the disease with the autosomal recessive allele that confer the BB's immune defect (7). Thus, it appears that in most cases the immunodeficiency is necessary for disease development. It should be mentioned that Like et al reported identification of a handful of immunocompetent animals in their colony in which diabetes apparently occurred (8). The significance of this observation is difficult to assess without an indepth evaluation of the immune system of such animals.

A second observation implying that the absence of a lymphoid population is relevant to disease predisposition is found in work studying cells bearing the RT6 alloantigen. Greiner et al first noted that diabetic BB lymphocytes were devoid of the population defined by anti RT6 antibodies (9). These normally comprise 50% of CD4+ and 70% of the CD8+ T cell subsets. Estimating the role of these cells in an autoimmune setting was initially difficult due to the paucity of information concerning the function of RT6+ lymphocytes in the normal immune system. However, subsequent studies demonstrated that diabetes could be induced in a non-immunodeficient, non diabetes prone subline of BB rats by selective depletion of RT6+ cells by monoclonal antibody immunotherapy. Thus it is tempting to speculate that RT6+ cells, which are lacking in diabetic BB rats, might normally play a role in suppressing autoimmunity.

Perhaps the most convincing evidence suggesting that the absence of normal immune regulation might be an important facet of BB diabetogenesis is found in work attempting to study the effect of immune reconstitution on the diabetogenic response. Two such strategies have been successfully utilized: 1) transfusions in the prediabetic period and 2) neonatal bone marrow transplantation.

Rossini et al first determined that whole blood transfusions from non-diabetes prone rats effectively prevented diabetes if administered in the prediabetic period (10). Further study of this model determined that the lymphocyte population within the whole blood inocula was apparently the protection conferring component. Moreover it was possible to demonstrate the presence of donor derived lymphocytes in the BB recipients weeks after completing the transfusion regimen indicating that immune chimerism had induced.

This documentation of donor strain lymphocytes implied that the BB had not rejected the transferred cells and suggested that the normal lymphocytes immunologically reconstituting the BB recipient might be serving a regulatory function. Subsequent work by the same group of investigators utilized lymphocyte populations fractionated into T cell subsets (10). Administration of relatively pure CD4+ T cells were fully capable of disease prevention. One drawback of this model is that it does not permit transfer of cells from a variety of donor strains. For example, whether MHC incompatible lymphocytes could also prevent disease in this model could not be effectively assessed because the BB recipient would mount an immune response and reject the foreign transfused cells. The use of lymphocyte transplantation to BB rats in the neonatal period circumvents this difficulty as described below.

The second protocol of immune intervention, bone marrow cell (bmc) transplantation to neonates has been a major focus of work in our laboratory. We have previously reported that injection of diabetes prone neonatal (< 24 hours of age) BB rats with WF(RT1^{u}MHC compatible with BB but differing in minor antigens) bmc strikingly reduced the incidence of spontaneous diabetes (11). These studies suggested that, for unknown reasons, transplantation of bmc from normal rats altered the BB's immune system in such a way to afford near complete protection from spontaneous diabetes.

We next investigated possbile mechanisms of the observed protection. It seemed likely that normal bone marrow could mature in BB rats, reverse the immunological abnormalities, and thereby shortcircuit autoimmune diabetogenesis. This was first tested by studying the immune status of tolerant BB rats by standard assays of immune function (12).

Diabetic BB rats are known to be severely T-lymphopenic as assessed by FACS analysis. Immunologically tolerant BB rats however display partial immune reconstitution as shown in Table 1. Both the CD4+ and CD8+ T cell subsets are found to be increased in number compared to levels observed in non tolerant diabetics. However, even tolerant rats are not fully restored when compared to normal (Lewis) rats. In addition we observed improved function of lymphocytes from tolerant hosts in _in vitro_ T cell dependent assays such as the MLR as compared to non tolerant diabetics.

TABLE 1

TWO COLOR IMMUNOFLOURESCENT ANALYSIS OF PERIPHERAL BLOOD LYMPHOCYTES

% Positive Cells[*]

Lymphocyte donor	Th (OX19$^+$, OX8$^-$)	NK (OX19$^-$, OX8$^+$)	Tc/s (OX19$^+$, OX8$^+$)
Lewis	45.3 ± 4.2	5.8 ± 3.2	19.6 ± 4.2
BB diabetic	5.4 ± 2.4	17.7 ± 10.4	1.6 ± 1.5
Tolerant BB diabetic	16.4 ± 3.5	13.6 ± 7.9	10.5 ± 3.8

* Mean percentage of positively stained cells ± Standard Deviation.

These results again support the hypothesis that the immune defect is an important prerequisite for diabetes, and that if reversed, autoimmunity can be avoided. A more precise understanding of the cellular components involved and the mechanisms by which they act should not only further our understanding of the disease process, but also, might suggest logical strategies for immune intervention during the prediabetic period in humans.

The first question we addressed was which component of the bone marrow inocula was responsible for disease prevention. We hypothesized that the T lymphocyte was a probable candidate because this cell type is the most profoundly reduced in immunodeficient BB rats. Unfractionated normal WF bone marrow could potentially supply BB recipients with T cells from either of 2 sources: 1) from T cell progenitors/stem cells that would develop into mature T cells following transfer and 2) from T cells that had already matured fully in the WF bmc donor animal and contaminated the bmc preparation. Differentiating these alternatives was of added interest because the former hinged on whether normal WF stem cells would develop normally in an abnormal BB milieu.

To digress momentarily, this particular issue was addressed in part by previous studies performed on our laboratory that examined adult irradiation chimeras (13). In these experiments BB marrow was transferred to lethally irradiated WF rats or in the reciprocal transfer. WF marrow was transplanted to irradiated BB recipients. The results of these experiments indicated that the marrow, not the irradiated recipient, determined the chimera's immune phenotype. For example, BB marrow produced an immunodeficient WF host and WF marrow fully reconstituted an irradiated BB recipient. The question addressed in the neonatal tolerance model differs importantly in that the BB recipient of the WF marrow is not irradiated.

Returning to the tolerance model, we therefore produced a bmc preparation devoid of contaminating mature T lymphocytes. This was accomplished by the use of standard techniques, as described previously (14). FACS analysis of the bmc preparation confirmed that 5% of cells expressed the T cell specific cell surface antigen CD5(OX-19$^+$). When T depleted WF marrow was injected into diabetes prone BB rats at birth, although a full state of immune tolerance developed, protection from autoimmunity did not result, as shown in Table 2. In addition, we found that transfer of 50×10^6 WF lymphocytes at 40 days of age in rats tolerant of T depleted marrow did not alter the course of the disease. Thus, already mature T lymphocytes are required for protection in this system, and they are apparently necessary at an early time point, at least prior to 40 days of age.

TABLE 2

EFFECT OF DEPLETING T LYMPHOCYTE FROM THE
MARROW INOCULA ON DIABETES INCIDENCE

Neonatal injection	Injection at 40d	# diabetic/total studied(%)	
		Injected	Controls
WF	None	2/58(3.4)	19/61(31.1)
WF T depleted	None	23/54(42.6)	22/52(42.3)
None	WF LNC	4/7 (57.1)	--
WF T depleted	WF LNC	18/51(35.2)	--

One possible explanation for the absence of disease prevention by T depleted marrow transfer ·was that normal mature WF T lymphocytes did not undergo normal maturation from the transplanted WF marrow stem cell following introduction into the BB environment. Indirect evidence supporting of this hypothesis is found in Table 3. As already mentioned, BB rats rendered tolerant of unfractionated WF bmc displayed at least partial restoration of their immune profiles, both quantitatively and functionally. However, BB rats injected at birth with marrow depleted of mature T lymphocytes showed no improvement in T cell number by FACS analysis. We infer from these data that T cell progenitors present in WF bone marrow are not able to develop successfully into mature T cells when relocated to immunodeficient BB rats. Further, it seems likely that this inability to mature normally is responsible for the ineffectiveness of T depleted marrow in disease prevention.

TABLE 3

THE EFFECT OF T DEPLETED WF MARROW TRANSPLANTATION
ON BB'S IMMUNODEFICIENCY

		% LNC Labelled With			
Status of BB	mAb:	OX19	W3/25	OX8	OX6
BB		28 ± 2	30 ± 2	6 ± 1	66 ± 4
BB tol WF(-T) bmc		26 ± 3	27 ± 3	7 ± 2	56 ± 4

We next sought to define the mechanism of action of protection conferring T cells upon transfer to the BB neonate. Specifically, we examined whether cells of the marrow inocula needed to share MHC antigens with the BB host (recall that the WF marrow utilized thus far is MHC compatible with BB --- both being RT1^u) (15). To study this issue, we utilized marrow harvested from a panel of bmc donor strains, some of which differed from the BB in the MHC antigens they expressed. As shown in Table 4, three bmc preparations were found to be successful in disease prevention: WF, (WF x Lew)F$_1$, and the congenic strain BN.B2. Each of these carriers at least one RT1^u haplotype. In contrast, none of the three MHC incompatible bmc preparations employed (Lewis, BN and the congenic BN.B1) was found to provide any degree of disease prevention.

TABLE 4

NEONATAL INOCULATION WITH MHC COMPATIBLE AND INCOMPATIBLE
BONE MARROW CELLS

BMC donor	RT1	# diabetic/total studied (%)	
		Injected	Control
Wistar Furth (WF)	u/u	2/58(3.4)	19/61(31.1)
BN. B2	u/u	2/30(6.7)	10/23(43/5)
(WF x Lew)F$_1$	u/1	10/38(26.3)	7/30(23.3)
Lew	1/1	21/34(61.8)	12/27(44.4)
BN	n/n	10/35(28.6)	12/40(30.0)
BN.B1	1/1	12/30(40.0)	10/28(35.7)

These data suggest that MHC compatibility is a prerequisite for the ability to inhibit or down-regulate the autoimmune potential of BB rats. Two possible mechanisms for this requirement were considered. First, it was possible that antigenic determinants expressed by $RT1^u$ lymphocytes were required. For example, the process of tolerance induction to certain $RT1^u$ specific or genetically closely linked antigenic determinants resulted in deletion or inactivation of autoreactive BB lymphocytes; simply stated, the phenotype of the marrow inocula was essential. Second, the alternative possibility was that it was essential for the transferred T cells to function in an $RT1^u$ restricted manner. Under this constraint, only cells that matured in a host in which the thymus expressed $RT1^u$ MHC gene products would be capable of $RT1^u$ restricted interactions and disease prevention. These possibilities were distinguished employing lymphocytes from radiation chimeras in which cell phenotype or restriction capacity were independently manipulated.

We first demonstrated that lymph node cells from both WF and (WF x Lew)F_1 animals would also result in a high level of protection from autoimmunity. This result was expected since the lymph node compartment contains a much greater percentage of T lymphocytes than does bone marrow. We next constructed two groups of animals in which the lymphoid populations of each were phenotypically identical but differed with respect to their MHC restriction specificty (16). This was accomplished by maturing (WF x Lewis)F_1 T depleted marrow cells in either WF or Lewis irradiated hosts. In the former case, all T cells should be educated to recognize antigen in the context of $RT1^u$ MHC molecules and, in the case of the latter only in the context of $RT1^l$ MHC molecules; in both instances lymphocytes found in the lymph nodes and spleen should be entirely of the F_1 bmc donor and therefore phenotypically identical. Lymph node and spleen cells from both types of chimeras were assessed for disease protection capacity by injection into BB neonates. The results are shown in Table 5. (WF x Lew)F_1 T cells educated in WF hosts, and therefore restricted to $RT1^u$, were fully capable of preventing autoimmunity. In contrast, BB rats injected with (WF x Lew)F_1 T cells that had matured in a Lewis host, and thus became restricted to $RT1^l$, were afflicted with diabetes as frequently as as untreated BB rats or recipients of MHC incompatible marrow. We conclude from these data that it is the ability to recognize antigen in the context of $RT1^u$ encoded MHC molecules and not the marrow phenotype which is relevant to disease prevention. These findings may indicate that a regulatory interaction of the protective T cells with autoimmune BB cells is necessary to effect protection.

TABLE 5

PROTECTION IS DEPENDENT ON LYMPHOCYTES RESTRICTED FOR ANTIGEN RECOGNITION IN THE CONTEXT OF $RT1^u$ MHC ANTIGENS

LNC/Spl cell donor	# Diabetic/total (%)
WF	0/49 (0)
(WF x Lew)F_1	0/13 (0)
(WF x Lew)F_1 -- WF	2/38 (5.2)
(WF x Lew)F_1 -- Lew	10/28 (36.7)

In summary, the observation that diabetic BB rats are immunodeficient suggested that the absence of normal immunoregulatory mechanisms might be a pivotal predisposing factor to autoimmunity. Compelling evidence supporting this contention was obtained using a system of neonatal bone marrow cell transfusion (neonatal tolerance induction). Protection from diabetes was found to be conferred by mature T lymphocytes present in the bone marrow cell inocula. Moreover, we determined that a prerequisite for T cell efficacy was that they recognize antigen in the context of RT1^u MHC molecules. This finding suggests that the protection conferring T cells must be able to interact productively with malregulated lymphocytes present in the diabetic BB host. Finally, in all cases in which protection from diabetes was accomplished, at least partial restoration of the BB immune function was observed. We conclude that the BB's immune defect contributes significantly to disease pathogenesis and that strategies employing host immunomodification during the prediabetic period can successfully halt disease progression.

REFERENCES

1. Banting, F.G., Best, C.H., 1922, The internal secretion of the pancreas. J. Lab. Clin. Med. 251–266.

2. Opie, E.L., 1900–1901, The relation of diabetes mellitus to lesions of the pancreas. J.Exp. Med. 5:527–540.

3. VonMeyenburg, H., 1940, Ueber "Insulitus" bei diabetes. Schweiz Med. Wochenschr. 21:554.

4. Irvine, W.J., 1980, Immunological Aspects of Diabetes Mellitus: A Review (including the salient points of NDDG report on the classification of diabetes). In Immunology of Diabetes, Irvine, W.J., ed. Edinburgh, Teviot Scientific Publications, p. 1.

5. Stiller, C.R., Dupre, J., Gent, M., Venmer, M.R., Keown, P.A., Laupacis, A., Martell, P., Rodger, N.W., Groffemed, B.V., and Wolfe, B.J.J., 1984, Effect of cyclosporine immunosuppression in insulin dependent diabetes-mellitus of recent onset. Science 223:1363–1367.

6. Marliss, E.B., Nakhooda, A.F., Poussier, P., Sima, A.A.F., 1982, The diabetic syndrome of the BB Wistar rat: possible relevance to type I (insulin-dependent) diabetes in man. Diabetologia 22:225–232.

7. Fuks, A., Colle, E., Ono, S., Prud'homme, G., Seemayer, T., and Guttman, R.D., 1988, Immunogenetic studies of insulin-dependent diabetes in the BB rat. In: Frontiers in Diabetes Research, (Shafir, E., and Renold, A.E., eds.) London, John Libbey, p. 29.

8. Like, A.A., Guberski, D.L., and Butler, L, 1986, Diabetic biobreeding/worester (BB/Wor) rats need not be lymphopenic. J. of Immunol. 3254–58.

9. Greiner, D.L., Mordes, J.P., Handler, E.S., Angelillo, M., Nakamura, N., Rossini, A.A., 1987, Depletion of RT6.1+ T lymphocytes induces diabetes in resistant Biobreeding/Worcester (BB/W) rats. J. Exp. Med. 166:461–75.

10. Mordes, J.P., Desemone, J., Rossini, A.A., 1987, The BB rat. Diabetes/Metabolism Reviews 3:725–750.

11. Naji, A., Silvers, W.K., Bellgrau, D., Barker C.F., 1981, Spontaneous diabetes in rats: destruction of islets is prevented by immunological tolerance. Science 213:1390- 1392.

12. Naji, A., Silvers, W.K., Kimura, H., Bellgrau, D., Markmann, J.F., and Barker, C.F., 1983, Analytical and functional studies on the T cells of untreated and immunologically tolerant diabetes prone BB rats. J. Immunol. 130:2168-2172.

13. Francfort, J.W., Naji, A., Silvers, W.K., and Barker, C.F., 1985, The influence of T-lymphocyte precursor cells and thymus grafts on the cellular immunodeficiencies of the BB rat. Diabetes, Vol. 34, No. 11:1134-38.

14. Brayman, K.L., Markmann, J.F., Barker, C.F., and Naji, A., 1988, Immunoprediction of diabetes and evaluation of pancreatic islet transplantation during the prediabetic period. Surgery 4:445-451.

15. Brayman, K.L., Markmann, J.F., Silvers, W.K., Barker, C.F., and Naji, A., 1987, The immunoregulation of autoimmune diabetes in BB rats is MHC-restricted. Diabetes 36 (Suppl. 1):65A.

16. Brayman, K.L., Markmann, J.F., Barker, C.F., and Naji, A., 1988, Prevention of diabetes in BB rats requires lymphocytes functionally restricted to MHC-compatible thymic determinants. Diabetes 37 (Supp. I): 55A.

PREVENTION OF DIABETES-RELATED RETINAL MICROANGIOPATHY
WITH ALDOSE REDUCTASE INHIBITORS

¶W. Gerald Robison, Jr.

Section on Pathophysiology, Laboratory of Mechanisms of Ocular Diseases
National Eye Institute, National Institutes of Health
Bethesda, Maryland

One of the most significant breakthroughs in research on diabetes since the advent of insulin was the discovery, in animal models, that the polyol pathway involving aldose reductase is responsible for tissue complications similar to those occurring in diabetic patients (1). Under diabetic conditions polyol accumulates in cells from the activity of aldose reductase which would normally remain inactive. The accumulation of intracellular polyol and associated loss of myo-inositol somehow result in alterations in cell function and eventual cell death, though the mechanisms are not thoroughly understood and may vary from tissue to tissue.

Significant amelioration of ocular complications is provided by treatment of diabetic patients and animal models with aldose reductase inhibitors (1). Several potent inhibitors of aldose reductase have been found to be effective in preventing the early, diabetes-related alterations in the retinal microvasculature of experimental animals, and are now being tested in clinical trials for their efficacy in halting or delaying diabetic neuropathy and retinopathy. Utilization of aldose reductase inhibitors is a novel approach which would potentially provide a very effective diabetic therapy to be used in addition to insulin.

Diabetic retinopathy is not so much a neuropathy as it is an angiopathy with primary effects in the microvasculature. The characteristic early changes involve the integrity of the vessel walls: thickening of capillary basement membranes; loss of pericytes; and microaneurysm formation (2,3). As with many other ocular and systemic complications of diabetes which occur in spite of insulin treatment, recent evidence indicates that the polyol pathway is involved in the etiology of these capillary wall lesions. The present report examines current data related to the prevention of diabetes-induced retinal microangiopathy by aldose reductase inhibitors.

PATHOLOGY

Capillary Basement Membrane Thickening

Obvious thickening of retinal capillary walls has been observed consistently in long-term diabetics and animals models of diabetes (3). The amount of thickening is generally more than that which results from hypertension or the normal aging process alone. It occurs in the basal laminae, or so-called basement membranes. These "membranes" consist mainly of extra-cellular collagen type IV, but also contain several glycoproteins such as laminin, fibronectin, entactin, and nidogen, as well as many polyanionic proteoglycans, heparan sulfate being the most prominent (4). Basement membrane material ensheathes the capillary and separates the pericytes and endothelial cells from each other and from adjacent tissues, except in certain areas where cell-membrane-to-cell-membrane contacts are made. Pathophysiologists have long considered capillary basement membrane thickening to be of utmost significance in diabetic vasculopathy of essentially all tissues.

In the human retina, excessive basement membrane thickening in microvessels of diabetics has been reported repeatedly. Recent studies (3) have confirmed the observations of early investigators, and have quantified the thickening by modern techniques (Fig.1).

Quantification of capillary basement membrane thickening has been surrounded by controversies and confusion owing to the many different techniques of tissue preparation and methods of measurements used in early studies. Utilization of modern techniques should eventually resolve essentially all the confusion (3,5). However, the precise measurement of basement membrane thickness is difficult at best, and there is still no universally accepted method. Even in normal capillaries the basement membrane is not the same thickness throughout the perimeter of a capillary viewed in cross section. In diabetics and models of diabetes, including galactosemic animals, there is extraordinary irregularity within the same capillary. Bundles of collagen, vacuoles, focal thickenings, and surface irregularities are common in such basement membranes. Where should the measurement or measurements be made to give a true average thickness? None of the manual methods which have been developed fully accounts for all the variables. Only regions of endothelial cell basement membrane free from overlying pericyte cytoplasm as seen in transection were utilized in most studies. This makes such methods inadequate for retinal capillaries because much of the endothelial cell basement membrane in these vessels is surrounded by pericyte cytoplasm and would thus be eliminated from measurement. Also measurements of basement membrane thickness in areas where focal lesions (fibrillar collagen deposits, vacuolization) or focal thickenings occur would not be reflected by any of the manual methods of basement membrane measurement.

Several recent studies using computer planimetry permit inclusion of all the variables in a reproducible manner (3,5). Since suitable computers, digitizing tablets, and programs are now commonly available, standardization from laboratory to laboratory of precise methods for measurement of basement membrane thickness should be possible. However, the accuracy of these computer methods will be of no avail unless only high quality micrographs of capillaries cut very close to a 90° angle are utilized.

Another complicating variable which continues to plague studies on capillary basement membrane thickness is the variation in location from which tissue is obtained for analysis. Except where very extraordinary differences occur, studies by electron microscopy are required for quantification. The important compromise made in turning to ultrastructural studies is the tremendous decrease in sample size and potential increase in sampling error. One way to minimize the sampling error is to take samples from precisely the same region within each tissue from individual to individual. The retina provides one of the best opportunities for precise localization of tissue samples. First, the region of the retina can be clearly defined. Robison and Nagata (3) took samples only from the superior temporal quadrant within 1.0 mm of the optic nerve. Second, the

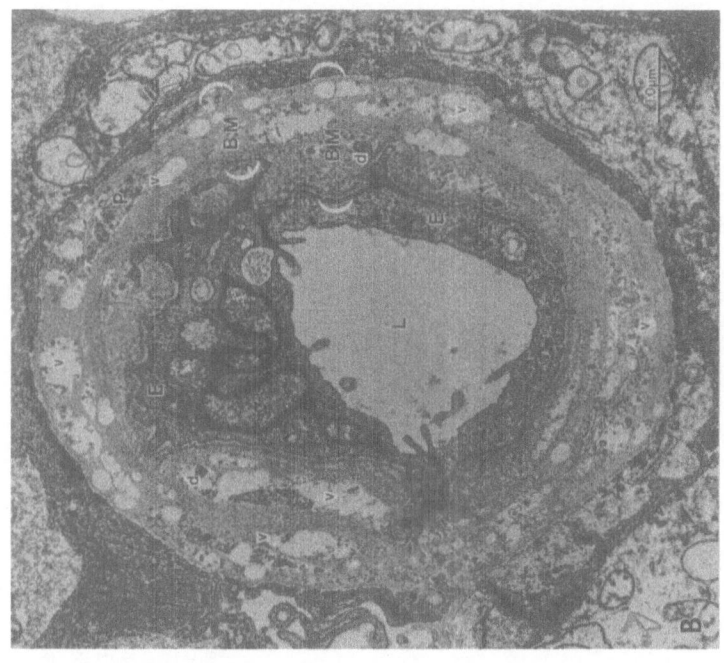

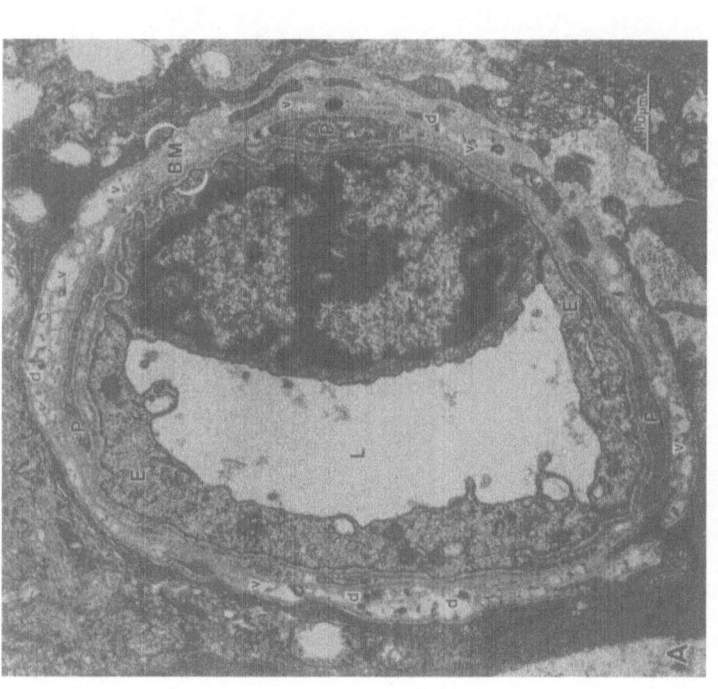

Figure 1. Retinal capillary basement membrane thickening in human diabetes. Ultrastructure of transected retinal capillaries of the superior temporal sector near the macula from: A) a 71-year-old, non-diabetic man and B) a 68-year-old man who had non-insulin-dependent diabetes for 36 years. Note, in the diabetic, the striking thickening of the basement membrane (BM and parenthesis), multiple layers of basement membrane, the many intercalated vacuoles (v), the dense particulate inclusions (d), and the apparent partial loss of pericyte cytoplasm. In the nondiabetic capillary there are various extentions of pericyte cytoplasm (P) embedded in the basement membrane. Endothelial cells (E) delimit the lumen (L) completely and, in turn are surrounded by a sheath of basement membrane. (X21,000: bar = 1.0 micrometer).

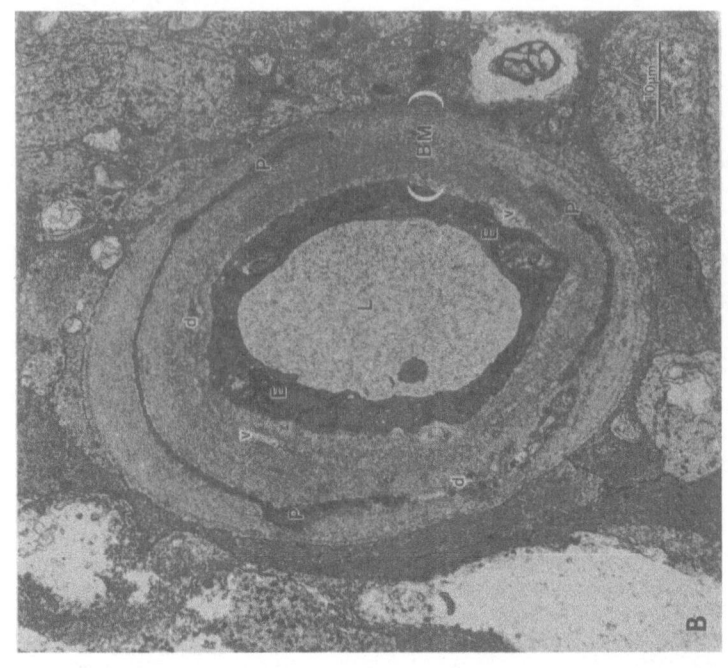

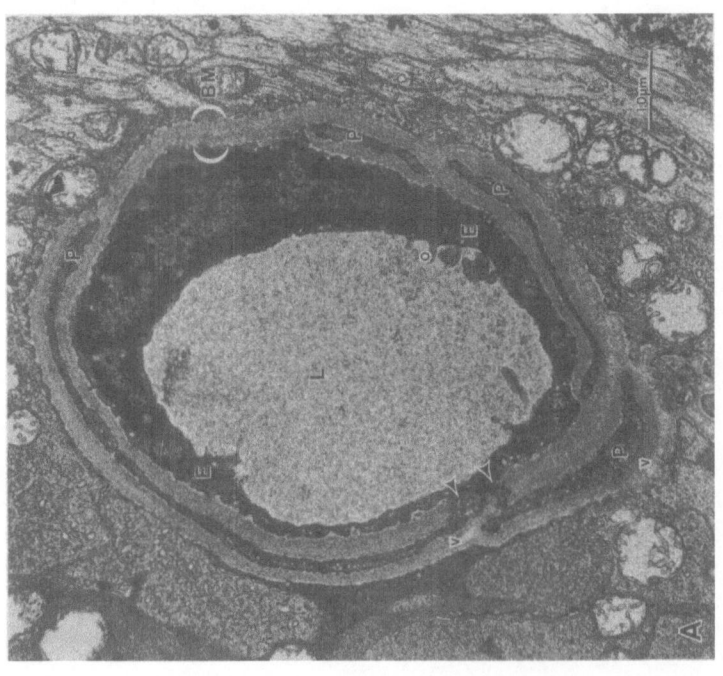

Figure 2. Prevention of diabetes-like thickening of basement membrane in galactose-fed rats. Transected retinal capillary bed (nerve fiber/ganglion cell layer) of rats fed for 88 weeks A) a control diet, B) a 50% galactose diet, or C) a 50% galactose diet with 0.04% tolrestat added. Note the comparative thicknesses of basement membranes (BM and parenthesis) which surround the endothelial cells (E) and encase the pericytes (P). Vacuoles (v), and dense inclusions (d) are typical characteristics of the capillary basement membranes of the galactose-fed rats, whereas cell-membrane-to-cell membrane contacts (arrowheads) between pericytes and endothelial cells are approximately twice as common in normal and tolrestat-treated rats. L = lumen; o = endothelial cell process; rbc = red blood cell. (X21,000: bar = 1.0 micrometer).

layers within the retina can be easily distinguised and should be analyzed separately. Several investigators have reported that the capillary basement membranes in the nerve fiber and ganglion cell layers of rat retinas are thicker than those in the inner or outer plexiform layer. Although it would be relatively simple to employ modifications which would permit extra precision, decrease variability, and make basement membrane studies of the retina more comparable among laboratories, few technical updates have been employed. Sampling differences probably account for much of the variability in data reported from different laboratories.

Aldose reductase appears to be involved in diabetes-related basement membrane thickening. A diabetic-like thickening of retinal capillary basement membranes has been induced by galactose feeding in dogs (2) and has been prevented by inhibitors of aldose reductase in rats (3). The galactose rat model was used to mimic the diabetes-related thickening of basement membranes and test the effects of aldose reductase inhibitors administered orally. Weanling male, Sprague-Dawley rats were given a normal diet or a 50% galactose diet with or without an aldose reductase inhibitor (0.04% tolrestat) for 88 weeks. Portions of the central retina in the superior temporal sector near the optic nerve were dissected and processed for electron microscopy. Micrographs were taken of capillaries of the inner capillary bed (nerve fiber/ganglion cell layer). Only vessels of capillary size (5-8 micrometers) which were transected at close to a 90 degree angle from their long axis, so that the cell outlines were clearly distinguishable, were chosen for analysis.

Figure 2A shows an ultrastructural transection of a typical capillary of the inner capillary bed from the control group after 88 weeks of normal diet. The lumen is delimited by an endothelial cell. This is covered by basement membrane, the pericyte, and more basement membrane, as in human retinal capillaries. Note the normal basement membrane thickness. By contrast, Figure 2B shows the marked basement membrane thickening which typically occurs in the retinal capillary walls of rats fed a 50% galactose diet for 88 weeks. Note the multiple layers, intercalated vacuoles, and dense material, as seen in capillaries of human diabetics. Only thin remnants of mural cell cytoplasm are present. As with previous experiments (3), computer planimetry was used to quantify the thickening of basement membrane. The average capillary basement membrane thickness was approximately threefold normal values after 88 weeks of galactose feeding. The thickening was prevented by adding tolrestat (0.04%), a potent inhibitor of aldose reductase, to the diet for the total period of the galactose insult (Figure 2C). There were no significant differences in the capillary basement membrane thicknesses between the control rats and those fed 50% galactose plus an aldose reductase inhibitor. These results are consistent with reports of capillary basement membrane thickening in streptozotocin diabetic rats which has also been prevented with aldose reductase inhibitors when utilized.

The significance of capillary basement membrane thickening under diabetic conditions is not well understood. However, basement membrane changes may induce the observed decrease in the normal numbers of contacts between pericytes and endothelial cells (Figure 2) which may be important in contact inhibition. This may influence the normal control of the proliferation of endothelial cells, and thus be important in the development of the proliferative stages of diabetic retinopathy.

Pericyte Loss from Retinal Capillaries

A selective loss of pericytes from the walls of retinal capillaries is the earliest reported histopathological sign of retinal microangiopathy in long-term diabetics (6). After several years of diabetes, but before clinical signs of diabetic retinopathy, the normal 1:1 ratio of endothelial

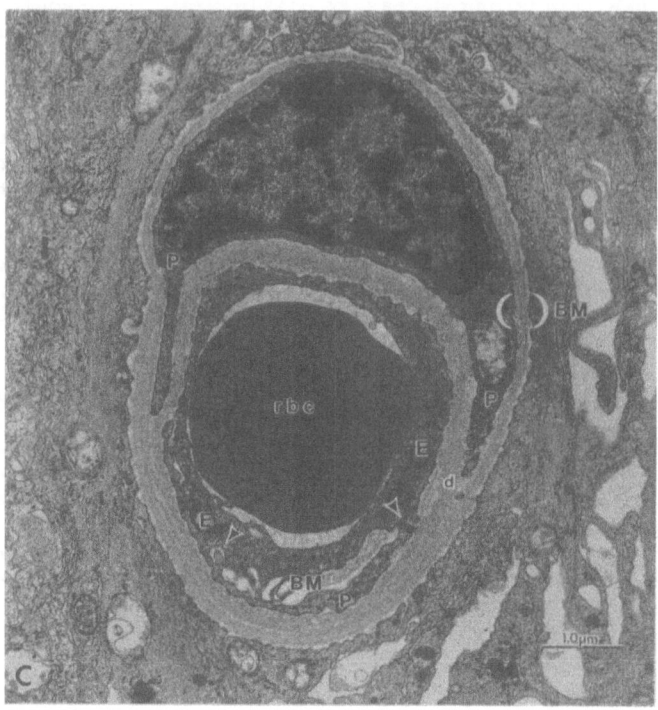

Figure 2 (C).

to mural cells nuclei in the capillaries of the central retina is increased in spite of insulin treatment. This occurs concomitantly with the appearance of pericyte "ghosts" which are bulged regions of the basement membrane sheath of the capillary surface, containing only remnants of degenerated pericyte organelles. Loss of these potentially contractile cells is believed to result in loss of capillary tone, increased capillary diameter, and decreased regulation of the dynamics of the microcirculation. Loss of pericytes eventually leads to a decreased number of cell-membrane-to cell-membrane contacts between pericytes and endothelial cells. Loss of such cell contacts and their probable role in contact inhibition may initiate the subsequent microvasculature changes of diabetic retinopathy such as proliferation of endothelial cells, formation of microaneurysms, and hemorrhages.

Aldose reductase is involved in the loss of pericytes from retinal vessels under diabetic conditions. The presence of aldose reductase has been demonstrated in retinal capillaries and their cellular derivatives. Immunoreactive amounts of aldose reductase are present in the pericyte cytoplasm which surrounds the endothelial cell tube of the retinal capillaries in both human and dog (7). Capillaries isolated from canine retinas (8) as well as pericytes grown from human retinal vessels (9) accumulated polyol when incubated in high hexose concentrations. Polyol production was prevented in the presence of the aldose reductase inhibitors sorbinil (Pfizer) or tolrestat (Ayerst), respectively. When pericytes cultured from retinal capillaries of the rhesus monkey were incubated in a high glucose medium, they showed a threefold increase in sorbitol concentration and an increased cell death compared to similar cells grown under low glucose conditions (10). Since aldose reductase is active in cultured human pericytes, these cells, like lens cells, may be susceptible to high polyol concentrations, thus implicating a role of aldose reductase in the degeneration of pericytes. Pericyte loss may result in the subsequent micro-angiopathies common to the retinal capillaries of long-term diabetics.

Prevention of Diabetic Retinopathy

Galactosemic animals provide useful models for understanding the role of aldose reductase in the development of various complications of diabetes, including diabetic retinopathy. Insulin, which has been shown in and of itself to stimulate production of excess basement membrane proteins and proteoglycans, is not altered in galactose-fed models (2). Though already suggested in diabetics and diabetic models, the galactosemic models make it clear that high serum sugar levels alone can account for significant basement membrane thickening, pericyte loss, and microaneurysm formation (2). Whatever mechanisms may be involved, they must somehow be related to an increased flux of sugars through the polyol pathway, since the various aldose reductase inhibitors have in common only their unique ability to block the polyol pathway and to concomitantly prevent basement membrane thickening and other complications.

Recent findings indicate that the galactose-fed rat is a better model for diabetic retinopathy than previously suspected. Microaneurysms, which have been reported occasionally in diabetic rats, have been found in rats fed a diet with 50% galactose for 28 months, and preliminary results suggest that they are prevented with an aldose reductase inhibitor (W. Gerald Robison, Jr., 1988, unpublished data).

In dogs, long-term galactosemia not only results in thickening of capillary basement membranes but also in capillary pericyte loss, formation of microaneurysms, hemorrhaging, cotton wool spot development, capillary non-perfusion and atrophy, and varicose capillaries (2). All these conditions mimic very closely those found in diabetic dogs as well as in patients. In diabetic dogs such changes can be elicited in 3 to 5 years. On the other hand, dogs fed dry ration containing 30% galactose develop clinically visible retinopathy after only 32 months. Recent findings (11) indicate that loss of pericytes can be detected as early as 21 months, and microaneurysms as early as 27 months, in Beagle dogs fed 30% galactose from 10 months of age. Both are prevented with aldose reductase inhibitors. Therefore, the galactosemic dog provides a new and very promising model for diabetic changes in the human eye. No other animal model develops retinopathy to the extent dogs do. Now that such galactose models are available, the etiology of diabetic retinopathy can be worked out in detail under tightly controlled conditions, and the benefits of aldose reductase inhibitors can be assessed. The evidence to date suggests that aldose reductase inhibitors delay or prevent diabetic retinopathy. Soon definitive evidence will be provided as the results of experiments with animal models and the findings from clinical trials become available.

SUMMARY AND CONCLUSIONS

Before any clinical signs of diabetic retinopathy can be detected, two major histopathological lesions occur in the walls of retinal capillaries: basement membrane thickening; and loss of intramural pericytes (mural cells). A decrease in the number of pericyte to endothelial cell junctions also occurs under diabetic conditions and may result in subsequent proliferation of endothelial cells and microaneurysm formation. Aldose reductase inhibitors prevent all these diabetic microangiopathies of the retina in animal models of diabetes and are presently being tested in clinical trials on diabetic retinopathy. Utilization of aldose reductase inhibitors is a novel approach which would potentially provide a very effective diabetic therapy to be used in addition to insulin.

ACKNOWLEDGMENTS

The authors wish to thank Anne B. Groome for her technical assistance, the National Disease Research Interchange (Philadelphia, Pennsylvania) for supplies of human donor eyes, and Dr. Dushan Dvornik of Ayerst Laboratories Laboratories Research, Inc. for supplies of tolrestat (Ayerst AY-27, 773).

REFERENCES

1. Kinoshita, J.H., 1986, Aldose reductase in the diabetic eye, XLIII Edward Jackson Memorial Lecture. Amer J Ophthamol 102: 685-692.

2. Engerman, R.L., Kern, T.S., 1986, Hyperglycemia as a cause of diabetic retinopathy. Metabolism 35: 20-23.

3. Robison, W.G., Jr., Nagata, M., 1988, Aldose reductase in mural cell loss and retinal capillary basement membrane thickening. In Polyol Pathway and Its Role in Diabetic Complications. Sakamoto, N, Kinoshita, J.H., Kador, P.F. and Hotta, N., Eds. Amsterdam, Elsevier Science Publishers (Biomedical division): 267-275.

4. Timpl, R., Dziadek, M., 1986, Structure, development, and molecular pathology of basement membranes. International Rev Exp Pathol 29: 1-112.

5. McEwen, T.A.J., Chakrabarti, S., and Sima, A.A.F., 1987, A rapid reproducible method for determination of basement membrane thickness in biological structures. Comput Biol Med 17: 193-197.

6. Cogan, D.G. and Kuwarbara, T., 1967, The mural cell in perspective. Arch Ophthalmol 78: 133-139.

7. Akagi, Y., Terubayashi, H., Millen, J., Kador, P.F., Kinoshita, J.H., 1986, Aldose reductase localization in dog retinal mural cells. Current Eye Res 5: 883-886.

8. Kern, T.S., Engerman, R.L., 1985, Hexitol production by canine retinal microvessels. Invest Ophthalmol Vis Sci 26: 382-384.

9. Hohman, T.C., Nishimura, C., Robison, W.G., Jr., 1988, Aldose reductase and polyol in cultured pericytes of human retinal capillaries. Exp Eye Res (in press).

10. Buzney, S.M., Frank, R.N., Varma, S.D., Tanishima, T. and Gabbay, K.H., 1977, Aldose reductase in retinal mural cells. Invest Ophthalmol Vis Sci 16: 392-396.

11. Kador, P.F., Akagi, Y., Terubayashi, H., Wyman, M., Kinoshita, J.H., 1988, Prevention of pericyte ghost formation in retinal capillaries of galactose-fed dogs by aldose reductase inhibitors. Archiv Ophthalmol (in press).

DISCUSSION

F. SCOTT: Dr. Grodsky, in your thymidine treatment, do you think that you're simply supplying thymidine nucleotide by the salvage pathway and bypassing an inhibition of denovo synthesis of nucleotides by Streptozotocin and allowing beta cell regeneration? Or, have you looked at that?

G. GRODSKY: We have no direct data on that question. The studies showing that you can protect with nicotinimide against partially pancreatectomized animals suggest that they are providing the NAD which will allow regeneration as a protective mechanism. So the actual mechanism of how these provide the nucleotides and how those nucleotides prevent the lesion is unknown.

F. SCOTT: I have just one more question if I might. How do you think this relates to the free radical mechanisms?

G. GRODSKY: Well, what I was trying to say is we have no evidence that Streptozotocin affects free radicals at all, so I doubt if that's the protective step. Years ago we attempted to show protective effect of free radicals, superoxide dismutase, but in our hands they never protected. These are in in vitro experiments. Alcohol, which is a pretty good quencher, has never protected. Just last week we finished a study with provacol which is another interesting free radical quencher and that has no effect on the Streptozotocin killing the cells. So my guess is it will not be in the free radical area that we are going to find this phenomenon going on. DNA nicking is a characteristic of Streptozotocin but that does not seem to be related to the cell death that occurs. I think its possibly related to methylation of proteins which occurs with Streptozotocin which can be blocked by nicotinimides, and right now we have more things that say no, that are negatives, than we do knowing what the actual mechanism is.

J. BARBOSA: We are conducting a trial using nicotinimide in humans and so far, we don't have the final results yet, but it appears that we are not going to confirm the report from France at all.

G. GRODSKY: How many patients?

J. BARBOSA: Well, in the open trial we have about 20. Now we are also doing a double blind, randomized trial. No fireworks whatsoever, I'm sorry to tell you that.

G. GRODSKY: No, no, I presented that because I think its something that obviously a lot of people have to check out and the Boston group is starting to study this effect of nicotinimide as well and I called them right before I left and they've only had 3, but they also haven't shown anything yet. So either it's going to be an unconfirmed study, which happens many times, or else there might be some possibility of working out proper dosages and things like that.

F. SCOTT: Dr. Robison, does lactose give the same effects as galactose?

Do very high lactose diets do the same thing?

W. ROBISON: Well, we have not tried a lactose diet. We tried glucose, too, and it works fine. The reason for using xylose in culture is because xylose or aldose reductase has a higher affinity. The reason we don't feed the animals xylose is because it causes diarrhea. I haven't tried lactose.

F. SCOTT: Well, lactose is, of course, the disaccharide of glucose and galactose, so you might think that it might have an effect.

W. ROBISON: It might.

H. LAUBE: Dr. Robison, would you like to take a guess why aldose reductase preferably accumulates in the pericytes?

W. ROBISON: Oh, because there's more there than in the endothelial cells. I hope you didn't feel there's none in the endothelial cell. Aldose reductase has been demonstrated in endothelial cells, but it's a much lower level. No one really knows what the normal function of aldose reductase is in the body. There are high concentrations of aldose reductase in the testes and in the seminal vesicles. It is not an antifertility drug. There's high aldose reductase in the collecting tubules of the kidney where the best evidence for normal function exists. The aldose reductase in the tubules of the kidney probably is there to control the osmotic pressure of those absorbing cells. There is aldose reductase in glomerular cells, too, but not as much as in the tubules, so that's the best clue for normal function and yet these drugs that are aldose reductase inhibitors are not causing problems in the kidney.

B. WAJCHENBERG: Dr. Robison, what would happen instead of using sorbinil if you would give, besides galactose, myoinositol?

W. ROBISON: The evidence that exists suggests that myoinositol is further down the pathway. That it's a secondary effect. That the primary effect is, in fact, damage to the cell membrane. Now, let me express some evidence for that. For instance, Dr. Kinoshita has been able to incubate lens in glucose, and have them become cataracts in situ. But, he can prevent that by simply controlling the osmotic pressure of the medium to the point that it equals the sorbitol that's accumulated in the lens. So, the first change is some type of an osmotic change which then leads to permeability of the membrane. Many amino acids, and other things, are lost including myoinositol from the cell. Now, Dr. Green and others have shown that you can treat some nerves with myoinositol and get a reversal, but you can do the same thing with aldose reductase inhibitor.

It's interesting that in rats, although we're causing retinopathy with the galactose feeding, they don't seem to be causing the same lesions in the kidney. We're causing a high sugar condition, which is something less than what diabetes is.

P. BENNETT: Dr. Robison, I'd like to push you a little bit more on the relationship of aldose reductase to basement membrane thickening per se. Would it be fair to say that at this moment in time you believe that the basement membrane thickening can be, perhaps, attributed entirely to the sorbitol aldose reductase problems? I'm sure you're going to say that's an over exaggeration, but I'd like you to try to explain the relationship there.

W. ROBISON: There is nothing known about the mechanism of why the basement membrane thickens under these galactosemic conditions. It is related to the aldose reductose pathway simply because you can inhibit it, and so if you have no aldose reductase activity, or less activity, you don't get the thickening. This has not been done with one, but with several aldose reductase inhibitors which are structurally entirely different.

B. WAJCHENBERG: Dr. Dupre, as practicing physicians we should not use cyclosporine, because it's experimental.

J. DUPRE: It's only appropriate to use such an experimental therapy in the context of a defined protocol which has been examined, which is addressing a specific question, and which is going to yield information to help answer these questions. I think that is our position.

J. BARBOSA: Dr. Dupre, as I'm doing a clinical trial with nicotinimide, I'm fully aware of the importance of duration of disease. But, the problem is how do you define duration of disease?

J. DUPRE: I think operationally what we've done is to date the duration of symptoms from nocturia. Quite frequently there are antecedent symptoms, sometimes vague, sometimes quite definite, but nocturia particularly in younger patients seems to be very well identified by the patient or the family and it does provide a data. That's the date that's been used empirically.

A. REDDI: I'm glad that Dr. Dupre mentioned about the renal function in these patients. We know that the cyclosporine causes both acute renal failure and, to some extent, chronic renal failure. And, it induces a type of glomerular lesion called focal segmental glomerulosclerosis. When you suppress or when you immunosuppress, these patients are prone to develop opportunistic infections, especially protozoal infections such as Pneumocystis pneumonia. Did you see any opportunistic infection during your follow-up for that one year period in any one of these patients?

J. DUPRE: To comment on your important comments about nephrotoxicity, we are, of course, familiar with this evidence. The argument we used for the acceptable safety of this drug includes the fact that in the large scale Canadian multi-center kidney transplant study there is actually no evidence of progressive impairment of the recipients of the kidneys in cyclosporine-treated patients. And, they maintain full reversibility of the functional effect. That was a very important component of our rationale. We're, of course, aware of the much more troublesome effects of cyclosporine in other transplant contexts which are, I maintain, not comparable with this one.

With regard to opportunistic infections, these have not been a problem in any single patient in these studies, nor in the rather large number of volunteer patients in the studies of immune diseases that are so well documented by the Sandoz Corporation, who are very careful in this regard and this extends now to approximately 4000 patients.

F. SCOTT: Dr. Greiner, in one of your slides you had figures showing that diabetes-prone irradiated animals were given diabetes-prone bone marrow and then diabetes-resistant irradiated animals were given diabetes-prone bone marrow, I believe. And, the incidence of insulitis in the diabetes-prone animals receiving the dibetes-prone bone marrow was 14%. The incidence in the diabetes-resistant animals was 40%. Do you think this difference is significant and can you speculate why it might be?

D. GREINER: I don't think the difference is significant. They're relatively small numbers, and I think if we increased the numbers of the animals in those experiments, which has been done, there would be no difference.

D. PYKE: The cultured islets lose their antigenicity by virtue of losing their macrophages. Two questions. One is, does the islet retain its biochemical endocrine function more or less perfectly? And, secondly, would there be other ways of hastening the process of its losing its antigenicity perhaps by monoclonal antibodies against the macrophages or whatever?

A. NAJI: Indeed, I think if the culture conditions are maintained properly the integrity of endocrine function of the islet cell is really maintained. When we use cultured islets and transplant them intraportally, in about 24 hours the recipient animals are normoglycemic. With respect to other methods the anti-IA, anti-class 2 plus complement works perfectly in the Murine model of deleting the antigen presented cells of the passenger leukocytes of the islets. But, unfortunately, it does not work very well in the rat and the reason is that the molecule does not get into the core of the islet complex to remove all the antigen presenting cells.

S. EFENDIC: Is it possible to prevent development of manifest diabetes in the BB rat if you treat the rat in the prediabetic state?

A. NAJI: Yes. If you treat the rat in the prediabetic state, less than 60 days of age, and start at about age 30 days with every day admini-stration of cyclosporin, there is almost 100% protection against diabetes.

H. GLEICHMANN: For how long did you observe your animals?

A. NAJI: 275 days.

J. HOET: I'd like to ask you if the anti-insulin antibodies went down during the cyclosporine treatment?

J. DUPRE: We do not have the data in. We will have it for anti-insulin antibody. Islet cell antibodies were present in approximately 60% of these patients and the titers fell substantially and rapidly in the cyclosporin treated patients. But, not at the same rate in the placebo group. That's the only observation we have with regard to those antibodies.

VII.   PREVENTION OF DIABETES

REGULATORY T CELL CONTROL OF AUTOIMMUNE DESTRUCTION OF BETA CELLS

IN THE BB RAT

¶Dale L. Greiner*, Marianne Angelillo*, John P. Mordes+,
Eugene S. Handler+, Christopher F. Mojcik*, Naoto Nakamura+,
and Aldo A. Rossini+

*Department of Pathology, University of Connecticut Health Center,
Farmington, CT; +Department of Medicine, University of Massachusetts
Medical School, Worcester, MA

Type I insulin-dependent diabetes mellitus (IDDM) in humans appears to be an autoimmune-mediated disease process that selectively destroys the pancreatic beta cells (1). Numerous lines of evidence support the concept of an autoimmune pathogenesis of IDDM. A mononuclear cell infiltration of the islets of Langerhans (insulitis) is observed in diabetics, consisting predominately of Ia+ activated T cells and monocytes. Islet cell autoantibodies are readily detectable in the serum of people with IDDM, and lymphocytes from acutely diabetic children can kill human insulinoma cells in vitro. Furthermore, IDDM appears to have a genetic component that is strongly associated with the major histocompatibility complex, and patients with IDDM have a high incidence of other autoimmune disorders (1).

In order to study the mechanisms involved in the autoimmune destruction of pancreatic beta cells, and to allow experimental manipulation of the disease process, investigators have turned to animal models of IDDM for study. Clearly, an appropriate animal model should have a close analogy to the human syndrome with respect to the clinical, biochemical and morphological characteristics of IDDM. A few such animal models exist, including the multiple dose streptozocin model, the non-obese diabetic (NOD) mouse and the spontaneously hyperglycemic BB rat (2). There are many similarities between the diabetic syndrome observed in the BB rat and Type I diabetes in humans (Table 1). This report will discuss the use of the BB rat model of IDDM to identify and characterize a regulatory T cell population that prevents the autoimmune destruction of pancreatic beta cells.

THE BB RAT

The diabetes-prone BB/Wor (DP) rat spontaneously develops IDDM at about 90 days of age. The disease occurs with a frequency of approximately 40-70% in both males and females and is not associated with obesity. Diabetic rats become ketoacidotic and absolutely dependent upon exogenous insulin for survival (1,2). There are many lines of evidence suggesting that IDDM in BB/Wor rats is autoimmune in origin (1,2). Acutely diabetic BB/Wor rats

Supported in part by grants DK-36024 and DK 25306 from the National Institutes of Health and by a grant from the Juvenile Diabetes Foundation, International.

TABLE I

COMPARISON BETWEEN IDDM AND BB RAT DIABETES[1]

	IDDM	BB RAT
Insulitis	+	+
Insulin Dependence	+	+
Ketoacidosis	+	+
Cytotoxic Cells to Islets	+	+
MHC Association	+	+
Islet Autoantibodies	+	+
Equal Sex Distribution	+	+
Prevention by Immunosuppression	+	+
Spontaneous Onset	+	+
Non-association with Obseity	+	+
Other Autoimmune Disorders	+	+

[1] See references 1,2

invariably display a moderate to severe insulitis, with concurrent destruction of the beta cells. As in humans, the cell infiltrate consists predominately of IA[+] T cells and monocytes. Additionally, IDDM in BB/Wor rats is closely associated with the class II region of the major histocompatibility complex, islet autoantibodies are detected in the serum of diabetic and prediabetic BB/Wor rats and DP rats have a high incidence of other autoimmune related disorders, including thyroiditis.

The cellular basis for IDDM in BB/Wor rats has been demonstrated. Concanavalin A activated spleen cells from acutely diabetic DP rats can adoptively transfer diabetes to histocompatible recipients (1,2). In addition, immunomodulatory procedures such as neonatal thymectomy, total lymphoid irradiation, administration of anti-T cell antibodies and normal bone marrow allografts into neonatal or irradiated DP recipients can prevent diabetes.

A striking immunological feature of DP rats is the severe T cell lymphopenia (2). Reduced numbers of the W3/25[+] helper/inducer (CD4) T cell subset are observed, while the OX8[+]/OX19[+] cytotoxic/suppressor (CD8) T cell subset appears to be totally absent (2). DP rats display deficient T cell mediated immune responses, most likely the direct result of the severe T cell lymphopenia.

In parallel with the development of the DP strain of rats, a diabetes-resistant BB/Wor (DR) strain of rats has also been derived. DR rats have a spontaneous incidence of diabetes of < 1%, have normal numbers of T cells and display normal T cell functional responses. However, low-dose irradiation or cyclosphamide induce diabetes in DR rats (2). Alternatively, lymphocyte transfusions from DR rats to DP rats are able to prevent diabetes in the DP recipients (3). The protection from diabetes following lymphocyte transfusion in the DP rat is associated with the restoration of normal ratios of CD4[+] and CD8[+] T cell subsets and with normal in vitro proliferative responses to mitogens (1-3).

TABLE II

CELL DISTRIBUTION AND FUNCTIONS OF RT6$^+$ CELLS[1]

Cell Distribution

      70% of peripheral T cells

      45% of W3/25+ helper/inducer (CD4+) T cell subset

      70% of OX8+ suppressor/cytotoxic (CD8+) T cell subset

      Absent on thymocytes and bone marrow lymphocytes

      Restricted to the T cell lineage

Functions

    RT6+ T cells

        Proliferate in response to mitogens

        Proliferate in response to allogeneic stumulation

        Secrete IL-2

        Participate in induction of Graft-versus-Host reaction

    RT6- T cells

        Cytotoxic T cell activity

        Mediate delayed type hypersensitivity

[1] See reference 5

The above observations suggest that a regulatory T cell population is absent or defective in DP rats and that DR rats have regulatory T cells that can prevent diabetes. Replacement of functional regulatory T cells in DP rats by lymphocyte transfusions prevents diabetes, while non-specific depletion of the putative regulatory cell population in DR rats by immuno-suppression procedures allows the expression of diabetes. These observations are of special importance in light of our recent demonstration that a major subset of peripheral T cells which express the RT6 peripheral T cell alloantigen are absent in DP rats, while normal numbers of RT6$^+$ T cells are observed in DR rats (4; also see below).

DEVELOPMENT AND FUNCTION OF RT6$^+$ T CELLS

The RT6 antigen in the rat is a 21,000 molecular weight non-glycosylated T cell restricted antigen that is linked to the cell membrane via phosphatidylinositol (5). Presently, there is no known mouse or human homologue of RT6. Approximately 70% of peripheral T cells in the rat express RT6, with approximately 45% of helper/inducer (CD4$^+$) T cells and 70% of suppressor/cytotoxic (CD8$^+$) T cells being RT6$^+$ (Table II) No bone marrow lymphocytes or thymocytes express RT6 (5).

RT6$^+$ T cells appear late in ontogeny and do not reach maximal levels in the peripheral lymphoid tissues until 6-8 weeks of age (5). Not surprisingly, since RT6$^+$ T cells are found in both CD4$^+$ and CD8$^+$ T cell subsets, a variety of functions have been ascribed to the RT6$^+$ T cell population (see Table 2).

TABLE III

POSSIBLE ROLE(S) OF RT6[+] T CELLS IN PATHOGENESIS OF BB RAT IDDM

<u>DP BB/Wor Rat</u>

> Absence of RT6[+] T Cells
>
> Protection from diabetes following lymphocyte transfusion; protection associated with persistance of RT6[+] T cells
>
> Lymphocyte transfusion protection:
>
> > age, cell dose dependent
> >
> > associated with appearance of RT6[+] T cells in recipients
>
> Transfer of diabetes to irradiated recipients DP marrow:
>
> > associated with inability of marrow to generate RT6[+] T cells in recipients

<u>DR BB/Wor Rat</u>

> Normal numbers of RT6[+] T cells, resistance to diabetes
>
> Depletion of RT6[+] T cells:
>
> > Induces diabetes, age dependent
> >
> > Removes protective cells in lymphocyte transfusions
> >
> > Renders non-diabetic DR rats susceptible to passive transfer of diabetes
>
> DR bone marrow transfer of resistance to diabetes to irradiated DP recipients:
>
> > associated with generation of RT6[+] cells in the recipients

ABSENCE OF RT6[+] T CELLS IN DP BB/WOR RATS

Since DP rats are lymphopenic and have a number of T cell functional defects, we investigated the development of RT6[+] T cells in the DP rat. Surprisingly, no RT6[+] T cells were detected in the peripheral lymphoid tissues of young pre-diabetic, older non-diabetic or in acutely diabetic DP animals (4). In contrast, normal numbers of RT6[+] T cells were apparent in the normolymphocytic DR rat at all ages studied. Furthermore, since RT6[+] T cells comprise approximately 70% of the peripheral T cell population in rats and since DP rats lack 60-80% of their peripheral T cells, we have postulated that the T cell lymphopenia in DP rats is due in part, if not entirely, to the absence of the RT6[+] T cell subset (2,4). To investigate directly whether the lack of RT6[+] T cells in DP rats has a role in determining their susceptibility to diabetes, lymphocyte transfusion, bone marrow adoptive transfer experiments and <u>in vivo</u> depletion studies of RT6[+] T cells have been performed.

PROTECTION FROM DIABETES FOLLOWING LYMPHOCYTE TRANSFUSION IS

ASSOCIATED WITH ENGRAFTMENT OF RT6[+] T CELLS

Spleen and lymph node cell transfusions from normal DR rats or histo-compatible WF strain rats into 30 day old unirradiated DP recipients prevents the development of diabetes. Using monoclonal antibodies to RT6, the periphereal lymphoid tissues of the lymphocyte transfused unirradiated DP recipients were examined for the presence of donor-origin RT6[+] T cells 4-6 months after spleen cell transfusion (6). In each of the non-diabetic transfusion-protected DP recipients, donor origin RT6[+] T cells were readily detected in the peripheral lymphoid tissues. In contrast, in 4 of the transfused DP recipients that subsequently became diabetic, no RT6[+] T cells were observed (6). Furthermore, transfusion of lymphohemopoietic tissues that lack RT6[+] T cells, such as bone marrow and thymus, fail to generate RT6[+] T cells in unirradiated DP recipients and further fail to protect DP rats from diabetes (Rossini, unpublished observations).

The protective effect mediated by transfusions of RT6-containing lymphoid populations appears to be both cell dose and recipient age dependent. Protection from diabetes can routinely be achieved by a single infusion of 200×10^6 WF or DR spleen cells into 30 day old DP recipients, but not by infusion of 50×10^6 spleen cells (7). The protective effect of the lymphocyte transfusions and the susceptiblity to diabetes correlate directly with elevated or deficient numbers, respectively, of donor-origin RT6[+] T cells that are detected in the DP recipients. In addition, there appears to be a critical time period when this protective effect can be mediated by lymphocyte transfusions. Transfusions of DR or WF spleen and lymph node cells into 30-45 day old DP recipients protects from diabetes, while lymphocyte transfusions at 60 days of age fails to influence the frequency or time of onset of diabetes (7). However, engraftment of donor-origin RT6[+] T cells occurs in all ages of transfused DP recipients as demonstrated by subsequent immunofluorescence analysis. Thus, the ability to intervene and alter the development of the disease process by lymphocyte transfusion is only successful during a time period prior to the onset of diabetes in DP rats: less than 0.5% of DP rats develop diabetes prior to 60 days of age, and greater than 85% of all diabetics are observed between 60 and 120 days of age (2). This observation is similar to the results obtained following intervention with the immunomodulatory agent, cyclosporin A, which is also effective only if employed during the preclinical phase of the disease syndrome in the BB/Wor rat, i.e. prior to 60 days of age.

DEPLETION OF RT6[+] T CELLS IN DP RATS INDUCES DIABETES

If in fact the lack of RT6[+] T cells in DP rats is an important factor in their susceptibility to diabetes and that RT6[+] lymphocytes from DR rats are the regulatory T cells that protect DP rats from diabetes, it would follow that removal of RT6[+] T cells in DR rats would: 1) remove the regulatory population that prevents diabetes in this strain and; 2) remove the DR lymphocyte population that protects DP rats from diabetes following transfusion of DR lymphocytes. These postulates were tested experimentally (8).

Following selective depletion for four weeks of RT6[+] lymphocytes in 30 day old DR rats using the lymphocytotoxic anti-RT6.1 monoclonal antibody DS4.23, approximately 50% of the RT6-depleted DR rats become diabetic (8). No diabetics were observed during the first 14 days of monoclonal antibody treatment, and the mean age of diabetes onset was 49 days of age. In addition, approximately 40% of the non-diabetic RT6-depleted DR rats displayed evidence of insulitis, while insulitis only rarely occurs in untreated DR rats.

As observed in the lymphocyte transfusion experiments, the effect of depletion of RT6$^+$ T cells in DR rats was age dependent. Thus, RT6 T cell depletion for four weeks starting at 60 days of age in DR rats did not induce the development of diabetes. Furthermore, injection of anti-RT6.1 into RT6-deficient DP rats did not alter the time course, age of onset or frequency of diabetes. Next lymphocytes from RT6-depleted DR rats were tested for their ability to protect DP recipients from diabetes in lymphocyte transfusion experiments. In contrast to spleen cells from untreated DR rats, RT6-depleted DR spleen cells not only failed to protect DP recipients from diabetes, but in fact accelerated the onset of diabetes (8).

DEVELOPMENTAL BASIS FOR THE LACK OF RT6$^+$ T CELLS IN DP RATS

To investigate the cellular basis for the transfer of susceptibility for diabetes by DP bone marrow cells (9), syngeneic and reciprocal bone marrow adoptive transfer experiments were performed between irradiated histocompatible WF and DP rats (10). DP bone marrow was unable to generate RT6$^+$ T cells in irradiated WF recipients, even though DP-origin thymocytes and RT6- peripheral T cells were present in the irradiation chimeras. In contrast, WF bone marrow was able to generate both WF-origin thymocytes and RT6$^+$ and RT6- peripheral T cells in irradiated DP recipients. Furthermore, no evidence for the presence of autoantibodies to RT6$^+$ T cells (or to their precursors) that would prevent the development of RT6$^+$ T cells in the DP rats were observed in a series of control experiments. These results suggest that the absence of RT6$^+$ T cells in DP rats is due to defects intrinsic to the development of DP prothymocytes, and is not due to the lack of accessory cells, or to the presence of inhibitory cells or autoantibodies that would prevent the development of RT6$^+$ T cells.

CONCLUSIONS

In conclusion, the susceptibility of DP rats to diabetes appears to be due, at least in part, to the absence of the RT6$^+$ regulatory T cell population. Replacement of RT6$^+$ T cells in young, prediabetic DP rats by lymphocyte transfusion prevents the development of diabetes. Alternatively, depletion of RT6$^+$ T cells in DR rats allows the expression of diabetes. The effect of the RT6$^+$ regulatory T cell population appears to be age dependent, and these regulatory T cells must be present during the pre-clinical phase of the diabetes syndrome in order to mediate their protective effect. Moreover, since DP marrow can transfer the susceptibility for diabetes to irradiated recipients, our present results suggest that an important predisposing factor for IDDM is the inability of DP prothymocytes to generate RT6$^+$ T cells have an important role in preventing the autoimmune destruction of beta cells in BB/Wor rats.

REFERENCES

1. Rossini, A.A., Mordes, J.P., Like, A.A., 1985, Immunology of insulin-dependent diabetes mellitus. Ann. Rev. Immunol. 3: 291-322.

2. Mordes, J.P., Desemone, J., Rossini, A.A., 1987, The BB rat. Diabetes/Metabolism Reviews 3: 725-750.

3. Rossini, A.A., F ustman, D., Woda, B.A., Like, A.A., Szymanski, I., Mordes, J.P., 1984, Lymphocyte transfusions prevent diabetes in the Bio-Breeding /Worcester rat. J. Clin. Invest. 74: 39-46.

4. Greiner, D.L., Handler, E.S., Nakano, K., Mordes, J.P., Rossini, A.A., 1986, Absence of the RT6 T cell subset in diabetes-prone BB/W rats. J. Immunol. 136: 148-151.

5. Greiner, D.L., Mordes, J.P., Angelillo, M., Handler, E.S., Mojcik, C.F., Nakamura, N. Rossini, A.A., 1988, Role of regulatory RT6[+] T cells in the pathogenesis of diabetes mellitus in BioBreeding/Worcester (BB/Wor) rats. In Frontiers in Diabetes Research: Lessons from Animal Diabetes II. Renold, A. & Shafrir, E., Eds., London, John Libbey & Co. In press.

6. Rossini, A.A., Mordes, J.P., Greiner, D.L., Nakano, N., Appel, M.C., Handler, E.S., 1986, Spleen cell transfusion in the Bio-Breeding/ Worcester rat: Prevention of diabetes, major histocompatibility complex restriction, and long-term persistence of transfused cells. J. Clin. Invest. 77: 1399-1401.

7. Mordes, J.P., McKeever, U., Handler, E.S., Greiner, D.L., Burstein, D., Rossini, A.A., 1988, Immune modulation of autoimmune diabetes in the BB rat. In Frontiers in Diabetes Research: Lessons from Animal Diabetes II. Renold, A. & Shafrir, E., Eds., London, John Libbey & Co. In press.

8. Greiner, D.L., Mordes, J.P., Handler, E.S., Angelillo, M., Nakamura, N., Rossini, A.A., 1987, Depletion of RT6.1[+] T lymphocytes induces diabetes in resistant BioBreeding/Worcester (BB/W) rats. J. Expt. Med. 166: 461-475.

9. Nakano, K., Mordes, J.P., Handler, E.S., Greiner, D.L., Rossini, A.A., 1988, The role of the host immune system in the BB/Wor rat: Predisposition to diabetes resides in the bone marrow. Diabetes. In press.

10. Greiner, D.L., Mordes, J.P., Handler, E.S., Nakamura, N., Angelillo, M., Rossini, A.A., 1987, Prothymocyte development in diabetes-prone BB rats: Description of a defect that predisposes to immune abnormalities. Transplant. Proc. 19: 976-978.

PREVENTION OF DIABETES IN THE BB RAT BY INJECTION OF MAJOR

HISTOCOMPATIBILITY COMPLEX- (MHC-) COMPATIBLE BONE MARROW CELLS

Joanne Scott, *, Victor H. Engelhard, +,
and David C. Benjamin +

Departments of Pediatrics*, Pharmacology*, and Microbiology+
University of Virginia School of Medicine
Charlottesville, Virginia

The emerging consensus that Type I diabetes mellitus has an autoimmune etiology has led to speculation that it could be prevented or cured by man-ipulation of the immune system. A concise understanding of the role of the immune system in the pathogenesis of Type I diabetes is crucial to devising preventive measures. Our understanding of the events that precede the onset of Type 1 diabetes comes mainly from the study of animal models. The avail-ability of these models has prompted efforts to gain better understanding of the fundamental nature of autoimmune diseases in general, and of Type 1 diabetes in particular, through extensive studies of their immunologic abnormalities.

The spontaneously diabetic BB rat is the best-characterized rodent model of autoimmune (Type 1) diabetes mellitus (1,2, for reviews). The disease in this non-obese animal model rapidly progresses to ketoacidosis and death if not treated with exogenous insulin. The diabetic syndrome in BB rats shares many features with the human disease: (a) mononuclear cell infiltration of the pancreatic islets (insulitis), (b) selective destruction of the pancreatic beta cells, (c) genetic control involving loci of the major histocompatibility complex (MHC), and (d) multiple organ-specific abnormali-ties of humoral immunity, including antibodies directed against the surface of the pancreatic beta cell. The BB rat also manifests severe T-lymphocyto-penia, present at time of weaning, with reductions of both T-helper/inducer (T_h/T_i) and T-cytotoxic/suppressor (T_c/T_s) cell populations. These animals also have decreased lymphocyte response to mitogens and to alloantigens.

The BB rat provides an excellent model for testing potential therapeutic modalities aimed at immune intervention in the prophylaxis or early treat-ment of Type 1 diabetes. Procedures that result in the removal or inacti-vation of lymphoid cell populations have been shown to prevent diabetes in the BB rat, e.g., neonatal thymectomy (3), injections of antilymphocyte serum (4), or injections of cyclosporin (4). Such findings suggest that the disease can be prevented by destroying or modulating the population of ef-fector cells responsible for beta cell destruction. Procedures that result

These studies were sponsored in part by a Pilot Feasibility Grant awarded by the University of Virginia Diabetes Research and Training Center, by a grant from the American Diabetes Association, and by the National Institutes of Health grant RO1-AM 34984.

in the addition of lymphoid cell population, e.g., lymphocyte transfusions from diabetes-resistant line of BB rats (5), also have been shown to prevent diabetes in susceptible animals. Such findings suggest that the absence of a specific population of lymphoid cells may play a key role in disease susceptibility.

In an earlier study by Naji and co-workers, neonatal inoculation of diabetes-prone BB rats with bone marrow from a normal MHC-compatible strain of rat significantly reduced the incidence of diabetes (6). However, it is well established that normal bone marrow contains a significant population of mature T-cells, which most probably enter the bone marrow parenchyma as part of the normal recirculating lymphocyte pool. If the defect(s) in the BB rat leading to diabetes and/or to the T-cell lymphopenia resides in the lymphoid stem cells, transplanting only stem cells (depleted of mature T-cells) from diabetes-resistant animals into diabetes-prone animals should prevent the onset of diabetes and/or correct the T-cell abnormalities. Our laboratory constructed a series of bone marrow chimeras (7,8) in an attempt to address this question. It is well established that neonatal animals can be made chimeric through the injection of bone marrow from either MHC-compatible or MHC-disparate animals. In adult rats, the recipients must be lethally irradiated prior to repopulation with bone marrow cells, to prevent rejection of the allogeneic donor cells; in neonatal rats, such irradiation is unnecessary. Our studies involved the construction of both neonatal (7) and adult (8) chimeras.

NEONATAL BONE MARROW CHIMERA STUDIES:

Procedure : Within 36 hours after birth, 88 diabetes-prone BB rats were inoculated intraperitoneally with bone marrow from MHC-compatible Wistar-Furth (WF) rats. In one-half of the animals, the bone marrow inoculum was depleted of mature T-lymphocytes by treatment with rabbit anti-rat thymocyte antiserum plus guinea pig complement, as described previously (7). The inoculated animals remained with their mothers until weaning, after which they were maintained under conditions identical to those of other animals in the colony. All animals were observed for > 140 days. Beginning at ∼ 50 days of age, urinary glucose and ketone levels were determined weekly, and rats were classified as diabetic on the basis of positive, sustained glycosuria. Each overtly diabetic rat was subsequently maintained, until day of sacrifice, on a single daily dose of PZI insulin, with the dose dependent upon daily assessment of glycosuria and ketonuria. At time of sacrifice, the rats were lethally anesthetized with methoxyflurane, in accordance with a protocol approved by the University of Virginia Animal Care Committee. Prior to cardiac arrest, intracardiac puncture allowed collection of peripheral blood in EDTA for leukocyte counts and differentials.

Cytofluorographic analyses of spleen cells were performed on a fluorescence-activated cell sorter (FACS) by incubation with murine-derived monoclonal antibodies to surface antigens W3/13 (T-cells and neutrophils), OX19 (T-cells), W3/25 (T_h/T_i cells and macrophages), and OX8 (T_c/T_s and Natural Killer cells), followed by incubation with a fluorescein isothiocyanate-conjugated (FITC) $F(ab')_2$ fragment of goat anti-mouse immunoglobin G (IgG). Lymphocyte function was assessed by 5-day mixed lymphocyte reactions (MLRs) using allogeneic (Fisher) rat spleen cells as stimulators, and 3-day concanavalin A (ConA) stimulation assays. The above procedures have been described previously (7).

Statistics: Probability values for differences in incidence of diabetes between experimental groups were calculated by X^2-analysis. For leukocyte and lymphocyte counts, and for lymphocyte in vitro function,

TABLE I

DIABETES INCIDENCE AND LYMPHOPENIA IN BB RATS NEONATALLY INJECTED
WITH WF BONE MARROW

Animal Group	Incidence of Diabetes[*]	Leukocytes/μl	Lymphocytes/μl
WF controls	----	8,670 $\pm$ 752 (10)	7,441 $\pm$ 601 (10)
BB controls	68% (76/111)	5,204 $\pm$ 785 (12)	3,551 $\pm$ 539[†](12)
Neonates given untreated (whole) WF bone marrow	23%[‡] (10/44)	6,734 $\pm$ 1,186 (16)	4,936 $\pm$ 786[§](16)
Neonates given T-cell-depleted WF bone marrow	75%[‖](33/44)	4,363 $\pm$ 820 (11)	3,053 $\pm$ 542[¶](11)

Animals are as described in the text. Leukocyte/lymphocyte counts are expressed as means $\pm$ SEM. Analyses were conducted at time of death, ⌁150 days of age or within 2-3 wk after onset of diabetes. Number in parentheses indicates number of rats examined.
[*]Number of diabetics/total number of rats. [†]$p < 0.0001$ compared with WF controls.
[‡]$p < 0.005$ compared with BB controls. [§]$p < 0.02$ compared with BB neonates given T-cell-depleted bone marrow; $p < 0.006$ compared with WF controls. [‖]NS ($p > 0.10$) compared with BB controls. [¶]$p < 0.0001$ compared with WF controls; NS ($p > 0.37$) compared with BB controls.

groups were compared by analysis of variance (with general linear model) accompanied by a Duncan's multiple-range test (α set at 0.05).

Results: As illustrated in Table 1, the incidence of diabetes in the recipients of untreated (whole) WF bone marrow was significantly reduced compared with BB controls ($p < 0.005$), with only 10 of the 44 (23%) inoculated BB neonates becoming diabetic by 140 days of age. These animals showed a significant improvement in lymphocyte counts, regardless of whether or not they became diabetic. In contrast, among the BB neonates inoculated with T-cell-depleted bone marrow cells, 33 of 44 (75%) became diabetic; this is not significantly different from the 68% incidence in control BB rats ($p > 0.10$). These rats still exhibited profound lymphopenia, with lymphocyte counts significantly lower than counts in the BB recipients of untreated (whole) WF bone marrow. Inoculation of T-cell-depleted WF bone marrow did not significantly affect T-cell subset distributions (data not shown). These results indicate that transfer of T-cell-depleted bone marrow not only did not change the incidence of diabetes but also did not correct the lymphopenia.

TABLE II
LYMPHOCYTE IN VITRO FUNCTION* IN BB RATS
NEONATALLY INJECTED WITH WF BONE MARROW

Animal Group	Mixed Lymphocyte Response	Response to Concanavalin A
Untreated BB controls	2,865 ± 399 (5)	22,084 ± 2,435 (15)
Neonates given untreated (whole) WF bone marrow	15,606 ± 4,883 (6)	50,927 ± 8,126 (8)

Animals are as described in the text and in Table 1. Spleen cells were plated in the presence of either 10 μg/ml ConA or allogeneic spleen cells, in medium containing 5% horse serum. Responsiveness was assessed by the subsequent incorporation of ^{3}H-thymidine. Number in parentheses indicates number of rats examined. *Data are expressed as means ± SEM of cpm of ^{3}H-thymidine.

The results of lymphocyte functional analyses are shown in Table 2. Splenic lymphocytes from BB rats given untreated (whole) WF bone marrow demonstrated significantly increased in vitro responsiveness compared with lymphocytes from control BB rats. Comparable studies on BB recipients of T cell-depleted bone marrow were not performed.

BONE MARROW IRRADIATION CHIMERA STUDIES:

Procedures: A series of bone marrow irradiation chimeras were constructed, using various combinations of normal (WF) or BB rat recipients and bone marrow donors. Since the bone marrow recipients were adults (> 37 days of age), each recipient was given 800 rads whole-body irradiation prior to bone marrow inoculation. Within 6 hours of irradiation, recipients were mildly anesthetized with methoxyflurane and were given an intracardiac injection of 5 x 10^7 (excluding erythrocytes) viable T-cell-depleted bone marrow cells. A total of 52 diabetes-prone BB rats were inoculated with WF bone marrow (designated WF → BB chimeras), ranging in age from 40-109 days of age. Seven adolescent WF rats were inoculated with WF bone marrow, as irradiation controls, and were designated WF → WF "chimeras." Twenty-one adolescent diabetes-prone BB rats were inoculated with bone marrow from overtly diabetic BB donors, as additional irradiation controls; these recipients were designated BB → BB "chimeras."

All bone marrow recipients were kept for at least 2 months in a dual-flow cleanroom furnished with HEPA filters (Lab Products, Maywood, NJ); all animals were observed for at least 140 days post-inoculation, or until onset of diabetes. Animals were maintained, and diabetes was diagnosed, in the same manner as in the neonatal bone marrow chimera studies, as previously described (7). Animals were sacrificed, and assessments were made of peripheral blood lymphopenia, splenic T-cell subset distributions, and

TABLE III

DIABETES INCIDENCE AND LYMPHOPENIA IN BB RAT BONE MARROW IRRADIATION CHIMERAS

Animal Group	Incidence of Diabetes[*]	Leukocytes/μl	Lymphocytes/μl
WF controls	---	10,151 $\pm$ 705 (18)	8,616 $\pm$ 625 (18)
WF rats injected with WF bone marrow (WF→WF chimeras)	0% (0/ 7)	9,230 $\pm$ 741[†] (5)	7,647 $\pm$ 738[†] (5)
BB rats injected with WF bone marrow (WF→BB chimeras)[‡]	0%[§](0/32)	10,780 $\pm$ 1,047[∥](18)	9,101 $\pm$ 904 [∥](18)
BB rats injected with BB bone marrow (BB→BB chimeras)	24%[¶](5/21)	5,305 $\pm$ 414[**](19)	3,215 $\pm$ 299[**](19)
Untreated BB littermates of the irradiation chimeras	38% (8/21)	5,233 $\pm$ 539 (21)	3,452 $\pm$ 359 (21)

Animals are as described in the text. Leukocyte/lymphocyte counts are expressed as means $\pm$ SEM. Analyses were conducted at time of death, ⌒150 days of age or within 2-3 wk after onset of diabetes. Number in parentheses indicates number of rats examined. [*]Number of diabetics/total number of rats. [†]NS (p > 0.44) compared with WF controls. [‡]Only those WF →BB chimeras irradiated and inoculated at < 44 days of age are included in this table. [§]p < 0.007 compared with BB→BB littermates. [∥]NS (p > 0.25) compared with WF and WF→WF controls. [¶]NS (p > 0.5) compared with litter-matched untreated controls. [**]p < 0.0001 compared with WF controls; NS (p > 0.61) compared with untreated BB littermates.

lymphocyte in vitro function, as described for the neonatal bone marrow chimeras. In addition, a monoclonal antibody to the RT-7.2 T-cell differentiation alloantigen (9) was used to document the persistence of donor-origin lymphoid cells in the WF → BB chimeras. The RT-7.2 antigen is expressed on WF T-cells, B-lymphocytes, and thymocytes, but is totally missing on BB rat lymphoid cells. Cells were analyzed on the FACS in a manner similar to that for the other monoclonal antibodies, as described previously (8).

Statistics: Probability values for differences in incidence of diabetes between experimental groups were calculated using the Fisher's Exact test. For leukocyte and lymphocyte counts, T cell subset distributions, and lymphocyte in vitro function, groups were compared by analysis of variance (with general linear model) accompanied by a Duncan's multiple-range test (α set at 0.05).

Results: As illustrated in Table 3, irradiated WF recipients of WF bone marrow (WF → WF chimeras) did not develop disease. The incidence of diabetes in BB → BB chimeras was not significantly different (p > 0.5) compared with their litter-matched controls. In irradiated BB rats that had received T cell depleted WF bone marrow (WF → BB chimeras), spleen cells

TABLE IV

T-LYMPHOCYTE SUBSET DISTRIBUTIONS IN BONE MARROW IRRADIATION CHIMERAS

Animal Group	N	Cell Type (% of Total)			
		T-cells (OX19$^+$)	T-cells (W3/13$^+$)	T_h/T_i (W3/25$^+$)	T_c/T_s/NK (OX8$^+$)
WF controls	19	38.7 $\pm$ 1.4	45.9 $\pm$ 1.3	25.1 $\pm$ 0.5	22.5 $\pm$ 0.8
WF→WF chimeras	6	43.1 $\pm$ 0.5	44.4 $\pm$ 1.7	28.1 $\pm$ 0.3	20.3 $\pm$ 0.5
WF→BB chimeras[*]	13	17.5 $\pm$ 2.2[†]	31.8 $\pm$ 1.5[‡]	16.1 $\pm$ 0.9[†]	11.7 $\pm$ 0.9[§]
BB→BB chimeras	15	5.9 $\pm$ 0.6[‖]	25.5 $\pm$ 2.2[‖]	12.8 $\pm$ 0.9	9.2 $\pm$ 0.8
BB controls	18	6.0 $\pm$ 0.6	27.9 $\pm$ 1.4	10.2 $\pm$ 0.7	6.5 $\pm$ 0.7

Rats are as described in the text and in Table 3. Spleen cells were analyzed on a fluorescence-activated cell sorter. Results are expressed as means $\pm$ SEM of the percent of total viable leukocytes with the indicated phenotype. [*]Only those WF→BB chimeras irradiated and inoculated at < 44 days of age are included in this table. [†]$p < 0.003$ compared with BB or BB→BB controls; $p < 0.001$ compared with WF or WF→WF controls. [‡]$p < 0.01$ compared with BB→BB controls; $p < 0.0001$ compared with WF or WF→WF controls. [§]$p < 0.04$ compared with BB→BB controls; $p < 0.007$ compared with BB controls; $p < 0.0001$ compared with WF or WF→WF controls. [‖]NS ($p > 0.29$) compared with BB controls; $p < 0.001$ compared with WF or WF→WF controls.

were positive for the RT7.2 differentiation alloantigen, verifying the persistence of donor-origin lymphoid cells and thus documenting the chimeric state. The overall incidence of diabetes in all 52 WF → BB chimeras was significantly reduced ($p < 0.001$) compared with untreated control BB rats (7/52, or 13%, vs. 113/184, or 61%, data not shown). When these data were examined more closely, it was seen that in animals that were less than 44 days of age at the time of bone marrow transfer, there was zero incidence (0/32) of diabetes. The total absence of diabetes in this latter group of animals, when compared with the BB → BB irradiation controls, was significant at the level of $p < 0.007$. Subsequent discussion of WF → BB chimeras will include only those animals irradiated and inoculated prior to 44 days of age. WF → WF irradiation controls had peripheral blood leukocyte and lymphocyte counts essentially identical to untreated WF control rats. Leukocyte and lymphocyte counts in the BB → BB chimeras were depressed and similar to those of the untreated BB control rats. In contrast, WF → BB chimeras were neither leukopenic nor lymphopenic. These results indicate that the transfer of T cell-depleted normal bone marrow into irradiated diabetes-prone BB rats completely corrected their peripheral blood lymphopenia as well as prevented the onset of overt diabetes.

Table IV shows the results of T cell subset analyses on spleen cells

TABLE V

MIXED LYMPHOCYTE RESPONSES* IN BB RAT BONE MARROW IRRADIATION CHIMERAS

| | Responder Cell Type | |
Animal Group	Spleen Cells	Lymph Node Cells
WF controls	$22,100 \pm 3,700$ (7)	$31,400 \pm 3,000$ (3)
WF→BB chimeras[†]	$20,600 \pm 4,200$[‡](10)	$30,700 \pm 3,000$[†](4)
BB→BB chimeras	$1,000 \pm 100$[§](16)	$5,300 \pm 1,800$[§](5)
BB controls	500 ± 200[‖](7)	$5,500 \pm 500$[‖](3)

Animals are as described in the text and in Tables 3 and 4. Spleen cells or lymph node cells were plated at 1×10^5 cells/well in the presence of 1×10^5 irradiated allogeneic (Fisher) spleen cells. Responsiveness was assessed by the subsequent incorporation of ^{3}H-thymidine. Number in parentheses indicates number of rats examined. *Data are expressed as means $\pm$ SEM of cpm of incorporated ^{3}H-thymidine. [†]Only those WF→BB chimeras irradiated and inoculated at < 44 days of age are included in this table. [‡]NS (p > 0.59) compared with WF controls; p < 0.0001 compared with BB controls. [§]NS (p > 0.94) compared with BB controls. [‖]p < 0.0001 compared with WF controls.

from the bone marrow irradiation chimeras. WF → WF irradiation controls had completely normal T cell subset distributions (essentially identical to WF controls). T cell subset distributions (essentially identical to WF controls). T cell subset distributions in the BB →BB chimeras were similar to the BB controls. Surprisingly, WF → BB chimeras did not show complete normalization of their subset distributions, despite the observation that these animals had normal leukocyte and lymphocyte counts in peripheral blood, and did not become diabetic. Although the fractions of cells in the OX19[+], W3/13[+], and WE/25[+] subsets were significantly increased compared to values in control BB rats, these subsets were still significantly decreased compared to WF and WF → WF control animals. THe proportion of OX8[+] cells was only slightly greater than that of BB → BB chimeras (p < 0.04).

The results of lymphocyte functional analyses are given in Table V. The table lists cpm of ^{3}H-thymidine incorporation in 5 day MLR assays. Lymph node cells and spleen cells from WF → BB chimeras showed complete restoration of responsiveness compared with WF control rats (NS, p > 0.60).

CONCLUSIONS AND THERAPEUTIC IMPLICATIONS

In our studies of neonatal bone marrow chimeras, we have shown significantly decreased incidence of diabetes and restoration of lymphocyte responsiveness after injection of MHC-compatible bone marrow from normal rats into neonatal diabetes-prone BB rats. However, we have also shown that injection of bone marrow pretreated with anti-T-cell antiserum plus complement had no effect on incidence of diabetes or on lymphocyte responsiveness. These results suggest that mature T cells in the bone marrow inoculum were responsible for the prevention of diabetes in such studies.

In our studies of adult bone marrow irradiation chimeras, we have shown that injection of T cell depleted bone marrow from normal MHC-compatible rats can completely prevent the expression of diabetes and can restore lymphocyte responsiveness. These findings suggest a defect in the BB rat lymphoid stem cell population. However, such treatment only partially restored the distributions of splenic T cell subsets of these animals, suggesting, as in the neonatal bone marrow chimera studies, a defect in the T cell differentiative environment. Interpretations of these studies with respect to identifying the sites of the defects within the immune system of this animal model are discussed more fully in the paper by Scott, et al., appearing elsewhere in this volume. Briefly, however, these studies suggest that there are two defects in the BB rat associated with the expression of diabetes, one occurring at the level of the bone marrow stem cell, and the other residing within the T cell differentiative environment.

What are the therapeutic implications of these animal studies to Type I diabetes in man? Justification for serious attempts at immunologic intervention in the prodromal period would require: (a) reliable markers for recognition of a population at high risk, and (b) a safe and effective method for prevention, to be used before the initiation of islet damage or at least prior to advanced islet destruction and hyperglycemia. Although HLA genotyping and islet cell antibody determinations are currently utilized, there remains an uncertainty about the predictive reliability of these markers. There are obvious concerns about subjecting to immunomanipulation individuals who are categorized as having an increased risk of diabetes but may in fact never become hyperglycemic. Of additional concern is our present lack of information on heterogeneity in the etiology of Type I diabetes. Until it is known which immunopathogenetic mechanism is responsible for end-stage beta cell failure in a given individual or family, therapeutic intervention may be contraindicated.

How would one envision, in future clinical trials, the treatment of an individual, reliably identified as "prediabetic," with bone marrow from a normal MHC-compatible donor? Unfortunately, the most common choice of bone marrow donor, an HLA-identical sibling, would in this case be inappropriate, since the sibling too would be at high risk for development of the disease. A major complication, even in bone marrow transplantation from HLA-identical siblings, is graft-versus-host (GVH) disease. Despite the use of immuno-suppressive agents such as methotrexate, cyclophosphamide, corticosteroids, antilymphocyte globulin, cyclosporin, or combinations of these agents given early after transplantation, moderate to severe acute GVH disease occurs in 35 to 75 percent of patients receiving bone marrow transplants from HLA-identical siblings, and it is fatal in up to one-half of affected patients (10). Treating the bone marrow of the donor ex vivo with anti-T-cell-anti-serum plus complement before inoculating the recipient can significantly reduce the potential for GVH disease. However, patients receiving T cell depleted bone marrow have been reported to have substantially higher risk of graft failure compared with those given untreated bone marrow (10). More important, our studies in the BB rat indicate that in order to prevent diabetes in that animal model by bone marrow engraftment in the newborn, mature T cells are needed in the bone marrow inoculum. If the human counterpart of this disease involves a defect in the T-cell differentiative environment, there would be a similar need for mature T cells in the inoculum.

Thus, although the construction of bone marrow chimeras provides an excellent opportunity to study, in the laboratory, the immunologic mechanisms associated with autoimmune expression in an animal model, it appears to have little direct clinical application to the prodromal period of Type I diabetes mellitus in man.

ACKNOWLEDGMENTS

PZI insulin was generously donated by Eli Lilly (Indianapolis, Indiana). We thank Dr. D.L. Greiner (University of Connecticut Health Center, School of Medicine, Farmington, Connecticut) for providing the monoclonal antibody RT-7.2.

REFERENCES

1. Naji, A., Silvers, W.K., Barker, C.F., 1983, Autoimmunity and Type I (insulin-dependent) diabetes mellitus. Transplantation 36: 355-361. [Review].

2. Rossini, A.A., Mordes, J.P., Like, A.A., 1985, Immunology of insulin-dependent diabetes mellitus. Ann Rev Immunol 3: 291-322. [Review].

3. Like, A.A., Kislauskis, E., Williams, R.M., Rossini, A.A., 1982, Neonatal thymectomy prevents spontaneous diabetes mellitus in the BB/W rat. Science 216: 644-646.

4. Like, A.A., Anthony, M., Guberski, D.L., Rossini, A.A., 1983, Spontaneous diabetes mellitus in the BB/W rat -- effects ofglucocorticoids, cyclosporin-A, and antiserum to rat lymphocytes. Diabetes 32: 326-330.

5. Rossini, A.A., Faustman, D., Woda, B.A., Like, A.A., Szymanski, I., Mordes, J.P., 1984, Lymphocyte transfusions prevent diabetes in the Bio-Breeding/Worcester (BB/W) rat. J Clin Invest 74: 39-46.

6. Naji, A., Silvers, W.K., Bellgrau, D., Anderson, A.O., Plotkin, S., Barker, C.F., 1981, Prevention of diabetes in rats by bone marrow transplantation. Ann Surg 194: 328-38.

7. Scott, J., Engelhard, V.H., Curnow, R.T., Benjamin, D.C., 1986, Prevention of diabetes in the BB rat. 1. Evidence suggesting a requirement for mature T cells in bone marrow inoculum of neonatally injected rats. Diabetes 35: 1034-1040.

8. Scott, J., Engelhard, V.H., Benjamin, D.C., 1987, Bone marrow irradiation chimeras in the BB rat: Evidence suggesting two defects leading to diabetes and lymphopoenia. Diabetologia 30: 774-781.

9. Greiner, D.L., Handler, E.S., Nakano, K., Mordes, J.P., Rossini, A.A., 1986, Absence of RT-6 T cell subset in diabetes-prone BB/W rats. J Immunol 136: 148-151.

10. Mitsyasu, R.T., Champlin, R.E., Gale, R.P., Ho, W.G., Lenarsky, C., Winston, D., Selch, M., Elashoff, R., Giorgi, J.V., Wells, J., Terasaki, P., Billing, R., Feig, S., 1986, Treatment fo donor bone marrow with monoclonal anti-T-cell antibody and complement for the prevention of graft-versus host disease. Ann Intern Med 105: 20-26.

THE INCIDENCE OF DIABETES IN BB RATS IS DECREASED

FOLLOWING ACUTE LCMV INFECTION

¶Thomas Dyrberg[*], Peter Schwimmbeck[+], and Michael Oldstone[++]

Hagedorn Research Laboratory[*], Gentofte, Denmark
University of Dusseldorf, Dusseldorf, West German [+]
Scripps Clinic and Research Foundation, La Jolla, California, USA[++]

BB rats are a well studied animal model of insulin dependent diabetes mellitus (IDDM). About 59-90% of animals spontaneously develop IDDM between 60-140 days of age, characterized by weight loss, glycosuria, hyperglycemia, and mononuclear infiltrations of the islets of Langerhans (1). The pathogenesis is believed to be immune mediated as they show a number of immune abnormalities, including autoantibodies to islet cells, lymphocytic infiltration, and injury to islets can be demonstrated before and during the onset of IDDM. The immune regulation is defective in the BB rats as indicated by reduced mixed lymphocyte reactions and reduced responsiveness to T-cell mitogens. Lymphopenia may accompany the course of disease but by itself it is not a prerequisite for development of IDDM. The immune pathogenesis can be passively transferred to non-diabetic animals by concanavalin A stimulated lymphocytes, and recently it has been shown that IDDM in BB rats can be prevented by treatment with monoclonal antibodies which recognize T-lymphocytes or natural killer cells (2).

Viruses can interfere with the function of the immune system either directly through viral replication in immune competent cells or indirectly by causing release of soluble immune modulators, e.g., monokines that may affect other uninfected cells (3). Viruses are generally known for the damage they do, however, the aim of the present study was to determine whether a virus could help control a disease through its ability to infect and alter lymphocyte function. Towards that goal we choose to study lymphocytic choriomeningitis virus (LCMV) and the BB rat model of IDDM. Previously it has been shown that LCMV clone13, which is a lymphotropic variant of LCMV Armstrong CA1371 establishes persistent virus infections in immunocompetent mice, by specifically suppressing the generation of LCMV specific, H2 restricted cytotoxic T-lymphocytes (4). The effect of this virus strain on rats in general or on BB rats specifically is unknown, although injection of adult rats with other strains of LCMV is not associated with persistent infection.

MATERIALS AND METHODS

Diabetes-prone (dp) and resistant (dr) BB rats obtained from the Worcester colony were weaned at 30 days of age. In each litter studied, 1-4 rats were given 1×10^7 pfu of LCMV clone13 by i.v. injection. The virus

This work was supported by NATO grant RG 86/0138

inoculated rats were separated from the remaining litter mates, and body weight and development of IDDM monitored from 45 to 200 days of age, 3 times a week. The virus, LCMV clone13 was propagated and checked for biological properties as described (4).

Intraperitoneal glucose tolerance tests were performed on non-diabetic dp and dr BB rats of approximately 200 days of age by standard method (1). For histologic analyses, rats with IDDM were sacrificed within one week after the onset of the disease and non-diabetic dr and dp BB rats were sacrificed between 200-250 days of age. Pancreatic insulin was extracted in acid ethanol and the insulin content measured by radio-immuno assay.

The presence of virus specific antibodies in serum was tested on LCMV infected cells by indirect immunofluorescence analysis and sera were also tested for their capacity to neutralize LCMV clone13 in vitro as described (5). Sera of uninfected animals were used as negative controls. To test for infectious virus, peripheral blood lymphocytes (PBL) were isolated and incubated in serial dilutions with a monolayer of Vero cells. The cells were overlayed with 1% Agarose in medium and stained with neutral red after 5 days and plaques counted 24 hours later. To test for the presence of viral nucleic acid sequences RNA was extracted from organs from infected and uninfected BB rats, applied to nitrocellulose filters and hybridized by standard method with a ^{33}P-labelled cDNA probe specific for the S segment of LCMV. As a positive control RNA was extracted from the spleens of mice persistently infected with LCMV clone13 and hybridized in parallel.

The T-lymphocyte subsets were analyzed by FACS using monoclonal antibodies for the following T-cell markers: W3/13, which labels all rat T-lymphocytes, W3/25 which labels helper T-cells, and OX8 which labels non-helper T-cells. Negative (only second anybody) and positive controls (PPL from Wistar rats) were included in each analysis.

RESULTS

In the present study we demonstrate that virus infection may help to modulate or cure a disease. Following inoculation of a lymphotropic virus into 30 days old dp BB rats, the incidence of spontaneous IDDM was markedly reduced. In 38 dp BB rats from 14 litters inoculated with LCMV clone13 the incidence of IDDM was only 14/38 (37%), with a median age of onset of IDDM of 109 days (range 77-220 days) (Fig 1). In contrast, 67/82 (82%) of control dp BB rats became diabetic by a median age of 103 days (range 65-237 days) (Fig 1). None of 8 dr BB rats inoculated with LCMV clone13 or of 50 control dr BB rats developed diabetes. The mean blood glucose levels at the onset of diabetes in virus inoculated rats were similar to those in uninfected dp BB rats (404±22 mg/dl versus 374±63 mg/dl, ±1 SD). Regularly monitored blood glucose levels in non-diabetic LCMV inoculated dp BB rats were equivalent to levels in non-diabetic control dp BB rats. The 37% of the LCMV inoculated dp rats that did develop IDDM were evenly distributed in the litters and were indistinguishable from the diabetic control dp BB rats in the biochemical parameters of IDDM.

Although LCMV inoculation of dp BB rats significantly reduced the incidence of IDDM, nevertheless, some early preclinical manifestations of beta cell damage were present. Thus, in the glucose tolerance test the mean 60 min value was significantly increased among 14 LCMV inoculated, non-diabetic dp BB rats (Table 1) and 11 of the 14 rats showed 60 min values above the mean +3SD of non-inoculated, dr BB rats (n = 10, 283 mg/dl). The histopathological analysis of virus inoculated dp BB rats that failed to develop diabetes showed a spectrum of morphological changes. Study of multiple tissue sections indicated that 4 out of 15 rats had completely normal islets and no signs of inflammation. The remaining rats had variable degrees of mononuclear cell infiltration, but in all cases inflammation was less severe than in the diabetic rats. Further, the pancreatic insulin levels in these rats were similar to those of non diabetic dp control BB rats and resembled those of uninfected dr BB rats (Table 1).

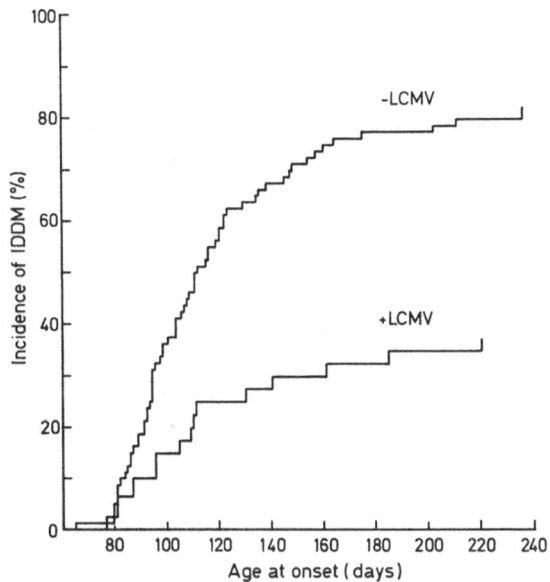

Figure 1. The incidence of diabetes in control (-LCMV) and in lymphocytic choriomeningitis virus clone13 inoculated (+LCMV) diabetes prone BB rats.
-LCMV: 82% incidence (67/82) of IDDM by 237 days, median age at onset was 103 days.
+LCMV: 37% incidence (14/38) of IDDM in rats inoculated with 1x10 pfu of LCMV clone13 intravenously by 30 days of age. Median age at onset was 109 days.

TABLE I

LCMV clone13 INFECTION DECREASES THE INCIDENCE OF DIABETES IN BB RATS

rats[a]	virus[b]	diabetes	serum glucose (mg/dl)[c]		pancreatic insulin (ng/mg)[d]	
			0 min	60 min		
dr BB	none	0/50(0%)	(n=10) 129(11)	166(39)	(n=3)	289(44)
dr BB	LCMV clone13	0/8(%)	(n=4) 131(16)	210(93)	(n=4)	227(69)
dp BB	none	67/82(82%)	(n=3) 152(29)	177(35)	(n=3)	217(22)
dp BB	LCMV clone13	14/38(37%)	(n=14) 163(18)	401(101)	(n=10)	203(49)

a) dr BB = diabetes-resistant BB rats
   dp BB = diabetes-prone BB rats
b) Rats were injected intravenously with 1x 10^7 pfu of lymphocytic choriomeningitis virus as described in the text.
c) Non-diabetic rats, approx. 200 days of age were injected i.e. with glucose, 2 g/kg bodyweight after 18 hours fast. Serum glucose was determined at 0 and 60 min, mean values and (SD) are shown.
d) The pancreas insulin content expressed as ng insulin per mg lyophilized pancreas in non-diabetic rats approx. 200 days of age. Mean values and (SE) are shown.

Although no illness was apparent in LCMV inoculated dp BB rats, their body weight was significantly lower from 14 days after injection compared to uninfected dp rats, and this difference was maintained throughout the study (Fig 2). However, the lower body weight itself cannot explain the reduced incidence of diabetes, since the animals were followed for more

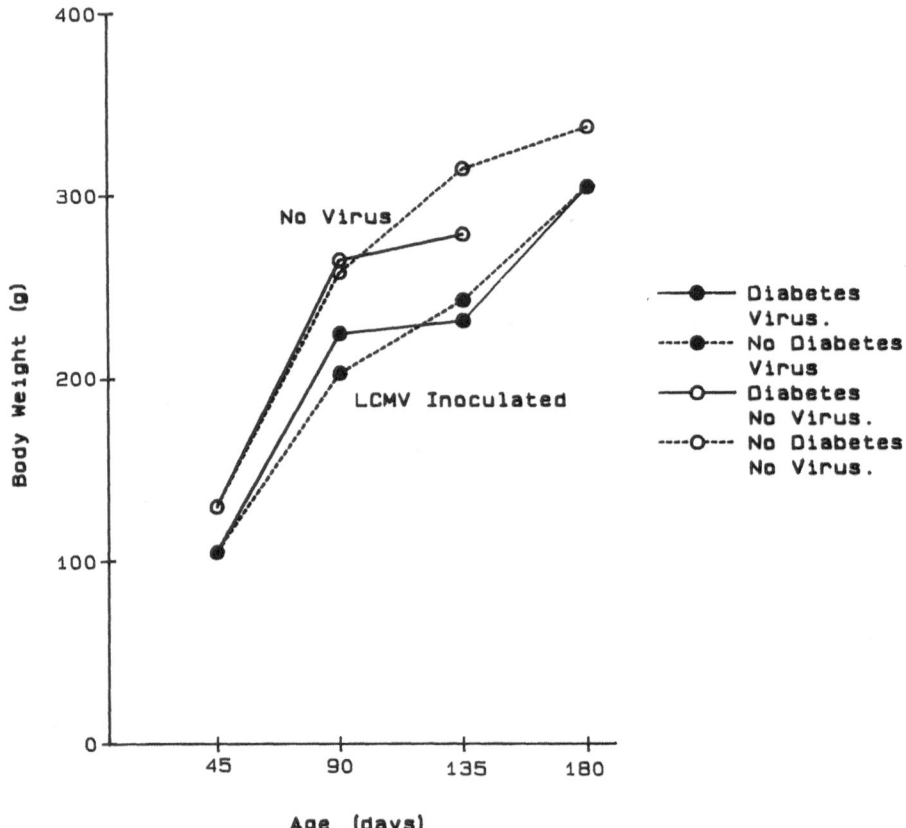

Figure 2. Body weight in diabetes prone BB rats with or without inoculation with lymphocytic choriomeningitis clone13.

than 200 days, and there was no difference in the body weight prior to onset of IDDM between animals that did or did not develop diabetes in either group of rats. LCMV inoculated rats appeared in good health during the observation period and the presence of normal pancreas insulin levels make it unlikely that the lower body weight masked a diabetic stage.

Reduction in the incidence of diabetes was associated with infection of infectious virus, since injection with UV-inactivated virus did not change the incidence of diabetes in dp BB rats (81%, 17/21) compared to uninoculated dp rats (82%, 67/82). The sera from virus inoculated BB rats (n=7) contained antibodies to LCMV from 7 days after inoculation and until the end of the study at 200 days. All sera neutralized LCMV when tested 170 days after viral inoculation. The prevention of IDDM virus was thus not followed by a general state of immune suppression since the infected dp BB rats could raise a specific humoral immune response against LCMV clone13 and did not develop secondary infections. These observations may indicate that LCMV clone13 prevents diabetes by a specific interference with the autoimmune response which cause the disease.

Virus could be recovered from lymphocytes by cocultivation on Vero cells up to 10 days after infection but not at 30 days or later. The virus was identified as LCMV by nucleic acid and immunochemical analysis; the titers of 10^2 to 10^5 infective centers /10^7 PBL indicated that less than 1% of the cells contained a full viral gene. To see if animals were persistently infected and whether cells or organs other than PBL had virus, we extracted RNA from several organs. By using LCMV specific probe for hybridization no viral transcript could be detected in the brain, kidney, pancreas, spleen or adrenals of infected BB rats. In contrast, RNA extracted from the spleen of a persistently infected mouse produced a strong signal under the same conditions.

The effect of virus infection on the T-lymphocyte subsets was studied by FACS analysis. As has previously been shown (6) we found that uninfected dp BB rats had a marked reduction in cytotoxic T- and helper T-lymphocytes. In contrast, analysis of dp BB rats 4 to 7 days after virus inoculation showed even lower levels of helper and suppressor/cytotoxic T-cells, but 14 days after infection the lymphocytes returned to normal levels or even higher and remained there for the entire observation period. Virus inoculated dr BB rats showed no changes in the T-cells subsets after infection when compared to uninfected rats.

DISCUSSION

Abrogation of diabetes in these experiments was associated with an acute infection of lymphocytes and with a marked decrease in all T-lymphocyte subsets. These observations suggest that the virus infection of lymphocytes may be directly related to the inhibition of IDDM, which is of particular interest because lymphocytes are thought to play a crucial role in the pathogenesis of IDDM (2). LCMV infection of BB rats could prevent diabetes through a number of ways. First, the particular variant of LCMV we used here is lymphotropic and may lyse selected subsets of lymphocytes responsible for making autoimmune responses at an early stage whereafter disease would not occure. These results are supported by our finding that LCMV can infect adult dp BB-rat lymphocytes in vitro (7). A second hypothesis is that LCMV persists in lymphocytes, at a low non-detectable level altering the lymphocyte function without destroying the cells, thus abrogating the autoimmune reaction causing IDDM. Interestingly, LCMV clone13 can cause a specific immune suppression (i.e. the failure to generate LCMV specific cytotoxic T-lymphocyte), when inoculated into adult immune competent mice (4). However, in conclusion our data suggests that LCMV virus does not persist in infected BB rats but that the clonal deletion of lymphocytes may be an important factor in preventing diabetes.

The observation that LCMV infection of BB rats decreases the incidence of IDDM is supported by recent studies in the spontaneously diabetic NOD mice (8). When these mice were infected with LCMV, IDDM was completely prevented and it was shown that a selective immune suppression was achieved by infection of lymphocytes. However, in contrast to the findings in BB rats where LCMV infection was acute and self-limiting, in NOD mice the virus caused a persistent infection.

Immunological responses can be altered upon infection of monocytes and lymphocytes by several RNA and DNA viruses. Depending on the time of infection, the viral agent and the immune status of the host, viruses have the ability to regulate the host's immune response based on their tropism for special cells of the immune system (3). This was shown in New Zealand mice, where infection with LCMV or polyoma virus, enhanced the humoral autoimmune response to DNA (9). To the contrary the lupus syndrome that normally occurs in New Zealand black mice was prevented by infection with lactate dehydrogenase virus (LDV) (10), which infects macrophages and changes lymphocyte functions. In conclusion, these data and the results presented in this paper suggest that virus and/or their products may be used to elucidate the mechanisms whereby some autoimmune diseases develop and be designed to provide help and not harm.

REFERENCES

1. Marliss, E., A. Nakhooda, P. Poussier, and A. Sima, 1982, The diabetic syndrome of the "BB" Wistar rat: possible relevance to type I (insulin-dependent) diabetes in man. Diabetologia 22: 225-232.

2. Like A.A., C.A. Biron, E.J. Weringer, K. Byman, E. Sroczynski and D.L. Guberski, 1986, Prevention of diabetes in Biobreeding/Worcester rats with monoclonal antibodies that recognize T. lymphocytes or natural killer cells. J Exp Med, 164: 1145-1159.

3. McChesney, M., and M.B.A. Oldstone, 1987, Viruses perturb lymphocyte functions: selected principles characterizing virus-induced immunosuppression. Annu Rev Immunol 5:279-304.

4. Ahmed, R., A. Salmi, L. Butler, J. Chiller, and M.B.A. Oldstone, 1984, Selection of genetic variants of lymphocytic choriomeningitis virus in spleens of persistently infected mice. J Exp Med 160: 521-540.

5. Doyle, M.V., and M.B.A. Oldstone, 1978, Interactions between viruses and lymphocytes. I. In vivo replication of lymphocytic choriomeningitis virus in mononuclear cells during both chronic and acute viral infections. J Immunol 121: 1262-1269.

6. Like A.A., and A.A. Rossini, 1984, Spontaneous autoimmune diabetes mellitus in the Bio Breeding/Worcester rat. Surv Synth Pathol Res 3: 131.

7. Schwimmbeck, P.L., T. Dyrberg and M.B.A. Oldstone, 1988, Abrogation of diabetes in BB rats by acute virus infection: association of viral-lymphocyte interactions. J Immunol 140: 3394-3400.

8. Oldstone, M.B.A., 1988, Prevention of type I diabetes in NOD mice by virus infection. Science 239: 500-502.

9. Tonietti, G., M.B.A. Oldstone, and F. Dixon, 1970, The effect of induced chronic viral infections on the immunologic diseases of New Zealand mice. J Exp Med 132: 89-109.

10. Oldstone, M.B.A., and F. Dixon, 1972, Inhibition of antibodies to nuclear antigen and to DNA in New Zealand mice infected with lactate dehydrogenase virus. Science (Wash. DC) 175: 784-786.

STRATEGIES FOR PRIMARY PREVENTION

OF NON-INSULIN DEPENDENT DIABETES MELLITUS

¶Jaako Tuomilehto

Department of Epidemiology
National Public Health Institute
Helsinki, Finland

Non-insulin dependent diabetes mellitus (NIDDM) is a disease with poorly understood natural history and severe long-term complications, and it is associated with large human and economic burden and costs. Epidemiologic data from various parts of the world suggest that NIDDM is increasing in most populations and in some of them it has already reached epidemic proportions (1). Diabetes seriously affects the quality of life because of its complications and the life of diabetic patients is clearly shortened. These facts make the question of preventing NIDDM important.

It has been asked whether sufficient data exist to commence large-scale prevention of NIDDM. However, in 1921 Dr. E.P. Joslin in his article The Prevention of Diabetes Mellitus (2) expressed his opinion in the following way: "...it is proper at the present time to devote time not alone to treatment, but still more, as in the campaign against typhoid fever, to prevention. The results may not be quite so striking or as immediate, but they are sure to come and to be important." During those nearly 70 years since Dr. Joslin's recommendations, the list of serious attempts for primary prevention of diabetes is rather brief (3). Dr. Joslin was particularly suggesting interventions against overweight. It is astonishing that despite all resources used in diabetes research – not even the hypothesis of weight control in the prevention of NIDDM has been scientifically tested in proper population-based studies by 1988. Uncertainty still may exist as to whether present data are sufficient for prevention of NIDDM, but very little is learned about prevention of NIDDM without trying it.

GENETIC SUSCEPTIBILITY

Type 2 diabetes has a strong familias aggregation and it has been estimated that almost 40% of the siblings of NIDDM patients could expect to develop diabetes assuming the maximum life expectancy of 80 years (4). Strong evidence of the importance of genetic factors has been obtained from twin studies which have shown that there is about 90% concordance in Type 2 diabetes (5). It can be argued that environmental factors unmask this susceptibility in genetically predisposed individuals but specific genetic markers or determinants still remain to be identified.

The research in the Pacific populations was supported by NIH grant ROI AM 25446.

Several markers independent of blood glucose concentration which have been proposed have failed to provide further understanding to this problem.

However, as little can be done to change genetic susceptibility, one of the major challenges in diabetes prevention remains by modifying some of the environmental factors identified to be associated with the risk of NIDDM in particular populations.

PREVENTION STRATEGIES

Primary prevention has been defined as all measures designed to reduce the incidence of a certain disease in a population, by reducing the risk of its onset. In other terms this means that the attributable risk related to certain risk factors is modified by influencing the levels of such factors. NIDDM is a multifactorial disease. Therefore, for preventive measures for NIDDM, to be effective in the population, they must be based on interventions on several potential risk factors simultaneously. This will also mean that univariate estimates of attributable risks of various risk factors must be interpreted with great caution.

Assuming that NIDDM is preventable, there are two components in the implementation of primary prevention:
(1)   a population strategy - for altering the life-style and those environmental determinants which are the underlying causes of NIDDM;

(2)   a high risk strategy - for screening for individuals at special high risk and bringing preventive care to them.

DETERMINANTS OF NIDDM

Central element to the planning of any NIDDM prevention activity is the definition of major behavioural and environmental determinants of NIDDM in the target population or in genetically susceptible individuals, which lead to a potential abnormality of glucose tolerance and to overt NIDDM.

In the following text data on putative risk factors of NIDDM are reviewed paying particular attention to their potential role in the primary prevention of NIDDM. For this it is important to determine the "population attributable risk." Using a univariate approach, the relative importance of different risk factors can be determined by calculating from incidence of the exposed (I_e) and nonexposed (I_o) populations and in the total population (I_p). Thus, the population attributable risk is:

$$\frac{I_p - I_o}{I_p} = \frac{P_e (RR - 1)}{1 + P_e (RR - 1)} \; ;$$

where P_e = prevalence of the risk factor in the population

RR = risk ratio $\dfrac{I_e}{I_o}$

The population attributable risk provides an estimate of the proportion of the disease that could be eliminated by eliminating the risk factor.

A. Study Materials

In addition to the existing data from the literature three major data sets were analysed for this report:

(1) Diabetes surveys in the Pacific Island populations in 1975-82 (1).

(2)   Diabetes surveys in Malta in 1981-83.

(3)   Cohort of Finnish men from the "Seven Countries Study" examined
during 1959-84 (6).

Survey methods in the Pacific population have been described in various reports by Prof. P. Zimmet and his coworkers (7).

In Malta, the original sample comprised 1100 households where 2945
people older than 15 years were identified and invited to the first survey examination in the beginning of 1981. Of 2149 responders, 86.7% were
found having normal glucose tolerance, 5.6% impaired glucose tolerance (IGT)
and 7.7% diabetes. Those with IGT and diabetes together with a sample of
250 subjects with normal glucose tolerance got an invitation to another,
more detailed examination which took place a few months later. All these
subjects invited to the second examination were then followed up for two
years, and the third examination was carried out in the spring of 1983.
Altogether 154 men and 159 women participated in the two-year follow-up
examination and had the necessary data available required for applying
the diagnostic criteria for diabetes.

Survey procedures of Finnish men are described elsewhere (6). Data
about diabetes at the first four examinations (1959, 1964, 1969 and 1974)
were based on clinical diagnosis only, whereas at 25 years in 1984 an oral
glucose tolerance test was done.

B.   Obesity and hyperinsulinemia

A strong, graded and consistent association has been demonstrated between obesity and NIDDM. As many as 80% of the NIDDM patients are obese
at the time of onset of the disease. The incidence of NIDDM increases ex-
ponentially with an increasing degree of obesity. The obese children of
diabetic parent(s) have a much higher risk of developing Type II diabetes
than obese persons with non-diabetic parents (8). Thus, the genetic
susceptibility and obesity seem to act synergistically. It is clear that
there is heterogeneity in the occurrence of obesity and in the impact of
obesity on diabetes between populations.

Vague proposed in 1956 that complications of obesity were more prevalent in android (excess fat in upper part of the body) than in gynoid (excess fat in gluteal-femoral parts of the body) obesity (9). This theory
has been replicated more recently many times. The findings from several
studies have suggested that this association is more pronounced in women
than in men. There is some evidence that subjects with predominantly upper body fat distribution are more insulin-resistant than equally heavy
subjects with predominantly lower body fat. Obese individuals exhibit
hyperinsulinemia after glucose, suggesting that obese individuals produce
excessive quantities of insulin after glucose challenge, but insulin is
in fact ineffective as glucose tolerance is relatively impaired even in
the face of massive hyperinsulinemia. Data from several studies have suggested that these populations at high risk for NIDDM have more hyperinsulinemia than can be accounted for by their adiposity alone.

In normal weight individuals, impaired glucose tolerance is a feature
of either impaired insulin secretion or insulin resistance. In the obese
with impaired glucose tolerance, however, insulin resistance is consistently present whereas impaired secretion is never found.

Among the Pacific Island populations and in Malta the vast majority
of the diabetic subjects were obese at the time of the survey. As a whole
70.9% of men and 80.6% of women had a body mass index (BMI($\geqslant$ 27.0 kg/m^2,

TABLE I

THE PROPORTION OF OBESE SUBJECTS AMONG DIABETIC SUBJECTS
IN MEN AND WOMEN AGED 20-59 IN 12 POPULATIONS WITH HIGH RISK OF DIABETES

Population	Number of diabetic subjects		Proportion of diabetic subjects with high BMI			
			BMI $\geq$27		BMI $\geq$29	
	MEN	WOMEN	MEN %	WOMEN %	MEN %	WOMEN %
Cook Islands	20	35	65.0	80.0	50.0	74.3
Niue	22	39	54.5	69.2	40.9	51.3
New Caledonia-Noumea	43	53	83.7	84.9	72.1	79.2
Fiji-Melanesian	13	29	53.8	79.3	30.8	55.2
Fiji-Asian Indian	65	78	21.5	56.4	9.2	37.2
Fiji-Lakeba	11	11	72.7	72.7	36.4	72.7
New Caledonia-Loyalty	9	18	66.7	66.7	33.3	55.6
Western Samoa	25	36	76.0	80.6	68.0	69.4
Tuvalu	3	13	100.0	92.3	100.0	92.3
Nauru	73	78	80.8	96.2	71.2	87.2
Kiribati	79	72	69.6	69.4	50.6	56.9
Nauru -82	140	168	92.9	92.3	84.3	88.1
Malta	40	62	57.5	80.6	42.5	67.7
Total	543	692	70.9	80.6	57.8	70.4

TABLE II

RISK OF DIABETES BY BODY MASS INDEX IN MIDDLE-AGED FINNISH MEN[1]

Initial body-mass index level (kg/m^2)	Diabetes at 25-year follow-up					
	40-49 yrs		50-59 yrs		Total	
	N	%	N	%	N	%
BMI <27.0 at baseline	227	18.5	102	32.5	349	22.8
BMI at 15 years						
<27.0	146	17.1	71	31.0	237	19.0
$\geq$27.0	81	21.0	31	35.5	112	25.0
BMI $\geq$27.0 at baseline	35	34.3	22	50.0	57	40.4
Total	262	20.6	124	35.5	386	25.4
Population attributable risk for BMI<27.0 at baseline	11.4%		8.5%		10.2%	
Population preventable fraction for BMI<27.0 both at baseline and at 15 years	21.4%		16.9%		18.9%	

[1] Only those subjects included whose fasting time before the oral glucose tolerance test was more than 3 hours and who were examined during the morning hours.

and 57.8% of men and 70.4% of women a BMI $\geqslant$ 29.0 kg/m^2)(Table I). Among Finnish men aged 40-59 the baseline BMI as a predictor of developing diabetes during the 25-year follow-up was stronger than the change in BMI during the follow-up (Table II). The effect of BMI on the risk of diabetes was clearer in the younger 10-year age group. High BMI, however, was not the main cause of diabetes in these men as the population attributable risk of high BMI at baseline was only about 10%. About 20% of diabetes of these men could have been prevented by keeping BMI all the time lower than 27 kg/m^2. Also among the Maltese the positive association between BMI and the risk of diabetes was only seen in subjects under 60 years of age (Figure 1).

C. Physical inactivity

Regular physical activity improves glucose tolerance in patients with non-insulin-dependent diabetes mellitus (NIDDM) by increasing insulin sensitivity. In non-diabetic people the positive effect of physical training on glucose tolerance seems to be only small. It has also been suggested that physical activity could partially prevent the deterioration of glucose tolerance with ageing. At present, epidemiological data on the role of physical activity in the etiology of NIDDM or in the worsening of glucose tolerance are still few but promising. Lower prevalence of diabetes was found in female former college athletes as compared with non-athletes using a questionnaire method, with a relative risk of 2.24 for the non-athletes (10). Results from cross-sectional studies suggest that physical inactivity is an independent risk factor of NIDDM.

In Malta, the age-standardized two-year risk of diabetes was consistently and inversely related to the level of physical activity (Table III). Among subjects with normal glucose tolerance at baseline those with low

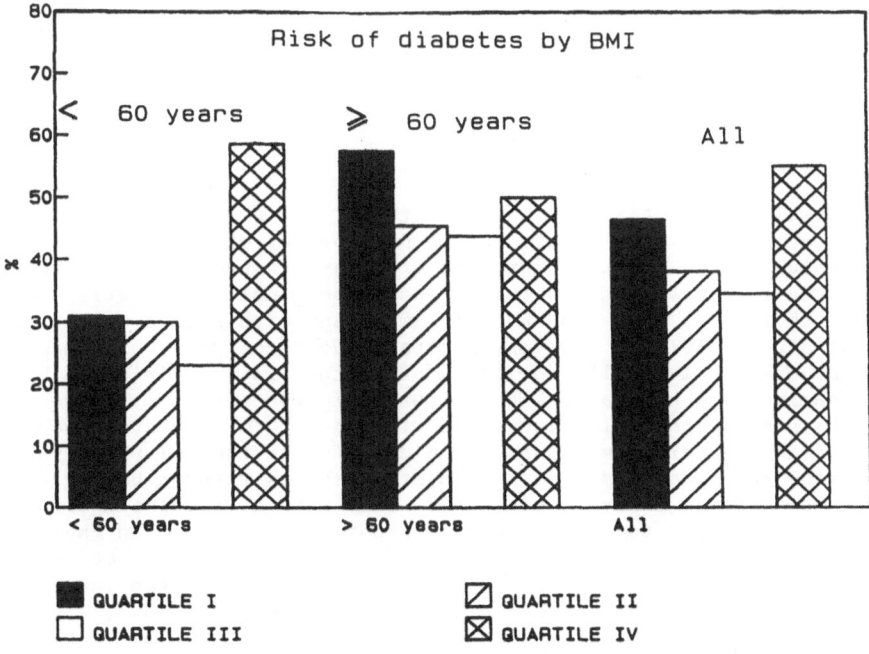

Figure 1. The risk of diabetes by body mass index (BMI) quartile during a two-year follow-up in people with impaired (IGT) or normal glucose tolerance at baseline (men and women together) in Malta.

TABLE III

RISK OF DIABETES IN MALTESE PEOPLE BY PHYSICAL ACTIVITY AND FAMILY HISTORY
OF DIABETES DURING A TWO-YEAR FOLLOW-UP IN MALTA

| Diabetes at follow-up | Baseline situation | | | | Total |
| | High or moderate physical activity | | Low physical activity | | |
	Family history negative (N)	Family history positive (N)	Family history negative (N)	Family history positive (N)	(N)
No	68	17	65	9	159
Yes	12	5	15	5	37
Total	80	22	80	14	196
Incidence of diabetes	15.0%	18.8%	22.7%	35.7%	18.9%
Risk ratio	1.00	1.25	1.51	2.38	
Population attributable risk for:					
- Low physical activity			11.7%		
- Family history of diabetes and low physical activity together			8.9%		

physical activity had a two-fold risk of diabetes during follow-up than
those with high physical activity. The risk was especially high in subjects with both a low physical activity and a family history of diabetes.

The population attributable risk for low physical activity was 11.7%
and when considering the family history simultaneously did not increase
but decreased it slightly, although the risk ratio increased. This dis-
crepancy reflects the relatively small population segment having these
two risk factors.

D. Impaired glucose tolerance

It is well documented that people with IGT may worsen to overt diabetes. IGT may be a critical stage in the development of NIDDM, because it
is detectable and treatment may prevent or delay its progression. IGT is
the first recognizable stage in the process from genetic susceptibility to
NIDDM, and therefore, it is potentially important with regard to the prevention of NIDDM. IGT is, however, a heterogenous category which might
contain not only individuals who indeed are either in transition to NIDDM
or at an early stage of disease, but also people who never will develop
NIDDM. The prevalence of IGT increases with age up to 65 years, when it
exceeds 20% in several populations. The duration of the IGT phase varies
markedly, and some people may develop overt diabetes without having diagnosed such an obvious intermediate stage. The rate of developing from IGT
to diabetes is about 2 to 3% per year in studies carried out in the UK and
USA. In the populations where the occurrence of diabetes was not very high
about half of those with IGT seem to return to normal in a ten years follow-up. In populations which have a higher prevalence of NIDDM, a greater
proportion of persons with IGT will develop NIDDM as shown in the Pima Indians and Nauruans.

In Nauru, IGT was associated with a four-fold risk of diabetes during
6 years (Table 4). At baseline about 20% had IGT, and the population attributable risk for developing diabetes was 42.5% suggesting that screening

TABLE IV

THE RISK OF DIABETES MELLITUS IN PEOPLE WITH NORMAL AND IMPAIRED (IGT)
GLUCOSE TOLERANCE DURING A 6-YEAR FOLLOW-UP IN NAURU AND DURING
A 2-YEAR FOLLOW-UP IN MALTA

Diabetes at follow-up	NAURU Glucose tolerance at baseline			MALTA Glucose tolerance at baseline	
	Normal	IGT	Total	Normal (N)	IGT (N)
No	201	38	239	117	40
Yes	14	13	27	18	14
Total	215	51	266	135	54
Incidence of diabetes	6.5	25.5	11.3	13.3%	25.9%
Risk ratio for IGT	3.92			1.95	
Population attributable risk for IGT during the follow-up	42.5%			8.9%	

for IGT could be useful. In Malta, the risk of diabetes among subjects
with IGT was two-fold. In the Maltese study population over 35 years of
age the prevalence of IGT was about 10%, and the population attributable
risk for developing diabetes was 8.9%. This indicates that in Malta by
screening for 100 only a small proportion of new cases of NIDDM could have
been potentially prevented.

E. Other risk factors

Other risk factors include gestational diabetes, hypertension, high
saturated fat intake and low fiber intake. There is uncertainty about
the prognostic significance of testing glucose tolerance in pregnant women.
The incidence of subsequent overt diabetes mellitus in women with gestational diabetes is quite high, about 3 to 5% per year which cumulatively
means in a 15 years follow-up 35-40%. Gestational diabetes in the mother
may mean an increased risk of the offspring for developing diabetes.

Hypertension is strongly associated with diabetes. In fact it is so
commonly associated with NIDDM and obesity that common underlying mechanisms have been suggested. Insulin resistance or hyperinsulinemia are present in the majority of hypertensives and could possibly explain the association between obesity, hypertension and glucose intolerance. It can be
argued that the hypertension and IGT are related, partially through genetic
factors and partially through dietary factors. Obesity per se is an important factor but is not sufficient to explain this association. Other important environmental factors are a high dietary fat intake and low dietary fibre intake. Moreover, commonly used antihypertensive agents may unmask glucose intolerance.

Within the male Adventist population in California, vegetarians had a
substantially lower risk of diabetes as an underlying or contributing cause
of death than non-vegetarians. The prevalence of self-reported diabetes was
also lower than in non-vegetarians. The reduced rates of diabetes could be
due to lower meat or saturated fat consumption.

INTERVENTION MEASURES TO PREVENT NIDDM

A. High risk approach

The potential for primary prevention of NIDDM exists in families in which a positive family history for NIDDM has been confirmed. persons between 40 and 65 years of age (in some populations up till 75) should be the main target group. All women with gestational diabetes should be considered to be at high risk. Hypertensive patients form another high risk group. Obese and physically inactive people should also be considered as additional risk groups, especially if the family history for diabetes is positive.

The best predictor of the development of diabetes in high risk groups is, apart from the genetic predisposition, the degree of glucose intolerance. Therefore, in populations with high risk for NIDDM, screening for IGT should probably be repeated at regular intervals. Subjects with IGT should be given individual health education counselling and care. Too little is known and too few controlled long-term intervention studies have been done to delay or prevent the worsening of diabetes in people with IGT. Therefore, it is not known which are the most efficient preventive measures to be employed. The recommendations concerning dietary and health behaviour changes listed below are not harmful and may have beneficial effects on general health in addition to the potential improvement in glucose metabolism.

The following actions are recommended for people at high risk for NIDDM:

1. Weight control when obese

2. Increase in physical activity.

3. Dietary regulation avoiding excessive energy intake and promoting high fibre intake.

4. Blood glucose lowering with oral antidiabetic agents.

5. Reduction of saturated fat intake.

6. Non-pharmacological treatment of hypertensive patients with a positive family history of NIDDM.

B. Population approach

The feasibility and effectiveness of reducing coronary disease rates through reduction of its main risk factors (smoking, elevated blood pressure and high serum cholesterol) has been demonstrated. Therefore, it is reasonable to assume that a healthier life style would also reduce the levels of the known risk factors if NIDDM. In fact, there is not much difference between the preventive measures for NIDDM and coronary heart disease at the community level. Because coronary heart disease is the major complication associated with NIDDM, any large-scale prevention program for NIDDM must be integrated with coronary heart disease prevention activities.

Even though it could be argued that uncertainty still exists as to whether large-scale prevention can be justified on the basis of existing data for NIDDM, very little is learned about prevention of NIDDM without trying it. Potentially enormous benefits can be achieved from community-based prevention programs aiming at balanced nutrition, reduction of smoking, promotion of physical activity and avoidance of obesity.

A number of colleagues have provided important data and significant input into the preparation of this manuscript. In particular I wish to thank Drs. P. Zimmet, A. Grech, A. Vassallo, A. Nissinen, J. Pekkanen and E. Wolf.

REFERENCES

1. Zimmet, P., 1982, Type 2 (non-insulin-dependent) diabetes - an idemiological overview. Diabetologia 22: 399-411.

2. Joslin, E.P., 1982, The prevention of diabetes mellitus. JAMA 76: 79-84.

3. Tuomilehto, J., Wolf, E., 1987, Primary prevention of diabetes mellitus. Diabetes Care 10: 238-248.

4. Kobberling, J., Tillil, H., 1982, Empirical risk figures for first-degree relatives of non-insulin-dependent diabetes. In: Kobberling, J., Tattersall, R., eds., The Genetics of Diabetes Mellitus. London: Academic Press, 201-210.

5. Barnett, A.H., Eff, C., Leslie, R.D.G., Pyke, D.A., 1981, Diabetes in identical twins - a study of 200 pairs. Diabetologia 20: 87-93.

6. Tuomilehto, J., Nissinen, A., Kivela, S-L et al., 1986, Prevalence of diabetes mellitus in elderly men aged 65 to 84 years in eastern and western Finland. Diabetologia 29: 611-615.

7. Zimmet, P., Taylor, R., King, H., 1982, Diabetes in the Pacific: An Epidemiological Perspective. Eschwage E., ed., Advances in Diabetes Epidemiology, INSERM Symposium, No. 22. New York: Elsevier.

8. Knowler, W.C., Pettit, D.J., Savage, P.J., Bennett, P.H., 1981, diabetes in Pima Indians: contributions of obesity and parental diabetes. Am J Epidemiol 113: 114-156.

9. Vague, J., 1956, The degree of masculine differentiation of obesities: a factor determining predisposition to diabetes, arteriosclerosis, gout and uric calculus disease. Am J Clin Nutr 4: 20-34.

10. Frisch, R.E., Wyshak, G., Albright, T.E., Albright, N.L., Schiff, I., 1986, Lower prevalence of diabetes in female former college athletes compared with nonathletes. Diabetes 35: 1101-1105.

C. HOWARD: Dr. Dyrberg, in some of the earlier studies when they were first beginning to show that viruses could cause diabetes in rodent models, that was based on those that survived, but there was often a high mortality. With your particular studies, did all the mice live or was it that you just studied those that survived the initial virus infection?

T. DYRBERG: No rats died following the virus inoculation.

H. LAUBE: Dr. Tuomilehto, I am quite aware that you are an epidemiologist. Nevertheless, I would like to confront you with some recent findings which suggest that many obese people, despite reducing their overweight, will continue to be at a high risk for becoming diabetic. Now, this may suggest that not overweight per se, but maybe a common metabolic disorder may underlie obesity and diabetes. Would you, as an epidemiologist, like to comment on that?

J. TUOMILEHTO: Sure. We all know that it is not obesity per se. There are many other factors and what I tried to explain was the amount of a disease that could be prevented probably through reduction of obesity in a population and the estimates from the data I used were very close to those estimates that Peter Bennett told us about. The proportion of insulin resistance in the Pima Indian population which can be accounted for by obesity alone was about 50%. And, the analysis that I did with several data sets also showed that between 10 and 20% of NIDDM could be presented. So, still there are about 80% left. But, the better markers or better indicators of obesity will definitely give us many good ideas and really one should try to see what can be done.

R. CAMERINI-DAVALOS: Dr. Dyrberg, in the virus infection study, did you follow the weight? Do you have data about the food intake?

T. DYRBERG: No, we did not monitor the body intake, but as I said the rats looked perfectly normal and were in good health. So, the only abnormality we could see was this decrease in body weight.

B. WAJCHENBERG: Dr. Tuomilehto, what would you suggest for treating patients because the major goal of this meeting is treating human beings. How can you treat obese patients for a long time?

J. TUOMILEHTO: I think that this is a very realistic question, and indeed there are other factors that play a major role. We have a Japanese population who are very well off and who are lean, who haven't got diabetes and so I can't see that it is impossible to achieve something which is healthy. And, then many other populations where the trend is towards better health. In the U.S. population, the amount of exercise is increasing and smoking rates are going down. People are changing all the time, but the question is whether medical people would like to be involved in this kind of change. It's not easy. And, there are many other factors that play a role. I have no answer to your question of what to do with the patients. Of course, the individuals do what they want to do and what the neighbors are doing, but I wanted to show you two different approaches and I do not believe that the so-called high risk approach is very efficient. I agree with you that it's almost impossible to change the patients' characteristics.

And, finally, I would like to say that what I tried to demonstrate was that we have to concentrate on the younger age groups, under 40-50 years of age, if we want to prevent it.